# SENSORY PHYSIOLOGY AND BEHAVIOR

# ADVANCES IN BEHAVIORAL BIOLOGY



*Recent Volumes in this Series*

Volume 5 • INTERDISCIPLINARY INVESTIGATION OF THE BRAIN
Edited by J. P. Nicholson • 1972

Volume 6 • PSYCHOPHARMACOLOGY AND AGING
Edited by Carl Eisdorfer and William E. Fann • 1973

Volume 7 • CONTROL OF POSTURE AND LOCOMOTION
Edited by R. B. Stein, K. G. Pearson, R. S. Smith, and J. B. Redford • 1973

Volume 8 • DRUGS AND THE DEVELOPING BRAIN
Edited by Antonia Vernadakis and Norman Weiner • 1974

Volume 9 • PERSPECTIVES IN PRIMATE BIOLOGY
Edited by A. B. Chiarelli • 1974

Volume 10 • NEUROHUMORAL CODING OF BRAIN FUNCTION
Edited by R. D. Myers and René Raúl Drucker-Colín • 1974

Volume 11 • REPRODUCTIVE BEHAVIOR
Edited by William Montagna and William A. Sadler • 1974

Volume 12 • THE NEUROPSYCHOLOGY OF AGGRESSION
Edited by Richard E. Whalen • 1974

Volume 13 • ANEURAL ORGANISMS IN NEUROBIOLOGY
Edited by Edward M. Eisenstein • 1975

Volume 14 • NUTRITION AND MENTAL FUNCTIONS
Edited by George Serban • 1975

Volume 15 • SENSORY PHYSIOLOGY AND BEHAVIOR
Edited by Rachel Galun, Peter Hillman, Itzhak Parnas, and Robert Werman • 1975

---

# SENSORY PHYSIOLOGY AND BEHAVIOR

Edited by

Rachel Galun

Department of Entomology
Israel Institute for Biological Research
Ness-Ziona, Israel

and

Peter Hillman, Itzhak Parnas, and Robert Werman

Unit of Neurobiology
Institute of Life Sciences
Hebrew University
Jerusalem

PLENUM PRESS · NEW YORK AND LONDON

Library of Congress Cataloging in Publication Data

"Oholo" Biological Conference on Sensory Physiology and Behavior, 19th, Ma'alot, Israel, 1974.
Sensory physiology and behavior.

(Advances in behavioral biology; v. 15)
Includes bibliographies and index.
1. Senses and sensation—Congresses. 2. Neuropsychology—Congresses. I. Galun, Rachel, 1926- II. Title.
QP431.037 1974 591.1'82 75-14130
ISBN 0-306-37915-5

Technical Editor:
Myra Kaye
Israel Institute for Biological Research
Ness-Ziona, Israel

Proceedings of the Nineteenth Annual "OHOLO" Biological Conference on Sensory Physiology and Behavior, held in Maalot, Israel, March 26-29, 1974


A Division of Plenum Publishing Corporation
227 West 17th Street, New York, N.Y. 10011

United Kingdom edition published by Plenum Press, London
A Division of Plenum Publishing Company, Ltd.
Davis House (4th Floor), 8 Scrubs Lane, Harlesden, London, NW10 6SE, England



Printed in the United States of America

## Organizing Committee

DR. YAACOV ASHANI, Israel Institute for Biological Research, Ness-Ziona
DR. AMNON BEN-DAVID, Israel Institute for Biological Research, Ness-Ziona
DR. RUTH CORETT, Israel Institute for Biological Research, Ness-Ziona
PROF. ANDRE DE VRIES, Tel-Aviv University, Tel-Aviv
PROF. ROBERT GOLDWASSER, Israel Institute for Biological Research, Ness-Ziona
PROF. NATHAN GROSSOWICZ, Hebrew University, Jerusalem
PROF. ALEXANDER KEYNAN, Hebrew University, Jerusalem
PROF. MARCUS A. KLINGBERG, Israel Institute for Biological Research, Ness-Ziona
PROF. ALEXANDER KOHN, Israel Institute for Biological Research, Ness-Ziona
PROF. HENRY NEUFELD, The Chaim Sheba Medical Center, Tel-Hashomer, Tel-Aviv University Medical School and Ministry of Health, Tel-Aviv
PROF. MICHAEL SELA, Weizmann Institute of Science, Rehovot

## Preface

In a recent book Arthur Koestler describes very cynically the superfluity of scientific meetings. He lists the various gatherings that are going to take place in one brief summer season in the Kongresshaus of a small Swiss village, ending the long list with three interdisciplinary symposia, titles of which contain the three words "Environment", "Pollution", and "Future" in three different permutations. By the same token, Koestler could list endlessly meetings on sensory physiology and behaviour or their synonyms, which have taken place all over the world on the national or international level in recent years.

The organizing committee of the Oholo conferences was very well aware of this situation when the topic for the 19th Conference was selected. However this field is relatively new in Israel - only in the last decade were several teams established in this country to carry out combined studies on sensory physiology and behaviour. They attracted ever-increasing numbers of students of zoology, physiology, medicine and psychology. The committee thought that the time was ripe to bring the Israeli students and scientists together with noted investigators from all over the world, to discuss and analyse the state of the art.

The Conference dealt with processing of information obtained through the various senses: visual, auditory, tactile, as well as the olfactory and gastatory senses.

More complex behavioural patterns were also analysed.

No attempt was made to relate these findings to human behaviour, although the act of terror which took place in Maalot, the site of this Conference, only several weeks after the meeting, may call for better understanding of human behaviour. We would like to perpetuate in this volume the memory of the 20 innocent schoolchildren who were killed in Maalot in May, 1974.

The editors gladly take this opportunity of expressing their thanks to the members of the program and organizing committees for their devoted work; to the members of the staff of the Israel Institute for Biological Research who gave so freely of their time, both outside and inside working hours; and to Mrs. Helen Bar-Lev for her skilled technical preparation of the manuscript of this book for printing.

No less thanks go to the participants, those from Israel and our guests from abroad, for making the Conference such a memorable and stimulating occasion. We especially are grateful to the Sessions Chairmen and the Moderator of the Round Table discussion.

We also wish to thank the management and staff of the Guest House at Maalot for their hospitality and care.

Finally, we are greatly indebted to the U.S. Army, European Research Office, for a grant in support of this Meeting.

Rachel Galun,
On behalf of the Editors

## Contents

# SENSORY PHYSIOLOGY AND BEHAVIOR

# WELCOMING ADDRESS

Amnon Ben-David

Israel Institute for Biological Research

Ness-Ziona, Israel

It gives me great pleasure to welcome the participants from Israel and abroad to this our 19th OHOLO Conference of 1973. After the tragic event of October, which for some time put in doubt whether we would be able to hold the Meeting, it gives me particular pleasure that we are gathered together here.

The OHOLO Conferences are intended to promote interdisciplinary understanding in specific fields in the forefront of scientific advance, by bringing together our local scientists and distinguished colleagues from abroad.

Our quiet and peaceful surroundings, be it the shores of Lake Kinnereth where our meetings were originally held at the OHOLO Education and Conference Center, or the mountain air of Galilee, here at Ma'alot, provide a relaxed atmosphere for informal discussion which has always contributed to the success of our annual OHOLO Conferences, initiated in 1954.

Our topic this year - SENSORY PHYSIOLOGY and BEHAVIOR - could occupy physiologists and behavioral scientists for much longer than three days of discussions. We hope that we can cover in the time as our disposal enough aspects of the topic as to bring them into sharper focus and perhaps awaken new ideas for future endeavours.

I hope that we shall have a pleasant and successful Meeting.

# DEVELOPMENTAL PLASTICITY IN THE CAT'S VISUAL CORTEX

C. Blakemore

Physiological Laboratory

Cambridge, England

## FEATURE DETECTION IN VISUAL SYSTEMS

In many species, the processing of visual information reaches a high level of complexity right in the retina itself. In rabbits (Levick, 1967), pigeons (Maturana and Frenk, 1963) and frogs (Lettvin, Maturana, McCulloch and Pitts, 1959), for example, retinal ganglion cells often demonstrate remarkable stimulus specificity. Within its receptive field (the region of receptors from which it receives information) each cell may require a quite specific visual stimulus to coax it into responding. Ganglion cells in these species sometimes require an edge at a particular orientation, an object moving in a particular direction or at a particular velocity, or even the complete absence of any pattern in the field, in order to make them respond.

Notably, those species with complex retinae have laterally placed eyes with rather little binocular overlap of the visual fields of the two eyes; but in cats and monkeys (with their frontal eyes and enormous binocular field) complex image processing seems largely to be delayed until the visual cortex - the first site in the geniculostriate pathway at which most neurones receive signals from both eyes. While the majority of ganglion cells and neurones of the lateral geniculate nucleus have straightforward round receptive fields with antagonistic surrounds (which only demand localized illumination or darkening), cortical neurones are almost always orientation-selective; they only respond when an edge or bar of a particular orientation appears in the receptive field (Hubel and Wiesel, 1962, 1968). The majority of them also have input from both eyes and it seems reasonable to suppose that image processing is delayed until the combination of simple messages from the two retinae, which are both viewing the same object in space.

Several workers have suggested, and provided evidence, that binocular cortical neurones in cats and monkeys play a part in stereoscopic vision (Barlow, Blakemore and Pettigrew, 1967; Joshua and Bishop, 1970; Hubel and Wiesel, 1970a). Each cell has very similar receptive field properties in the two eyes, but the two fields are not necessarily on exactly corresponding points, there is a limited variable disparity on the two retinae. Most neurones respond much more vigorously if stimulated by appropriate images falling on both receptive fields (as if the animal were viewing a single object at a particular distance from the eyes). The optimal disparity, and therefore the optimal distance, varies from one cell to another and thus the population of neurones may act as a system for the analysis of stereoscopic distance. The efficacy of this remarkable neural apparatus relies on the specific pattern-detecting properties of cortical cells, the similarity of these properties in the two eyes and the exact disparity-selectivity of each cell. Recent experiments have demonstrated that all of these properties are influenced by early visual experience and, indeed, the active modification of neural connections may be responsible for establishing the system for analysing retinal disparity.

## DEVELOPMENTAL INFLUENCES IN THE KITTEN'S VISUAL CORTEX

Genetic information alone is adequate to provide the majority of cortical neurones with connections from similar regions of both retinae: in the visual cortex of young kittens that have never had any visual experience, the majority of cells can be influences through both eyes (Hubel and Wiesel, 1963; Wiesel and Hubel, 1965; Barlow and Pettigrew, 1971; Blakemore and Van Sluyters, 1974). However, the receptive fields are diffuse, rarely strictly orientation-selective and never precisely "tuned" for retinal disparity (Pettigrew, 1974; Blakemore and Van Sluyters, in preparation). Visual experience early in life seems to refine crude innate specifications and, indeed, is capable of modifying the properties of cells quite drastically.

While depriving a kitten of patterned visual experience through <u>both</u> eyes simply leads to a general degradation in neuronal responsiveness (Wiesel and Hubel, 1965), covering <u>one</u> eye alone, even if only for a few days, causes virtually all cortical cells to abandon their connections from that eye (Hubel and Wiesel, 1970b). This loss of input occurs only after monocular deprivation between about 3 weeks and 3 months of age, and, within this "sensitive period", the changes are more or less reversed by covering the previously deprived eye and forcing the animal to use its originally inexperienced eye (Blakemore and Van Sluyters, 1974).

Inducing an artificial squint or deviation of one eye (strabismus) by sectioning one of the extraocular muscules of the eye also causes a specific reduction in the proportion of binocularly-driven cells and leaves two populations of neurones, some driven by the squinting eye, the others driven by the normal one (Hubel and Wiesel, 1965). However, small vertical misalignments of the visual axes, induced by rearing kittens wearing goggles with prisms of opposite power in front of the two eyes, can cause a remarkable compensatory change in receptive field organization. The cells usually remain binocular (if the prismatic displacement is not large) but each pair of receptive fields becomes, on average, vertically misaligned as if to correct for the misalignment of the retinal images of objects in space (Shlaer, 1971). Thus, during development, the disparity selectivity of each binocular cell is becoming refined (Pettigrew, 1974), and the optimal disparity may even be adjusted to match the alignment of the visual axes and to the most probable retinal disparity of the images of objects in the outside world.

The orientation selectivity of cortical neurones is also subject to a modifying influence. Kittens reared in conditions that restrict their visual experience more or less to edges of one orientation develop orientation-selective cortical neurones "tuned" almost exclusively to that orientation (Hirsch and Spinnelli, 1971; Blakemore and Cooper, 1970). These "environmental modifications" of orientation selectivity can also only occur as a result of visual stimulation within the 3 week to 3 month sensitive period (Blakemore, 1974) and they require only a few hours of exposure at the peak of this period, during the fourth week (Blakemore and Mitchell, 1973).

Thus, during the first few weeks of life, a number of crucial changes are occurring in the visual system of the kitten. The eyes change their orientation in the orbit and the two visual axes gradually become convergent rather than divergent (Pettigrew, 1974). Orientation selectivity is being refined and even modified as a result of visual experience. The binocularity of cortical cells is stamped in, their disparity selectivity is narrowed and their preferred disparities may even change to match the alignment of the retinal images.

## THE POSSIBLE FUNCTION OF ORIENTATIONAL MODIFICATION

It can be contended that environmental modification of preferred orientation would bestow important selective advantages on an animal, since it might match the detection properties of its visual system to the predominant features in its visual world. Indeed, cats reared in environments of one orientation have slight but definite acuity deficits with regard to stimuli of the opposite orientation (Blakemore and Cooper, 1970; Muir and Mitchell, 1973). However there are two important objections to this concept:

1) The acuity deficits produced even by very prolonged exposure are really quite small. It would be difficult to imagine how a subtle change in the population of orientation-detecting neurones (caused by slight differences in the probability of certain orientations in the normal visual environment) could have any noticeable effect on sensitivity or acuity.

2) One could argue that some very important stimuli in an animal's visual world (for instance, the shape of a dangerous predator) are likely to occur very rarely, not very commonly. To lose the ability to detect such stimuli would be disastrous.

There might be an alternative reason for binocular animals to possess the ability to change the preferred orientation of their cortical cells. In order to play their proposed role in the analysis of retinal disparity, these cells must be capable of "recognising" the two images of a single object in the two eyes, in order to signal its disparity. The fact that the optimal orientation of cortical cells is always very similar in the two eyes means that they will only respond optimally when the two images of a single contour (having the same angle on the two retinae) appear on the receptive fields. But it seems an intolerable burden on genetic information alone to specify for each cortical cell exactly what its orientational preference will be, and to ensure that it is virtually identical in the two eyes. However, environmental modification of orientational preference could ensure that both receptive fields of each cortical cell adopt very similar orientations, for the two receptive fields will then be habitually stimulated by the two similarly orientated images of single objects in space.

Thus environmental modification of orientation selectivity, like developmental changes in binocularity and disparity selectivity, may be crucially involved in constructing the neural apparatus involved in stereoscopic vision.

## ACKNOWLEDGEMENTS

The work in Cambridge was supported by a grant from the Medical Research Council, London.

## REFERENCES


1. BARLOW, H.B., BLAKEMORE, C. & PETTIGREW, J.D. *J. Physiol.* *193:*327, 1967.
2. BARLOW, H.B. & PETTIGREW, J.D. *J. Physiol.* *218:*98, 1971.
3. BLAKEMORE, C. In: The Neurosciences: Third Study Program. F.O. Schmitt and F.G. Worden, editors. Cambridge, Mass. MIT Press, p. 105 (1974).
4. BLAKEMORE, C. & COOPER, G. *Nature* *228:*477, 1970.
5. BLAKEMORE, C. & MITCHELL, D.E. *Nature* *241:*467, 1973.
6. BLAKEMORE, C. & VAN SLUYTERS, R.C. *J. Physiol.* *237:*195, 1974.
7. HIRSCH, H.V.B. & SPINELLI, D.N. *Exp. Brain Res.* *12:*509, 1971.
8. HUBEL, D.H. & WIESEL, T.N. *J. Physiol.* *160:*106, 1962.
9. HUBEL, D.H. & WIESEL, T.N. *J. Neurophysiol.* *26:*994, 1963.
10. HUBEL, D.H. & WIESEL, T.N. *J. Neurophysiol.* *28:*1041, 1965.
11. HUBEL, D.H. & WIESEL, T.N. *J. Physiol.* *195:*215, 1968.
12. HUBEL, D.H. & WIESEL, T.N. *Nature* *225:*41, 1970a.
13. HUBEL, D.H. & WIESEL, T.N. *J. Physiol.* *206:*419, 1970b.
14. JOSHUA, D.E. & BISHOP, P.O. *Exp. Brain Res.* *10:*389, 1970.
15. LETTVIN, J.Y., MATURANA, H.R., McCULLOCH, W.S. & PITTS, W.H. *Proc. Inst. Radio Engr.* *47:*1940, 1959.
16. LEVICK, W.R. *J. Physiol.* *188:*285, 1967.
17. MATURANA, H.R. & FRENK, S. *Science* *142:*977, 1963.
18. MUIR, D.W. & MITCHELL, D.E. *Science* *180:*420, 1973.
19. PETTIGREW, J.D. *J. Physiol.* *237:*49, 1974.
20. SHLAER, R. *Science* *173:*638, 1971.
21. WIESEL, T.N. & HUBEL, D.H. *J. Neurophysiol.* *28:*1029, 1965.

# VISUAL INFORMATION PROCESSING: THE MANY-SPLENDORED PHOTORECEPTOR

Peter Hillman and Menachem Hanani

The Institute of Life Sciences
The Hebrew University of Jerusalem
Jerusalem, Israel

## INTRODUCTION

One of the most striking aspects of the visual sense of animals is its ability to encompass an intensity range of a thousand million or more and yet maintain a very high sensitivity to small temporal or spatial variations about the mean intensity to which the animal is exposed at any time. Part of this task of adaptation to light and dark is performed by mechanical control of the light intensity incident on the retina, through pupil contraction and screening pigment migration. In higher animals, adaptation is aided by the specialization of photoreceptor cells to different parts of the intensity range: rods for weak light and cones for strong. A third component, at least in higher animals, is maintained by processing beyond the photoreceptor, mainly in the retina: absorption of photons in only 1% of the rods for example, can reduce the overall sensitivity of the system by a factor of three (Rushton, 1965).

However, the largest part of the adaptation in all animals is due to the ability of the photoreceptor itself to adjust its "amplification" or sensitivity according to the average intensity of illumination. In general, of course, the amplification decreases with increasing intensity - that is, exposure to light, or increased light, reduces the amplification, and we shall restrict our treatment of *"adaptation"* to such reduction. The resulting non-linear dependence of response amplitude on stimulus strength enables the receptor to cover a very large stimulus range. In the barnacle, for instance, the upper end range is at least a factor of ten million greater than threshold (Fig. 1).

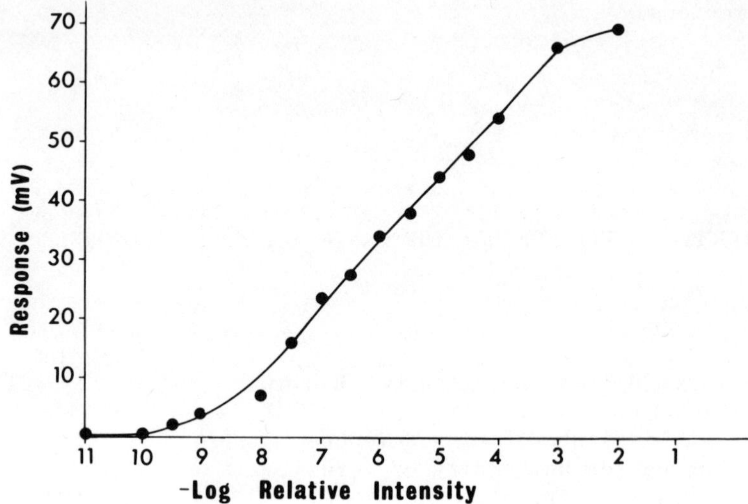


Fig. 1 The large range of stimulus intensity encompassed in the response of a single barnacle photoreceptor. The intracellular steady-state potential is plotted against the logarithm of the light intensity. A near-logarithmic dependence over 5 log-units is seen.

A few reports, however, have indicated that in certain preparations and under certain circumstances, exposure to light can *increase* the gain temporarily (Ruck and Jahn, 1954; Stratten and Ogden, 1971; Shaw, 1972 and DeVoe, 1972). We have found this *facilitation* to be particularly strong in the barnacle. In this preparation, both facilitation and adaptation appear normally to be present simultaneously, and we have found three parameters on which their relative strengths depend. These are: metabolic state, external $Ca^{++}$ concentration, and intensity of conditioning stimulus. This paper discusses these dependencies, and draws a parallel between the facilitation-adaptation balance and the excitation-inhibition balance between two antagonistic components of the transduction process previously seen in the barnacle (Hochstein, Minke and Hillman, 1973). The skeleton of a unified model for the two antagonistic pairs of processes is also presented.

## METHODS

Intracellular recordings were made as described in Hillman *et al.*, 1973. Cell sensitivity was tested at regular intervals before and after a conditioning stimulus by exposure to test flashes sufficiently weak as not to affect substantially the state of adaptation. The excised eyes were kept at 22±1°C in natural sea water or artificial sea water with 20 mM $Ca^{++}$ or, in "low-$Ca^{++}$" medium, with $Ca^{++}$ reduced to 0.5 mM, the remainder replaced by $Mg^{++}$. $Mg^{++}$ is believed to have no substantial effect on these cells (Millecchia and Mauro, 1969).

## OBSERVATIONS

Figs. 2a and b show examples of facilitation and adaptation in the same cell. The onset of both processes appears to be rapid, and recovery depended strongly on conditioning intensity, ranging from seconds at low intensities to minutes at higher intensities for both phenomena. The time course of recovery sometimes appeared to be biphasic, passing from an early facilitation to a later period of slight adaptation.

### "Metabolic" State

We have found a strong correlation between the facilitation/adaptation balance and the absolute sensitivity, resting membrane potential, and post-stimulus hyperpolarization (Koike, Brown and Hagiwara, 1971) of each cell. Strong adaptation appeared only in cells with high sensitivities, large membrane potentials and post-stimulus hyperpolarizations (Fig. 2a). On the other hand, strong facilitation (in normal sea water) was found only in cells with low sensitivities, lower membrane potentials and smaller post-stimulus hyperpolarizations (Fig. 2b). A decline in these three parameters with time in a single cell invariably paralleled a change-over from dominant adaptation to dominant facilitation.

### Conditioning Intensity

Fig. 3a shows the dependence on conditioning intensity of the ratio of the response to the test stimulus twenty seconds after the conditioning flash to that immediately before the flash. The two curves show a "high sensitivity" cell, in which adaptation (ratios

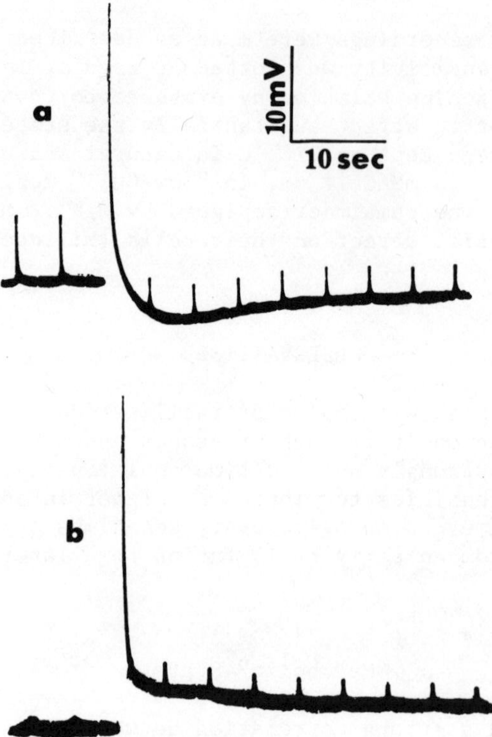


Fig. 2 Examples of facilitation and adaptation in the barnacle photoreceptor. Intracellular recordings from a barnacle photoreceptor at 22±1°C. Weak, brief test flashes were given at 5-second intervals to the cell after initial full dark-adaptation. About a third of the way through the traces, bright conditioning flashes were presented.

(a) illustrates the resulting adaptation observed in a cell of high sensitivity. Note the hyperpolarization following the conditioning flash.

(b) the facilitation observed in the same cell when in state of low sensitivity following the same conditioning flash as in (a) (see text).

Figs. 3a and 3b (below and on following page)

The effect of metabolic state and external $Ca^{++}$ concentration on the facilitation/adaptation balance. Abscissas: Logarithms of relative intensities of conditioning flashes. Ordinates: Ratios of amplitudes of responses to test flashes, presented about 20 sec after conditioning flashes, to amplitudes before conditioning flashes.

(3a) Lower curve: adaptation in a high sensitivity cell; upper curve: facilitation in a low sensitivity cell;

(3b) Lower curve: adaptation in another high sensitivity cell in a normal-$Ca^{++}$ medium; upper curve: responses of the same cell converted to facilitation in a low-$Ca^{++}$ medium. The effect was reversible.

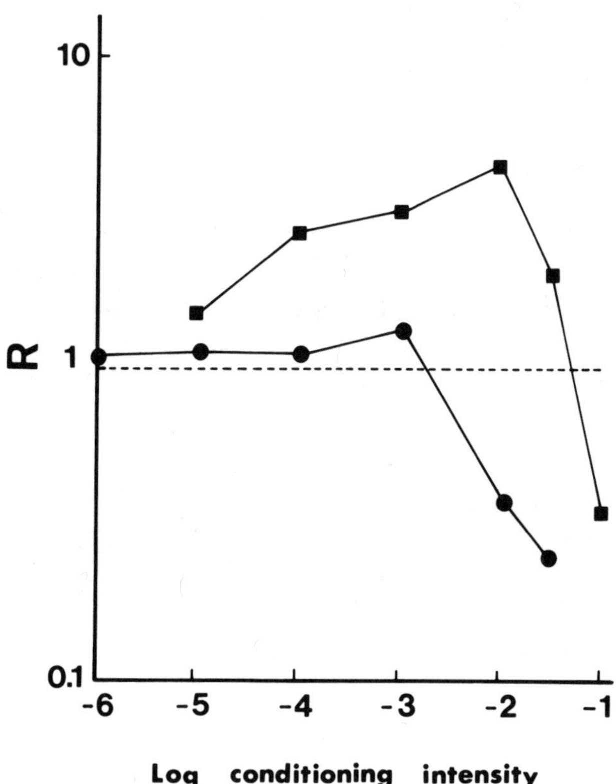


Fig. 3a

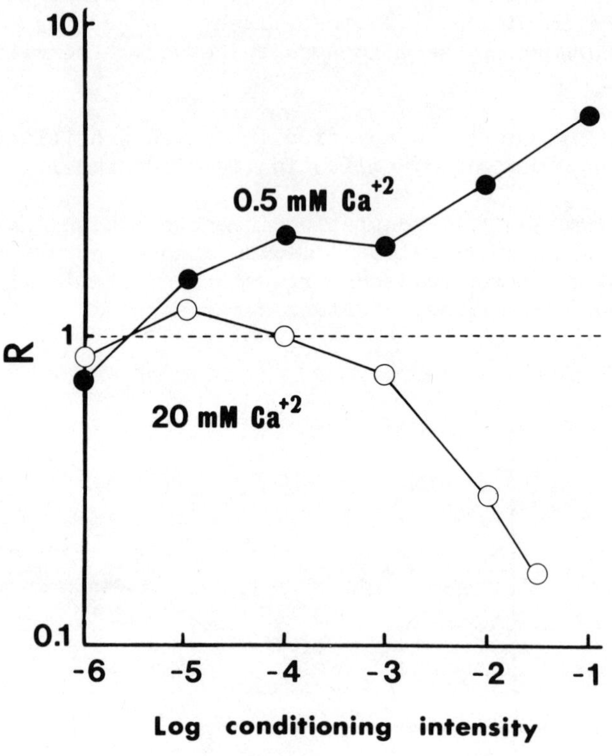

10
1
0.1
R
0.5 mM Ca+2
20 mM Ca+2
-6
-5
-4
-3
-2
-1
Log conditioning intensity


Fig. 3b

less than 1) is dominant, and a low sensitivity cell, in which facilitation is dominant.

### External $Ca^{++}$ Concentration

Fig. 3b illustrates the effect on a "fresh" cell of replacing the normal medium with a low-$Ca^{++}$ medium. The strong adaptation is converted into a strong facilitation. The effect was fully reversible.

## TWO PAIRS OF ANTAGONISTIC PROCESSES

It is clear that the facilitation and the adaptation are antagonistic in the sense that they are opposite effects on the same parameter. Whether they are two independent and antagonistic processes, or manifestations of a variation in the strength of a single process, is not yet clear. However, the biphasic dependences (passing from facilitation to adaptation or vice versa) on metabolic state, on stimulus intensity and on external $Ca^{++}$ concentration (and possibly on time) would be more easily explained by differential effects on two separate and opposing processes, and in particular by assuming that the adaptation process is more sensitive to all three parameters than is facilitation.

We call attention, therefore, to the parallel with the separate and antagonistic excitory and inhibitory processes described by Hochstein *et al.*, 1973. The excitatory process manifests itself directly as a residual post-stimulus $Na^+$-conductance increase or PDA (prolonged depolarizing afterpotential), and the inhibitory process as a suppression or prevention of this increase (anti-PDA), as opposed to the change in *sensitivity*, not accompanied by an appreciable conductance change, characterizing the facilitation/adaptation balance. The approximate coincidence of the time scales of the PDA/anti-PDA and facilitation/inhibition phenomena, seconds to minutes, is a first strong indication of a relationship, given that there are very few such time courses known in neural processes. However, the PDA and anti-PDA do not appear to depend strongly on cell metabolic state or on external $Ca^{++}$ concentration (our unpublished observations). The dependences on intensity also do not appear very similar, that of the PDA being roughly quadratic (Hillman, Hochstein & Minke, 1974) while that of the facilitation (presumably the parallel to the PDA) not exceeding linearity. Accordingly, we sketch a model, within the framework of the transduction process as a whole, which relates the PDA and the facilitation, but ascribes the adaptation to a process different from that of the anti-PDA and more sensitive to $Ca^{++}$ and metabolic state.

## NOTES FOR A MODEL

The model is based on the Hagins (1972) hypothesis of $Ca^{++}$ as an internal transmitter in photoreceptors, acting to *close* $Na^+$ channels normally open in the dark (See also: Szuts and Cone, 1973; Yoshikami and Hagins, 1973; and Brown and Lisman, 1974). We hypothesize for the present preparation: (1) There are ionic channels passing $Na^+$ and $Ca^{++}$ inwards; (2) There are *two* $Ca^{++}$-binding sites at each channel on the inside of the membrane, occupation of either of which closes the channels; (3) The internal $Ca^{++}$ concentration is kept low by a metabolically driven membrane pump (with mitochondria presumably serving as fast-acting internal buffer stores), and so rises when the "metabolic" state of the cell weakens; (4) The action of light is to remove $Ca^{++}$ ions from their channel sites, *and* either to put the pigment temporarily into a low-$Ca^{++}$-affinity state, resulting in a PDA, or temporarily into such a state that it *cannot* be transferred directly by light into the low-affinity state, resulting in an anti-PDA.

The *PDA* then arises from the conversion of most of the pigment into a state of low-$Ca^{++}$-affinity. The square dependence of the PDA amplitude on stimulus intensity is due to the necessity of affecting *both* $Ca^{++}$ sites to open a channel. During the *anti-PDA*, the pigment is in a state from which phototransitions lead only to high-$Ca^{++}$-affinity states. The *facilitation* is effectively a sub-threshold PDA, an increase in the number of low-$Ca^{++}$-affinity sites present in the cell at the time of test stimulation. The light adaptation is an increase and the dark adaptation a metabolically driven decrease in the $Ca^{++}$ concentration in the cell. The light-induced increase in this concentration arises from the opening of $Na^+$-$Ca^{++}$ channels and from release of $Ca^{++}$ from channel sites. In metabolically weak cells, the internal $Ca^{++}$ concentration is already so high, and thus the sensitivity is so reduced, that there can be little further light or dark adaptation, while facilitation is relatively unaffected.

## CONCLUSION

The photoreceptor is responsible for an imposing range of duties: To convert light into potential; to do so with a high degree of amplification; to vary this amplification over an enormous range according to need; and, to do all this as rapidly and efficiently as possible. In carrying out these duties, the photoreceptor exhibits a wide variety of phenomena. Fine control is apparently achieved by a delicate balance between opposing influences, of which we have discussed two pairs in this article.

It appears now to be possible to construct a model consistent with most of these phenomena, including the behaviorally vital dark-

and light-adaptation process. In this model, the amplification of the receptor depends on two factors, one being the internal $Ca^{++}$ concentration, which in turn depends on the light history (specifically the response history) and the "metabolic" state of the cell; and the other being the state of the pigment with respect to $Ca^{++}$ affinity, which depends only on the light history (especially wavelength).

## ACKNOWLEDGEMENT

Part of this work was supported by a grant from the Israel Commission for Basic Research.

## REFERENCES

1. BROWN, J.E. & LISMAN, J.E. *Fed. Proc.* *33:*434, 1974.
2. DE VOE, R.D. *Gen. Physiol.* *59:*247, 1972.
3. HAGINS, W.A. *Ann. Rev. Biophys. Bioeng.* *1:*131, 1972.
4. HILLMAN, P., DODGE, F.A., HOCHSTEIN, S., KNIGHT, B.W. & MINKE, B.J. *J. Gen. Physiol.* *62:*77, 1973.
5. HILLMAN, P., HOCHSTEIN, S. & MINKE, B. 1974. Submitted.
6. HOCHSTEIN, S., MINKE, B. & HILLMAN, P. *J. Gen. Physiol.* *62:*102, 1973.
7. KOIKE, H., BROWN, H.M. & HAGIWARA, S. *J. Gen. Physiol.* *57:*723, 1971.
8. MILLECCHIA, R. & MAURO, A. *J. Gen. Physiol.* *54:*310, 1969.
9. RUCK, P. & JAHN, T.L. *J. Gen. Physiol.* *37:*825, 1954.
10. RUSHTON, W.A.H. *J. Physiol. (London)* *178:*141, 1965.
11. SHAW, S.R. *J. Physiol. (London)* *220:*145, 1972.
12. STRATTEN, W.P. & OGDEN, T.E. *J. Gen. Physiol.* *57:*435, 1971.
13. SZUTS, E. & CONE, R.A. Quoted by Cone, *Exp. Eye Res.* *17:*507, 1973.
16. YOSHIKAMI, S. & HAGINS, W.A. Biochemistry and Physiology of the Visual Pigments. H. Langer (ed.), Springer-Verlag, Heidelberg, 1973.

# PHYSIOLOGICAL RESPONSES AND FUNCTIONAL ARCHITECTURE OF THE MONKEY VISUAL CORTEX

D. Hubel

Harvard Medical School

Boston, Massachusetts, U.S.A.

Over the last 15 years Torsten Wiesel and I have been engaged in a study of the normal visual cortex in cats and monkeys. We have attempted to learn how far one can come in understanding how the cortex is put together and what becomes of the visual information reaching it. Our main technique has been the recording of impulses from single cells while stimulating the retina with light, but we have also used a variety of anatomical methods.

Studies in the lateral geniculate body show that the information reaching the cortex is mainly coded in the form of concentric center-surround receptive fields, as described by Kuffler in 1951; each cell has its field center in the left retina or the right, but seldom, if ever, in both. There may be a weak interaction between the eyes: this has been established for the cat (Sanderson, Darian-Smith and Bishop, 1969) but is still not known for the monkey. In the cortex this information is radically transformed, not all at once, but probably in three or four more or less discrete stages. In the monkey, the first stage is represented probably by cells in layer IVC -- the region in which afferents from the geniculate terminate. These cells have not yet been studied in detail; their fields have circular symmetry and probably have a center-surround organization. Thus what difference, if any, exists between geniculate cells and these cells is not yet known.

The next stage occurs in layer IV, and the following two in the layers above and below it. "Simple" and "complex" cells have the property of responding to a short line segment only if the line crosses the receptive field in an appropriate orientation, which for a typical cell can be specified to the nearest few degrees. A line oriented on the retina at $90^{\circ}$ from the optimum is almost always ineffective, as is diffuse light. In many complex cells, an optimally oriented line stimulus swept across the receptive field produces a response only for one of the two directions of movement. Hypercomplex cells have properties similar to those of simple or complex cells, except that they respond only to lines of limited length.

Simple cells, like the concentric center-surround cells of layer IV, are practically always monocular. About 50% of complex cells and hypercomplex cells are binocular in the monkey. A binocular cell almost always has fields in the two eyes whose maps are similar and whose positions are quite precisely homologous. Many, and perhaps most, binocular cells respond consistently better to a stimulus to one eye than to the same stimulus to the other. It is as if binocular cells received qualitatively similar connections from the two eyes but with a greater density of connections from one eye. In a population of cells all degrees of dominance are represented, from total left eye dominance, through equality, to total right eye dominance.

These properties of simple, complex and hypercomplex cells may be understood in terms of simple circuits, in which excitatory and inhibitory influences at one stage converge on single cells at the next. In this model, a complex cell receives its input from many simple cells, and hypercomplex cells from many complex. This hierarchy is certainly not a rigid one -- it is clear, for example, that simple, complex and hypercomplex cells all may have axons leaving the cortex. There is also evidence that complex cells may receive some afferents direct from the lateral geniculate (Stone, 1972).

Over the past few years, we have been increasingly interested in examining the relationship between the physiology of the cortex and its architecture. Most of the connections between cortical cells are quite short, several millimeters or less, so that it is natural to expect cells that are close neighbors to have some common physiological characteristics. The groupings of cells by common function turns out to be highly patterned. Cells that are close neighbors always have their receptive fields on nearly identical parts of the retina. This is no surprise, for it has been known for a century that the visual fields are mapped in a systematic topographic manner on the striate cortex. In a vertical penetration through the cortex, however, there is a slight variation from cell to cell in position and size of fields, so that the retinal (or visual field) territory covered by the cells in such a penetration is several times larger than the size of any one field.

Neighboring cells practically always have similar receptive-field orientations. Here the spatial arrangement of groups of cells with similar preferred orientations is an unexpected one. In a perpendicular penetration through successive layers, the orientation of receptive fields remains constant. In a penetration parallel to the layers, the orientation generally changes in small regular discrete steps of $10^{\circ}$ or so, continuing clockwise or counter-clockwise for spans of $180-360^{\circ}$, with occasional reverses in the direction of rotation. Several lines of evidence make it clear that the regions of constant receptive field orientations have the form of parallel sheets which lie like slices of bread, perpendicular to the surface of the cortex. The sheets (or "columns", as they have been called) have a thickness of about 25-50 μ, so that to span a complete $180^{\circ}$ of orientation requires a movement, normal to the sheets, of about ½-1 mm. One complete set of sheets, making a complete cycle through $180^{\circ}$, we term a "hypercolumn".

One may regard each of these orientation columns as a discrete functional entity, since the cells within each column, all having the same receptive field orientation and roughly the same receptive field positions, are just the cells that one supposses are wired together in the circuits that we proposed to explain complex and hypercomplex properties.

If we compare the eye dominance of neighboring cells we find again that neighboring cells practically always prefer the same eye. Again, in a perpendicular penetration, all cells are highly likely to prefer the same eye. The neighborhoods within which a particular eye is dominant are once more slab-shaped, the cortex being subdivided into alternate left-eye and right-eye sheets, which are entirely independent of the orientation sheets. In this system, the regions are roughly ¼-½ mm thick. A complete set of ocular dominance sheets consists of two, one for each eye, and the thickness of such a set of two sheets, which we may call the ocular dominance hypercolumn, is thus again ½-1 mm. In both sets of columns, the thickness is apparently independent of position in the cortex.

This uniformity in size of the columns fits well with the uniformity of the histology of this area. Functionally, however, the striate cortex is in one respect far from uniform, for one millimeter of cortex corresponds to about $1/6^{\circ}$ in the foveal regions, and to about $6^{\circ}$ in the far periphery, the magnification falling off steadily as a function of distance of receptive fields from the fovea (eccentricity). But in parallel with this, receptive field size and the associated scatter in receptive field position (mentioned above) also increase with increasing eccentricity. Both variables, magnification and field size, change in such a way that a 2-3 mm displacement along the cortex is just sufficient to produce a shift in receptive field of about the same size as the fields themselves plus their scatter. This 2-3 mm is enough to span several column sets of each type. Consequently, a piece of cortex several mm on a side is enough comfortably to look after one region of visual field, whose size depends on eccentricity, in both eyes and in all orientations.

Thus despite the great difference in magnification over the striate cortex, and the equally great variation in field size, the structure is in a sense uniform functionally as well as histologically. Any region of cortex simply digests the information brought to it, presumably employing identical machinery throughout. This surely makes the development of the cortex much simpler than it would otherwise be. Any one 2-3 mm region is complex enough, but the whole structure, like a crystal, is at least to a first approximation a repetition of the same basic elements.

## REFERENCES

1. SANDERSON, K.J., DARIAN-SMITH, J. & BISHOP, P.O. *Vision Res.* *9:*1297, 1969.
2. STONE, J. *Invest. Ophthal.* *11:*338, 1972.

# THE QUESTION OF VARIATION IN TRANSMISSION IN THE VISUAL PATHWAY AS A RESULT OF ATTENTION TO AN AUDITORY OR A VISUAL STIMULUS

G. Horn
University of Bristol
Department of Anatomy
Bristol, U.K.

Attention is a difficult word to define but, amongst other meanings, the term implies a "...withdrawal from some things in order to deal effectively with others..." (James, 1890). This view relates specifically to human beings, but is commonly generalized to apply to a wide range of animals. The concept is one that, implicitly or explicitly, has been used frequently by neurobiologists interested in the neural mechanisms underlying attentive behaviour. One reason is that is poses specific problems. For example, does "...deal effectively (with some things)..." correspond to admitting to specific neuronal network signals elicited by the stimulus which is attended to; and does "...withdrawal from some things..." correspond to preventing signals elicited by stimuli that are not being attended to from gaining access to these networks? Work over the last decade suggests that, simple as these notions are, they are not implausible. Certain cells in the tectotegmental region of the rabbit brainstem respond briskly to a novel stimulus. If this stimulus is slowly repeated, the response declines. If a novel stimulus is presented, the cells may respond virogously while remaining unresponsive to the familiar stimulus - the pathway to the cell for one stimulus is closed, the pathway for the other open (Horn & Hill, 1964). At the behavioural level, a novel stimulus has a high probability of being perceived (Cherry, 1953); so it does not require a great leap of the imagination to suggest that cells of this type may play an important role in attentive behaviour (Horn, 1965). Recent evidence (Goldbert & Wurtz, 1972; Rizzolatti *et al.*, 1974) lends some support for this suggestion.

If switching attention from one stimulus to another entails a gating process, at what stage in the sensory transmission lines does the putative gate operate? For a variety of reasons it is sensible to study transmission in the primary afferent pathways, leading from receptors to the corresponding sensory area of the cerebral cortex, for evidence of such a gating operation. At various times in the past seventy years it has indeed been suggested that transmission in the primary visual pathways may be modified according to whether or not the animal attends to a visual stimulus (Tello, 1904; Berger, 1931; Adrian, 1944; 1954; Horn, 1952; Hernández-Péon *et al.*, 1957). This idea received indirect support from the findings that non-sensory fibres are present in the lateral geniculate nucleus (Tello, 1904; Shute & Lewis, 1963, 1967; Fuxe, 1965); that fibres pass from the visual cortex to the lateral geniculate nucleus (Beresford, 1962; Szentágothai *et al.*, 1966; Garey *et al.*, 1968); and that activity in the visual cortex and lateral geniculate nucleus (LGN) can be influenced by electrical stimulation of the mesencephalic reticular formation as well as by non-visual stimuli (Dumont & Dell, 1958; Akimoto *et al.*, 1961; Susuki & Taira, 1961; Hotta & Kameda, 1963; 1964; Jung *et al.*, 1963; Horn, 1965; Murata *et al.*, 1965; Godfraind & Meulders, 1969; Feeney & Orem, 1972; Horn *et al.*, 1972). In addition, the responses evoked in the visual pathways by "probe" stimuli, for example, light flashes or shocks applied directly to the optic pathways, change when the animal is presented with a novel stimulus (Hernández-Péon *et al.*, 1957; Horn & Blundell, 1959; Horn, 1960; Jane *et al.*, 1962; Walley & Urschel, 1972) and when there is a spontaneous change in the level of arousal (Bremer & Stoupel, 1956; Evarts *et al.*, 1965; Dagino *et al.*, 1965; Walsh & Cordeau, 1965; Malcolm *et al.*, 1970). However, although many efforts have been made in recent years to determine directly whether or not transmission changes with alterations in the state of attentiveness, the problem has still not been resolved (Horn, 1965; Worden, 1966; Näätänen, 1967). A major difficulty has been to distinguish changes in the level of attentiveness from other, less specific responses, such as the orienting reflex, or a general change in the level of arousal (Horn, 1965; 1975; Näätänen, 1967). It is not an easy matter to circumvent these difficulties convincingly, especially in experimental situations in which the animal is first required to attend to one stimulus and then to relinquish its attention to that stimulus whilst it attends to another. Fortunately, however, "attention-switching" behaviour is not the only way to study attention. An alternative method is to use a vigilance task (Mackworth, 1950; Broadbent, 1958; Moray, 1970). In a vigilance task an observer is required to pay attention in order to detect some event whenever it happens (Moray, 1970).

In a recent series of experiments (Horn & Wiesenfeld, 1974) the behaviour of six cats was studied in a vigilance task. Each cat was trained, in the light, to press a pedal on the floor of a training box (Fig. 1). A waiting interval of fixed or variable duration then followed, after which a stimulus (S), a spot of light or a tone, was presented for a short period of time. The cat gave a correct response if, during this time, it pressed a panel. The cat was then rewarded with food. After the cat behaviour had reached the required

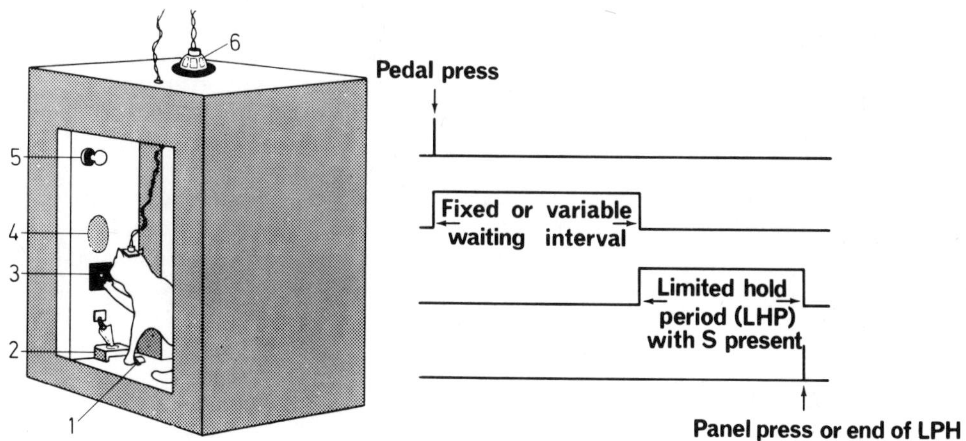


Fig. 1 Experimental system and behavioural sequence. *A*. Apparatus with door removed. 1. Pedal which was pressed when the cat made an observing response. 2. Food dish. 3. Hinged panel. If this was pressed in the presence of the stimulus (S) a reward (1 to 2 ml of a suspension of tinned cat food in milk or water ) followed immediately. Illustrated on the panel is the small spot of light, S, in the fixed and variable interval visual schedules. 4. Speaker used in the fixed and variable interval auditory schedules when S was a 4 k Hz tone. 5. Box light that was switched on only during the initial behavioural training. 6. Speaker used to delivery 70 dB (re $2 \times 10^{-4}$ dyne $cm^{-2}$) masking white noise continuously. All sides of the box, except the door and the front panel, were covered with a 2 cm thick layer of expanded polystyrene. The pedal (1) was close enough to the front of the box for the cat to press it without moving backwards. All cats were trained to press the pedal with the left paw and the panel with the right, enabling them to stand in one place during the whole sequence. *B*. Sequence of events in each trial. Read from above downwards, left to right. S. stayed on until either the panel was pressed, after which food was delivered, or the end of the limited hold period (LHP). This period was 3 sec for 4 cats and 5 sec for 2. These values were determined by assessing the behaviour of each cat during initial training; shorter periods increased the number of errors and disrupted performance (From Horn & Wiesenfeld, 1974).

criterion, the light was extinguished and all experiments were conducted in the dark. When an experiment had been completed using one stimulus, the cat was trained to respond to the other.

The latency of response following the onset of S was measured in the variable interval schedules. These schedules consisted of six interval lengths arranged in a quasi-random order. For five cats, the intervals ranged in multiples of 0.5 sec from 1.0 to 3.5 sec. In one cat, the intervals ranged from 0.8 - 2.8 sec in multiples of 0.4 sec. In a given trial, the probability of the stimulus occurring after the shortest waiting interval was 1/6. If S did not appear then, the probability of it occurring after the next interval was 1/5 and so on, such that the probability of S occurring after the sixth waiting interval was 1, provided S had not occurred earlier and provided also that the cat did not make an error by pressing the panel during the waiting interval. It was found (Fig. 2), that, in all, the longer latencies were associated with the shorter intervals. That is, as the probability of the stimulus occurring increased, the more quickly did the cat respond to the stimulus.

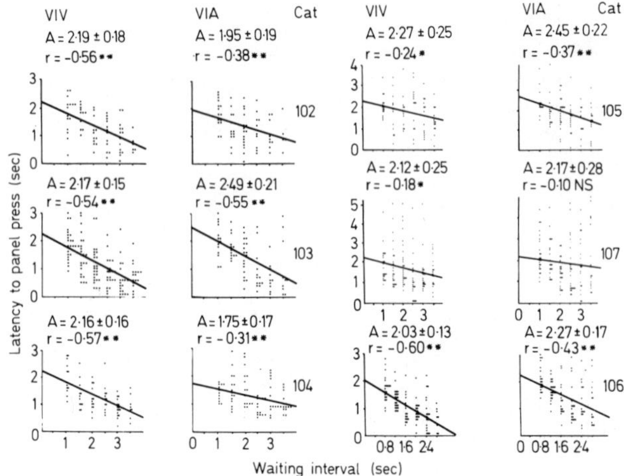


Fig. 2 Regressions of latency to press panel on length of waiting interval. Data for each cat and each condition, variable interval visual (VIV) and variable interval auditory (VIA), are shown. The cat number is given on the right of the corresponding 2 graphs. For each graph, the value of A of the equation $y = A + Bx$ is given, together with the standard deviation. The value of r, the Pearson correlation coefficient, is also given. The asterisks indicate the significance of this coefficient *p <0.05; **p <0.01; NS means not significantly different from zero. Note that the lengths of the waiting intervals used in the experiments with cat 106 are different from those intervals used for other cats (From Horn & Wiesenfeld, 1974).

Between the time the pedal and panel were pressed the optic tract (OT) was shocked once through implanted bipolar stainless steel electrodes. The responses of the LGN and visual cortex were recorded through monopolar recording electrodes. The time at which the shock was delivered was varied from one trial to the next. In the variable interval schedules, the shock to the OT, in any one trial, was given at the following times (in sec) after the pedal press: 0.0, 0.5, 1.0, 1.5, 2.0, 2.5, 3.0, 3.5 and at the time of the panel press, for all cats except cat 106 where all intervals except the last (preceding the panel press) were multiples of 0.4 sec. Naturally, the length of the waiting interval in a given trial imposed constraints on the timing of the OT shock. For example, for the waiting interval 1.0 sec the OT shock, if delivered at all, could only be given at the time of the pedal press, at 0.5 sec or at 1.0 sec. Apart from these constraints, the timing of the OT shocks varied independently of the length of the waiting interval. Twenty five responses for each of these shock intervals were recorded; responses obtained for intervals 3.0 and 3.5 sec were combined. There were thus 8 categories of evoked responses corresponding to the 8 shock intervals.

The peak to peak amplitudes of the t (presynaptic) and r (postsynaptic) waves of the LGN response and $C_1$ and $C_5$ of the cortical response (Fig. 3) were measured and standardised. $C_1$ is generated by activity in geniculo-calcarine radiation fibres and $C_5$ by postsynaptic cortical elements (Marshall *et al.*, 1943; Chang & Kaada, 1950; G.H. Bishop & Clare, 1952; Malis & Kruger, 1956; Bremer & Stoupel, 1956; Schoolman & Evarts, 1959).

It was found that the responsiveness of the LGN and visual cortex did not vary during the waiting interval in either of the fixed interval schedules or in the variable interval schedule in which S was a spot of light (VIV). However, in the variable interval schedule in which S was a tone (VIA), the responsiveness of the visual cortex, as indicated by the amplitude of $C_5$, to the thalamocortical input, declined as the length of the waiting interval increased (Fig. 4). No changes were observed at the LGN or in the presynaptic cortical response ($C_1$) in this schedule.

These results could be interpreted in several ways. For example, the responsiveness of the cortex at the shorter waiting intervals in the VIA condition may be greater than in the VIV condition: as the probability of the tone occurring increases, the responsiveness may fall to or below that of the VIV condition. It is possible to examine this question of relative changes in responsiveness by combining the corresponding data from the VIA and VIV schedules. An index of cortical responsiveness is given by the ratio of the amplitudes $C_5/C_1$. The measurements used to compute these ratios were the amplitudes of $C_5$ and $C_1$ of the cortical responses recorded in the longest experimental session analysed. The

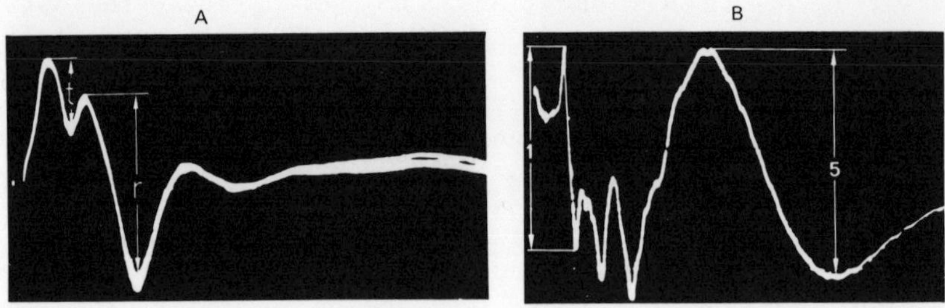


Fig. 3 Mean percentage changes in the amplitudes of $C_5$ and $C_1$, for all 6 cats during the VIA schedule. *A* - $C_5$. The mean amplitude of this component for each of the 8 categories of response in the VIA schedule was calculated for each cat and standardised against the overall mean of the 8 categories from that cat. This was done for each of the 6 cats. The percentage deviation of each of these mean values from the grand mean for all cats was computed. These deviations are plotted against evoked response category. The correlation coefficient for the regression fitted to data from categories 2 to 7 was $r = -0.66$ ($p < 0.001$). The slope was $B = -4.46 \pm 0.88$ (SD) which was significantly ($p < 0.001$) different from zero. *B* - $C_1$. The data were treated in the same way as those of $C_5$. The correlation coefficient, $r = -0.25$, was not significantly different from zero. Note the different scales of the ordinates in *A* and *B*. (From Horn & Wiesenfeld, 1974).

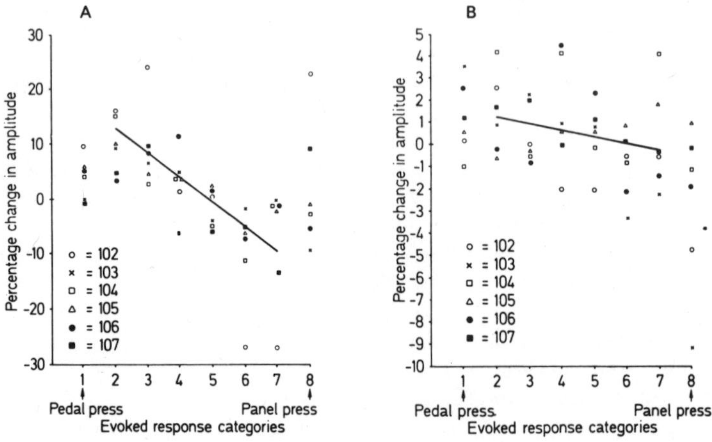


Fig. 4 Responses to shocks applied to the optic tract. *A*. LGN responses to 5 single shocks to the OT, superimposed. The presynaptic wave is labelled t and the postsynaptic wave, r. Scale 1 mv and 0.5 msec. *B*. Maximal cortical response to a single OT shock. Components 1 ($C_1$) and 5 ($C_5$) are labelled. Scale 200 μv and 2 msec. In both figures positivity at the recording electrode is represented as an upward deflexion of the trace (From Horn & Wiesenfeld, 1974).

ratios were calculated on data from five cats in which the amplitude of $C_1$ was stable throughout the waiting interval. The ratio was calculated for each of the response categories standardised. The means of these standardised values are plotted in Figure 5. Each value should approximate to zero if there is no effect of a waiting interval on cortical responsiveness, and the line fitted to the points should be horizontal. All the points derived from the VIV schedule

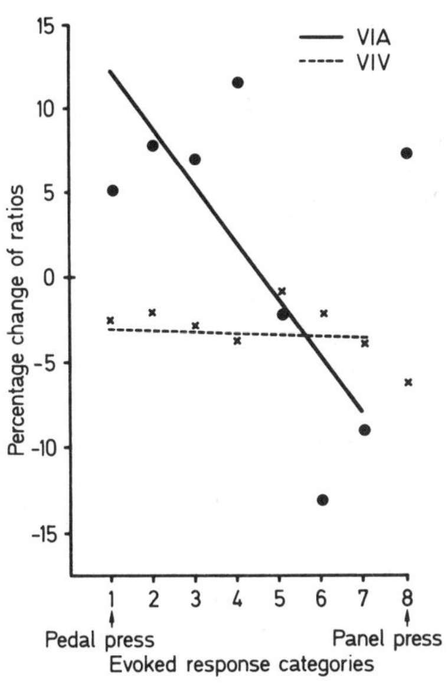


Fig. 5 Comparison of the averaged ratios, $C_5/C_1$, from the VIA and VIV schedules. For each cat, 8 ratios ($R_1$) corresponding to the 8 categories of shock interval, were calculated for the VIA and also for the VIV schedules. The overall mean ($\bar{R}$) of these 16 ratios was calculated together with the percentage deviation ($D_i$) of each $R_i$ from $\bar{R}$. The value of $D_i$ was calculated from the expression $D_i = (R_i - \bar{R}).10^2/\bar{R}$. The mean value ($\bar{D}_i$) was calculated for the 5 cats ($\bar{D}_i = \Sigma D_i/5$). These values are plotted against the evoked response category. Data from the VIA condition are plotted as filled circles, those from the VIV condition as crosses. Regression lines were fitted to data from evoked responses 1 to 7. For the VIA condition (solid line), the slope of the regression was B = -3.40 ± 1.07 (SD) which is significantly ($p < 0.01$) different from zero. The correlation coefficient was $r = -0.49$ ($p < 0.01$). For the VIV condition (broken line) B = -0.08 ± 0.76 and $r = -0.02$. Neither coefficient was significant. The mean percentage difference between the points for categories 2 and 6 in the VIA condition was 20.8% and was significant ($t = -6.17$, $p < 0.01$) (From Horn & Wiesenfeld, 1974).

are close to zero; those of evoked response categories 1 - 4 and 8 of the VIA data are above this value, and those from categories 5, 6 and 7 are below it. The standardised ratios in the VIA condition for evoked response categories 2, 3 and 4 combined are significantly ($t = 2.7$, $p < 0.05$) greater than the corresponding VIV values. The combined values from categories 6 and 7 in the VIA condition are significantly ($t = 2.83$, $p < 0.05$) less than those in the VIV condition.

In order to study the influence of changes in the level of arousal, as indicated by the state of the ECoG, on the responsiveness of the LGN and the visual cortex, the OT was shocked when the ECoG was synchronised and when it was desynchronised. Each cat was placed in the training box and maintained in darkness. The ECoG was considered to be desynchronised when it exhibited low voltage fast activity and synchronised when it contained high voltage slow (5 - 8 Hz) activity with no very slow waves (1 - 3 Hz) or spindles (12 - 15 Hz); the last two frequencies occurring in the drowsing or sleeping cat (Bradley and Elkes, 1957). Shocks were delivered to the OT once every 5 sec. Ten LGN and 10 cortical responses were analysed in the synchronised and in the desynchronised states of the ECoG. The amplitudes of the various components referred to above were measured and standardised. The results are summarised in Figure 6. There was a small (4%), but not significant, decrease in the size of the t component of the LGN response when the ECoG was desynchronised compared with the response evoked when the ECoG was synchronised. The postsynaptic LGN response and the presynaptic and postsynaptic cortical responses, however, were increased by 17%, 27% and 26% respectively. These percentage changes are not significantly different from each other. Thus, in the cat maintained in darkness,

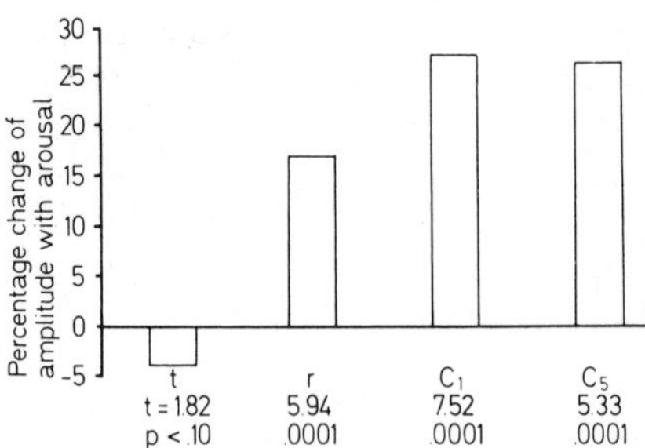


Fig. 6 Mean percentage change in the amplitude of the various LGN and cortical response components with changes in the ECoG. A positive value indicates that the amplitude of a component was greater when the ECoG was desynchronised (alert state) than when the ECoG was synchronised (non-alert state). The value of Student's t together with the associated values of p are given below each histogram (From Horn & Wiesenfeld, 1974).

changes in the state of arousal, as indicated by the state of the ECoG, profoundly affect transmission through the LGN but do not affect the responsiveness of the visual cortex to the input from the LGN.

## DISCUSSION

The results of the behavioural analysis were relatively simple in the variable interval schedules; the longer the waiting interval the more quickly did the cats respond to the stimulus. As the length of the waiting interval increased, electrophysiological changes were observed in the VIA schedule only. In the VIA schedule, cortical responsiveness decreased as the waiting interval increased. By comparing cortical responsiveness in the VIA with that of the VIV schedule it was found that, for the shorter waiting intervals, cortical responsiveness was higher in the VIA than the VIV condition (Fig. 5, evoked response categories 2-4, inclusive) then sharply declined and fell below that of the VIV condition (Fig. 5, evoked response categories 6 and 7).

There are no grounds for supposing that two variable interval tasks were of unequal difficulty; so there is no reason to suppose the animals were aroused to different extents in the two schedules. Nor is there any evidence that differences in eye movements or in the state of dark- adaptation during the performance of the auditory and visual tasks could have affected the amplitude of the evoked potentials (Wiesenfeld & Horn, 1974).

How are the behavioural changes related to vigilance? In the fixed interval schedules, the cats, after training, need not have attended to the stimulus to obtain a reward, but simply pressed the panel a set time after pressing the pedal. There may not, therefore, have been any changes in the level of vigilance during the performance of these tasks and it is of interest that no changes were observed in transmission through the LGN and the visual cortex. In the variable interval schedules, the cats did not know exactly when the stimulus would appear. However, the longer the interval that elapsed after the cat had pressed the pedal, the higher was the probability that the stimulus would occur. Such a distribution of stimulus events has been related to the subject's expectancy of the stimulus, expectancy increasing as stimulus probability increases (Elithorn & Lawrence, 1955; Audley, 1963; Thomas, 1970). Deese (1955) suggested that an observer's level of expectancy determines his vigilance level. Deese (1955) like Mackworth (1950) uses the term "vigilance" to mean a high state of readiness to respond to an event (Head, 1926). If Deese (1955) is correct, the vigilance of the cat in the present series of experiments should increase as the probability of the stimulus increased. Accordingly, the readiness of the cats to respond to the stimulus should have increased with the length of the waiting interval. The observed results are consistent with this prediction - the latency to respond shortened as the probability of the stimulus increased. If responsiveness increased with the lapse of time after the pedal press, the cats might have tended to press the panel in anticipation of the stimulus and so made more errors after the mean waiting interval (cf Deese, 1955) than before. This appears to have happened (Horn & Wiesenfeld, 1974). There is another factor that can usefully be considered when inferring the state of vigilance in these experiments. The cats had to withhold responding until the onset of the stimulus since a premature press was punished (that is, the cats failed to receive a reward on that trial). In order to minimise the risk of punishment, a higher level of attention to the occurrence of the stimulus may have been necessary during the longer than the shorter waiting intervals.

In order to interpret the significance of the electrophysiological changes, it is necessary to consider the physiological basis of the wave-forms that were measured. The response of the LGN to a shock applied to optic nerve or tract may contain two t waves (1 and 2 of P.O. Bishop and McLeod (1954) or (a) and (b) of Eisman *et al.*, (1967) respectively), and the corresponding r waves, depending on stimulus intensity and on the recording site in the LGN (Bishop & Evans, 1956; Eisman *et al.*, 1967). The response of the fast-conducting optic tract fibres is $t_1$, which has the shorter latency. We selected the recording site in the LGN to avoid contamination by $t_2$ and $r_2$. The fast-conducting fibres are the axons of ganglion cells which are, on the basis of a number of criteria, including their phasic response to standing contrast, referred to as Y or transient cells (Enroth-Cugell & Robson, 1966; Cleland *et al.*, 1971). The transient cells form a separate type from X or sustained cells which, among other characteristics, give a tonic response to standing contrast. The axons of sustained retinal ganglion cells are slow-conducting and activity in these fibres contributes to $t_2$ when the optic tract is shocked (Cleland *et al.*, 1971). The two types of retinal ganglion cells synapse with LGN cells having similar properties (Cleland *et al.*, 1971; Hoffman *et al.*, 1972), the $r_1$ and $r_2$ LGN waves probably corresponding to activity in the two types of postsynaptic cells (Fukada, 1973). Thus transient and sustained cells project separately to the visual cortex (Cleland *et al.*, 1971; Hoffman *et al.*, 1972; Stone & Dreher, 1973) and it is likely that component 1 of the cortical response to optic tract shock represents activity in the fast-conducting fibres (Clare *et al.*, 1969). Cells in the striate cortex may also be classified as transient or sustained (Ikeda & Wright, 1975) but it is of interest that cortical cells with slow-afferent cannot easily be excited by shocks applied to the optic tract (Stone & Dreher, 1973; Clare *et al.*, 1969). From these considerations it is clear that the LGN and optic radiation responses measured in the present study are due to activity in the transient fibre system and it is probable that the postsynaptic cortical response studied is due to cortical neuronal activity evoked by this system. It has been suggested that the transient system is concerned with the analysis of movement and the sustained system with the analysis of stationary patterns (Ikeda & Wright, 1972; Tolhurst, 1973; Kulikowski & Tolhurst, 1973).

During attention to vision, local ocular reflexes bring the image of an object sharply in focus on the retina and the movements of the two eyes, in a binocular animal, are coordinated. When the organism does not attend to vision there may be a loss of fixation so that images on the retina may not be sharply in focus and they are likely to fall on disparate regions of the retina of each eye. The input to the visual cortex from each eye would then be suboptimal (Hubel & Wiesel, 1962) for feature analysis. Under certain conditions of visual inattention, as when an organism is only moderately attentive to an auditory stimulus - a condition that may be met prior to the mean waiting interval in the present experiments - there might be some advantage in increasing the sensitivity of the visual cortex. Such an effect would increase the likelihood of the organism detecting a moving object even though the capacity of the visual system to identify the spatial characteristics of the object may be impaired. Such an arrangement might have survival value by allowing the animal to complete its response to the relatively easy non-visual tasks and then to switch its attention to the visual stimulus, locate it in space and examine its form in detail. In contrast, when a task is being performed which requires a high level of attention to a non-visual stimulus, an object moving in the visual field might, if it evoked a brisk discharge in the visual cortex, tend to distract the animal and so impair performance of the task. The possibility of this happening would be reduced if the responsiveness of the visual cortex were depressed. This depression occurs at the longer waiting intervals, at a time when attentiveness to the occurrence of the tone may be at its highest.

The failure to detect electrophysiological changes at the visual cortex during attention to vision is not entirely surprising. The recordings were made from the region of the striate cortex which receives the projection of the area centralis. If the responsiveness of this region to input from moving stimuli were depressed, the ability to discriminate any potentially dynamic aspect of the visual stimulus might be impaired, a consequence that could be disadvantageous to the animal. We cannot, of course, exclude the possibility that changes occur in the responsiveness of the visual cortex to input from a sustained system of fibres, which is likely to be involved in the analysis of stationary patterns. However, the techniques which we used to monitor transmission at the cortex are not well suited to such an analysis (Clare *et al.*, 1969; Stone & Dreher, 1973).

The physiological mechanisms that underlie the changes in responsiveness of the visual cortex to the input from the LGN are not known. It is possible that the changes are brought about by modifying inhibitory interactions between columns of cortical cells (Mountcastle & Powell, 1959; Benevento *et al.*, 1972; Blakemore & Tobin, 1972; Rose & Blakemore, 1974), an effect that might be mediated by the sensory fibres which project to the cortex (Shute & Lewis, 1963, 1967; Krnjević & Silver, 1965).

The electrophysiological results obtained in the behavioural tasks differ from the results obtained during "spontaneous" changes in the level of arousal as indicated by the state of the ECoG. When the ECoG was desynchronised there was a significant increase in the postsynaptic response of LGN relative to the response recorded when the ECoG was synchronised. The pre- and post-synaptic cortical responses were also increased, but these increases were not significantly different from that increase observed at the LGN; so that the cortical changes appear passively to reflect the LGN changes. Although changes in the responsiveness of the cortex to shocks applied to the thalamo-cortical fibres would be expected to accompany transitions in the state of the ECoG (Desmedt & LaGrutta, 1957; Evarts *et al.*, 1960; Palestini *et al.*, 1964; Dagnino *et al.*, 1965; Favale *et al.*, 1963, 1965; Walsh & Cordeau, 1965), such changes in cortical responsiveness may not be detected when the visual pathways are excited by shocking the optic tract (see, for example, Dagnino *et al.*, 1965; Walsh & Cordeau, 1965).

In the present series of experiments, then, changes in transmission at the LGN were observed during spontaneous changes in the level of arousal but not during the performance of any of the behavioural tasks. The direction of the changes occurring at the LGN during ECoG arousal is similar to that seen during low levels of attention to an auditory stimulus (VIA schedule) at the visual cortex - in each case there was an increased responsiveness to the optic tract shock - and the biological value of the change may also be similar. For example, when a cat becomes aroused, as in an orienting reflex, the lens of the eye accommodates for near vision. This happens whether the stimulus is non-visual or visual; and if visual, regardless of the distance of the object from the eye (Elul & Marchiafava, 1964; Horn, 1975). Such changes would not always be compatible with the optimum resolution of form. However, if the sensitivity of the visual system to movement is increased above the level found when the animal is drowsy, the ability of the organism to locate and direct its gaze to the moving object would also be increased. In the light of these considerations the orienting reflex might more appropriately be described as the "Where is it?" rather than the "What is it?" (Pavlov, 1955) reaction. When fixation is achieved, the image of the object might then be brought sharply into focus on the area centralis and so permit accurate analysis of the object's spatial characteristics.

Because changes in the state of attention are not directly observed but are inferred from the organism's behaviour and also, perhaps, from associated changes in the state of the nervous system (Brown, 1965; Thompson & Bettinger, 1970), difficulties in interpretation must inevitably arise. In this analysis, an attempt has been made to relate the behavioural and electrophysiological results of the present experiments in a particular, seemingly parsimonious, way and to infer the animal's state of attentiveness during the performance of the behavioural tasks. Other interpretations of these results are, of course, possible. But a change in the responsiveness of the visual cortex occurs during the performance of a task requiring attention to a visual stimulus and the change cannot in any simple way be accounted for in terms of such non-specific factors as changes in the level of arousal, the orienting reflex or eye movements.

## REFERENCES


1. ADRIAN, E.D. *Nature (London) 153:*360, 1944.
2. ADRIAN, E.D. The physiological basis of perception. In: Brain Mechanisms and Consciousness. (E.D. Adrian, F. Bremer & H.H. Jasper, eds.) Oxford: Blackwell, 1954.
3. AKIMOTO, H., SAITO, Y. & NAKAMURA, Y. Effects of arousal stimuli on evoked neuronal activities in cat's visual cortex. In: Neurophysiologie und Psychophysik des visuellen Systems. (R. Jung & H.H. Kornhuber, eds). Berlin-Göttingen-Heidelberg: Springer, 1961.
4. AUDLEY, R.J. Decision models in reaction time. In: Psychophysics and the Ideal Observer. Proc. 17th Int. Cong. Psychol. Amsterdam: North-Holland Publishing Co., 1963.
5. BENEVENTO, L.H., CREUTZFELDT, O.D. & KUHNT, U. *Nature New Biology 238:*124, 1972.
6. BERESFORD, W.A. *J. Hirnforsch. 5:*210, 1962.
7. BERGER, H. *Arch. Psychiat. 94:*16, 1931.
8. BLAKEMORE, C. & TOBIN, E.A. *Exp. Brain Res. 15:*439, 1972.
9. BISHOP, G.H. & CLARE, M.H. *J. Neurophysiol. 15:*201, 1952.
10. BISHOP, P.O. & EVANS, W.A. *J. Physiol. (London) 134:*538, 1956.
11. BISHOP, P.O. & MC LEOD, J.G. *J. Neurophysiol. 17:*387, 1954.
12. BREMER, F. & STOUPEL, N. *Arch. int. Physiol. 64:*234, 1956.
13. BROADBENT, D.E. Perception and Communication. London: Pergamon Press, 1958.
14. BROWN, J.S. Generalisation and discrimination In: Stimulus Generalisation (D.I. Mostofsky, ed.), pp. 7-23, Stanford: Stanford University Press, 1965.
15. CHANG, H.T. & KAADA, B. *J. Neurophysiol. 13:*305, 1950.
16. CHERRY, E.C. *J. Acoust. Soc. Amer. 25:*975, 1953.
17. CLARE, M.H., LANDAU, W.M. & BISHOP, G.H. *Exp. Neurol. 24:*400, 1960.

18. CLELAND, B.G., DUBIN, M.W. & LEVICK, W.R. *J. Physiol. (London) 217:*473, 1971.
19. DAGNINO, N., FAVALE, E., LOEB, C. & MANFREDI, M. *J. Neurophysiol. 28:*443, 1965.
20. DEESE, J. *Psychol. Rev. 62:*359, 1955.
21. DESMEDT, J.E. & LA GRUTTA, G. *J. Physiol. (London) 136:*20, 1957.
22. DUMONT, S. & DELL, P. *J. Physiol. (Paris) 50:*261, 1958.
23. EISMAN, J.A., HANSEN, S.M. & BURKE, W. *Vision Res. 7:*385, 1967.
24. ELITHORN, A. & LAWRENCE, C. *Quart. J. Exp. Psychol. 7:*116, 1955.
25. ELUL, R. & MARCHIAFAVA, P.L. *Arch. Ital. Biol. 102:*616, 1964.
26. ENROTH-CUGELL, C. & ROBSON, J.C. *J. Physiol. (London) 187:*517, 1966.
27. EVARTS, E.V., FLEMING, T.C. & HUTTENLOCHER, P.R. *Amer. J. Physiol. 199:*373, 1960.
28. FAVALE, E., LOEB, C. & MANFREDI, M. *Arch. Intern. Physiol. Biochim. 71:*229, 1963.
29. FAVALE, E., LOEB, C., MANFREDI, M. & SACCO, G. *Electroencephal. Clin. Neurophysiol. 18:*354, 1965.
30. FEENEY, D.M. & OREM, J.M. *Physiol. Behav. 9:*805, 1972.
31. FUKADA, Y. *Exp. Brain Res. 17:*242, 1973.
32. FUXE, K. *Acta Physiol. Scand. 64:Suppl. 247,*37, 1965.
33. GAREY, L.J., JONES, E.G. & POWELL, T.P.S. *J. Neurol. Neurosurg. Psychiat. 31:*135, 1968.
34. GODFRAIND, J.M. & MEULDERS, M. *Exp. Brain Res. 9:*183, 1969.
35. GOLDBERG, M.E. & WURTZ, R.H. *J. Neurophysiol. 35:*560, 1972.
36. HEAD, H. Aphasia. Cambridge University Press, 1926.
37. HERNÁNDEZ-PEON, R., GUZMÁN-FLORES, C., ALCAREZ, M. & FERNANDEZ-GUARDIOLA, A. *Acta Neurol. Lat.-Amer. 3:*1, 1957.
38. HOFFMAN, K-P., STONE, J. & SHERMAN, S.M. *J. Neurophysiol. 35:*518, 1972.
39. HORN, G. *Mermaid 18:*17, 1952.
40. HORN, G. *Brain 83:*57, 1960.
41. HORN, G. Physiological and psychological aspects of selective perception. In: Advances in the Study of Behavior, 1. (D.S. Lehrman, R.A. Hinde & E. Shaw, eds.) pp. 155-215, Academic Press, N.Y., 1965.
42. HORN, G. Attention and the orientation response. In: Experimental Approaches to Psychopathology. (M.R. Kietzman, S. Sutton & J. Zubin, eds.) Academic Press, N.Y., 1975.
43. HORN, G. & BLUNDELL, J. *Nature (London) 184:*173, 1959.
44. HORN, G. & HILL, R.M. *Nature (London) 202:*296, 1964.
45. HORN, G., STECHLER, G. & HILL, R.M. *Exp. Brain Res. 15:*113, 1972.
46. HORN, G. & WIESENFELD, Z. *Exp. Brain Res. 21:*67, 1974.
47. HOTTA, T. & KAMEDA, K. *Exp. Neurol. 8:*1, 1963.
48. HOTTA, T. & KAMEDA, K. *Exp. Neurol. 9:*127, 1964.

49. HUBEL, D.H. & WIESEL, T.N. *J. Physiol. (London) 160*:160, 1962.
50. IKEDA, H. & WRIGHT, M.J. *J. Physiol. (London)*, in press, 1975.
51. IKEDA, H. & WRIGHT, M.J. *J. Physiol. (London) 227*:769, 1972.
52. JAMES, W. The Principles of Psychology. London, Macmillan & Co., 1890.
53. JANE, J.A., SMIRNOW, G.D. & JASPER, H.H. *Electroencephal. Clin. Neurophysiol. 14*:244, 1962.
54. JUNG, R., KORNHUBER, H.H. & DA FONSECA, J.S. Multisensory convergence on cortical neurones. Neuronal effects of visual acoustic and vestibular stimuli in the superior convolutions of the cat's cortex. In: Progress in Brain Research, Vol. 1, Brain Mechanisms (G. Morozzi, A. Fessard & H.H. Jasper, eds.) Amsterdam: Elsevier, 1963.
55. KRNJEVIĆ, K. & SILVER, A. *J. Anat. (London) 99*:711, 1965.
56. KULIKOWSKI, J.J. & TOLHURST, D.J. *J. Physiol. (London) 232*:149, 1973.
57. MACKWORTH, N.H. Researches on the measurement of human performance. M.R.C. Special Report No. 268, pp. 1-156, H.M.S.O., 1950.
58. MALCOLM, L.J., BRUCE, I.S.C. & BURKE, W. *Exp. Brain Res. 10*:283, 1970.
59. MALIS, L.I. & KRUGER, L. *J. Neurophysiol. 19*:172, 1956.
60. MARSHALL, W.H., TALBOT, S.A. & ADES, H.W. *J. Neurophysiol. 6*:1, 1943.
61. MORAY, N. Attention: Selective Processes in Vision and Hearing. London: Hutchinson, 1970.
62. MOUNTCASTLE, V.B. & POWELL, T.P.S. *Bull. John Hopkins Hosp. 105*:173, 1959.
63. MURATA, K., CRAMER, H. & BACH-Y-RITA, P. *J. Neurophysiol. 28*:1223, 1965.
64. NÄÄTÄNEN, R. *Ann. Acad. Sci. Fenn. 151B*:1, 1967.
65. PALESTINI, M., PISANO, M., ROSADINI, G. & ROSSI, G.F. *Exp. Neurol. 9*:17, 1964.
66. PAVLOV, I.V. Selected Works. Foreign Languages Publishing House, Moscow, 1955.
67. RIZZOLATTI, G., CAMARDA, R., GRUPP, L.A. & PISA, M. *J. Neurophysiol. 37*:1262, 1974.
68. ROSE, D. & BLAKEMORE, C. *Nature 249: No. 5455*,375, 1974.
69. SCHOOLMAN, A. & EVARTS, E.V. *J. Neurophysiol. 22*:112, 1959.
70. SHUTE, C.C.D. & LEWIS, P.R. *Nature (London) 199*:1160, 1963.
71. SHUTE, C.C.D. & LEWIS, P.R. *Brain 90*:497, 1967.
72. STONE, J. & DREHER, B. *J. Neurophysiol. 36*:551, 1973.
73. SUSUKI, H. & TAIRA, N. *Jap. J. Physiol. 11*:641, 1961.
74. SZENTÁGOTHAI, J., HAMORI, J. & TÖMBÖL, T. *Exp. Brain Res. 2*:283, 1966.
75. TELLO, F. *Trab. Lab. Invest. Biol. Univ. Madrid 3*:39, 1904.
76. THOMAS, E.A.C. *Brit. J. Psychol. 61*:33, 1970.

77. THOMPSON, R.F. & BETTINGER, L.A. Neural substrates of attention. In: Attention: Contemporary Theory and Analysis (D.I. Mostofsky, ed.) pp. 367-401. New York: Appleton-Century-Crofts, 1970.
78. TOLHURST, D.J. *J. Physiol. (London) 231*:385, 1973.
79. WALLEY, R.E. & URSCHEL, J.W. *Physiol. & Behav. 9*:7, 1972.
80. WALSH, J.T. & CORDEAU, J.P. *Exp. Neurol. 11*:80, 1965.
81. WIESENFELD, S. & HORN, G. *Brain Res. 77*:211, 1974.
82. WORDEN, F.G. Attention and auditory electrophysiology. In: Progress in Physiological Psychology, 1. (E. Stellar & J.M. Sprague, eds.) New York:Academic Press, 1966.

# RETINAL AND CORTICAL CHANGES IN THE VISUAL SYSTEM OF PATTERN-DEPRIVED RATS[1]

U. Yinon, C. Shaw[2] and E. Auerbach
Vision Research Laboratory
Hadassah University Hospital
Jerusalem, Israel

## RETINAL CHANGES

Substantial electrophysiological changes in the visual cortex and lateral geniculate nucleus of cats result from unilateral pattern deprivation. The question arises whether these changes are secondary to those occurring in the retina. When retinal responses (ERG's) of visually deprived cats were examined, a diminution of the b-wave of the deprived eye was found in some studies. Baxter and Riesen (1961) showed a rapid recovery of the b-wave during exposure to normal light conditions in cats that had been dark-reared for 12 months. Similar depression and recovery of the ERG b-wave were obtained with adult cats visually deprived for a period of a few days to several weeks (Cornwell & Sharpless, 1968; Ganz *et al.*, 1968; Hamasaki & Pollack, 1972). Also, Hamasaki & Flynn (1973) found that children monocularly deprived for 1-6 months by eye patching showed a depression of the ERG followed by recovery after removal of the patch. No effects were observed in other studies in the cat (Wiesel & Hubel, 1963; Sherman & Stone, 1973) or in the monkey (von Noorden *et al.*, 1970). These inconsistencies led us to examine the effects of long term pattern deprivation on the rat retina. The rat was chosen as the experimental animal partially for technical reasons and because it is representative of a simple mammalian retina. A detailed report of our results is given elsewhere (Yinon *et al.*, 1974).

[1]Supported by Stiftung Volkswagenwerk under contract number 11 1538.
[2]Present address: Department of Zoology, Hebrew University of Jerusalem, Israel.

Eighteen rats were pattern-deprived by monocular lid suture between the eighth and fourteenth postnatal day, before natural eye opening, and were tested at 1.5 - 13.5 months of age. Twenty-one normal adult rats of various ages were used as controls. Animals were anaesthetized with urethane (135 mg/kg) and atropinized. The retinae were examined by ophthalmoscopy at the end of the deprivation period; no pathological conditions were noted. In most deprived rats, the dark adaptation period prior to testing was of 12 hours duration. A dim red light was used during opening of the sutures. Experiments were carried out in the dark. Stimuli consisted of white light flashes (Xenon, 10 μsec) with a maximum light intensity of $1.5 \times 10^6$ cp. Ag-AgCl ball electrodes of 1.0 mm diameter were used for corneal ERG recordings.

The deprived eye initially showed a considerable diminution in the b-wave amplitude of the ERG, followed by a slow recovery to near normal values (Fig. 1). These effects were noted for a wide range of deprivation periods between 1.5 and 13.5 months after birth and were not influenced by the duration of the deprivation. No differences in either a-wave amplitude or a- or b-wave latencies were found between the deprived and normal eyes (Fig. 2); nor were any significant differences noted in the b-waves of the control animals.

The above results are in accord with earlier data of Baxter & Riesen (1961) and Cornwall & Sharpless (1968), and Hamasaki & Pollack (1972).

## VISUAL CORTEX

Since most of the optic nerve fibers cross in the rat optic chiasm, binocular interaction is likely to be small, in accordance with the limited binocular field of vision. Despite the existence of commissural fibers between the two hemispheres, communication between them is negligible (Creel & Sheridan, 1966). Behavioral experiments on interocular transfer showed that application of the visual input in rats to one eye is largely limited to the contralateral hemisphere (Nadel & Buresova, 1968). Since it has been suggested that the deprivation effects in the cat visual cortex depend upon competition between inputs from the two eyes (Wiesel & Hubel, 1965), the relative independence of the two cortices of the rat has a certain advantage for studies where unilateral effects are under observation. Thus we were able to examine the assumption that competition is needed to produce deprivation effects.

We describe here experiments on visual-evoked potential (Yinon & Auerbach, 1973), the properties of neurons of the rat visual cortex and the effects on these, of monocular pattern deprivation. Preliminary studies on neural properties and retinotopic organization

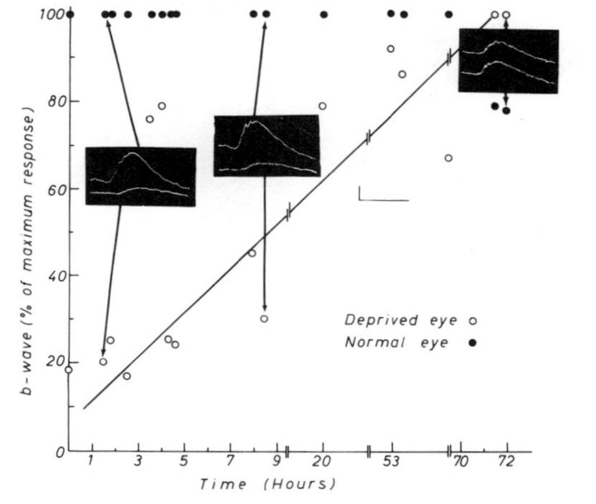


Fig. 1 Depression-recovery curve of the b-wave in a rat visually deprived for 11 months. The b-wave of the deprived eye was initially much smaller than that of the normal eye. Recovery to normal amplitudes is seen during the second and third days. Inset: ERG's at different times for each eye (arrows). Calibrations: 200 μV and 100 msec. Averaged responses (5-15) are plotted at different times after the beginning of the experiment. Stimulus intensity was 1.5 x $10^6$ cp. The decrease in both ERG's at the end of the experiment may be due to deterioration of the animal.

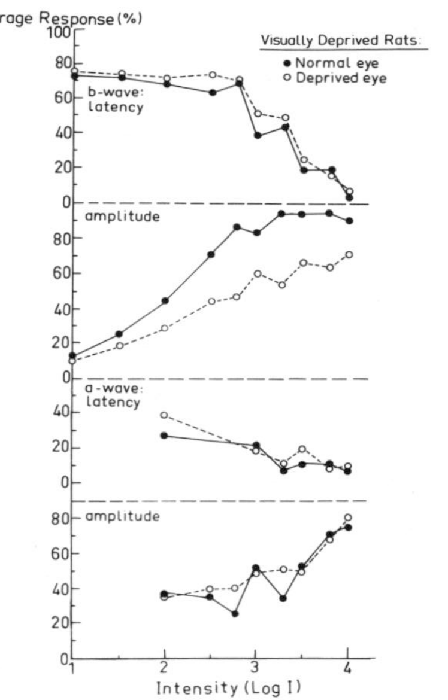


Fig. 2 ERG intensity-response curves for ten deprived rats. Each point represents the average percentage of the maximal response (2-10 experiments) of each animal. Differences are seen only in the b-wave amplitude.

of the rat visual cortex on the unit level have been published (Montero *et al.*, 1973; Shaw *et al.*, 1974).

Ball electrodes made of silver wire were used for recording visual evoked potentials (VEP's) and stainless steel microelectrodes served to record unit activity. For the VEP measurements, a diffuse light from a stroboscope was used, and for the unit activities, stationary spots or moving slits obtained from a slide projector. VEP's were averaged by a computer of average transients and action potentials were recorded by a tape recorder. Receptive fields were drawn on a tangent screen at a distance of 30-60 cm from the eye tested.

We will denote the hemisphere contralateral to the normal eye (and ipsilateral to the deprived eye) as the "normal" hemisphere and the other, contralateral to the deprived eye, as the "deprived" hemisphere.

In normal rats, most of the highest amplitude VEP's (80-100% of the maximum) were obtained in area 17 with contralateral stimulation (Fig. 3). The results provide physiological confirmation of Krieg's map (1946a, b). Areas 18 and 18a were much less responsive. The VEP's produced by stimulation of the ipsilateral eye were very low (Fig. 4). The fact that the binocular response (in the normal rat) is similar to the contralateral one supports the above mentioned findings on little binocular interaction in the rat visual system. These findings are basic to our approach in investigating separately the properties of the "deprived" and "normal" cortices of deprived rats.

Mappings were obtained from six deprived animals. The average VEP recorded in area 17 from the "normal" hemisphere of the deprived animal was greater by 26.7% than that from the corresponding area of the "deprived" hemisphere (Fig. 5). The duration of the deprivation period (70-170 days) does not influence the responsiveness of the "deprived" hemispheres.

Receptive fields of the units found in the rat visual cortex were large in comparison to those recorded by Hubel & Wiesel (1962) for cats (Fig. 6). The organization of most receptive fields was similar to that of complex cells of the cat visual cortex (Hubel & Wiesel, 1962), i.e. they could not be mapped into adjacent "on", "off" or "on-off" regions (Fig. 7).

We did not find differences in receptive field size and organization between "normal" and "deprived" neurons. However, only 13.3% of the cortical cells from "deprived" cortices (of 16 deprived animals) in comparison to 51.1% cells in "normal" cortices, were activated by specific visual stimuli such as light spots and moving slits.

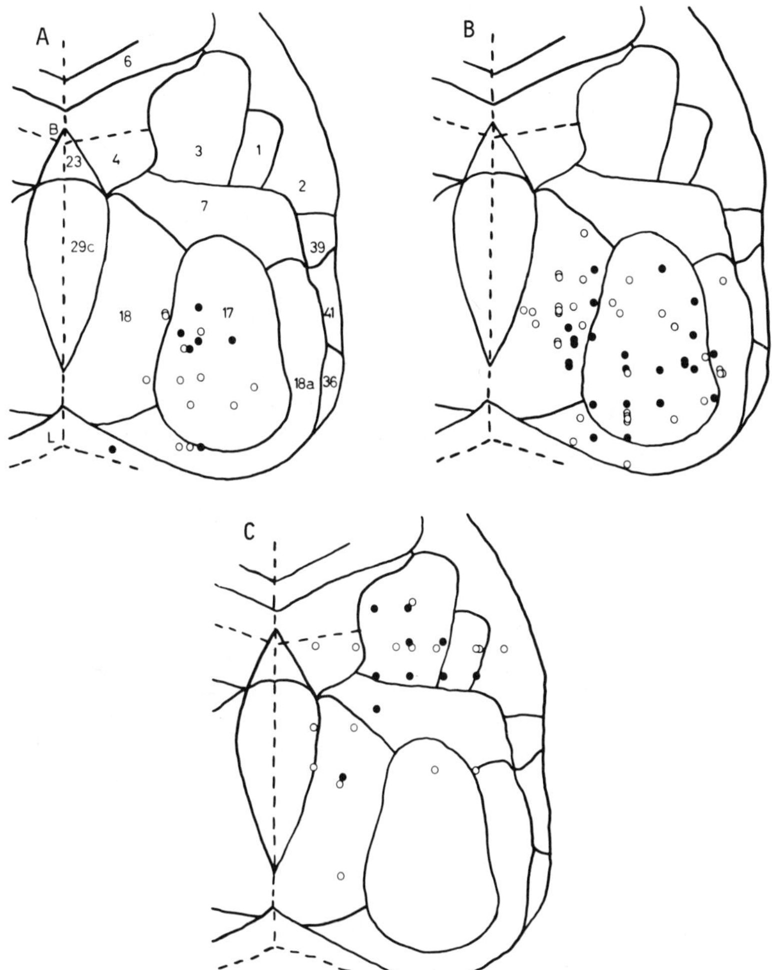


Fig. 3 Mapping of the contralateral visual response areas on the visual and other regions of the normal rat cerebral cortex. Each point represents 1-5 series of stimuli, each consisting of 50 average VEP's. The height of the principle positive potential was calculated as a percentage of the maximal response. Each map is based on data from 11 normal animals. Data from right (o) and left hemispheres (•) were superimposed. B - bregma, L - lambda. Cortical areas were redrawn and numbered after Krieg (1946a, b). A. Responses of 80-100% of maximal VEP amplitude. B. Responses of 40-60% of maximal VEP amplitude. C. Potentials that were not higher than the background activity. Note the concentration of the highest response in area 17 and smallest responses in non-visual areas.

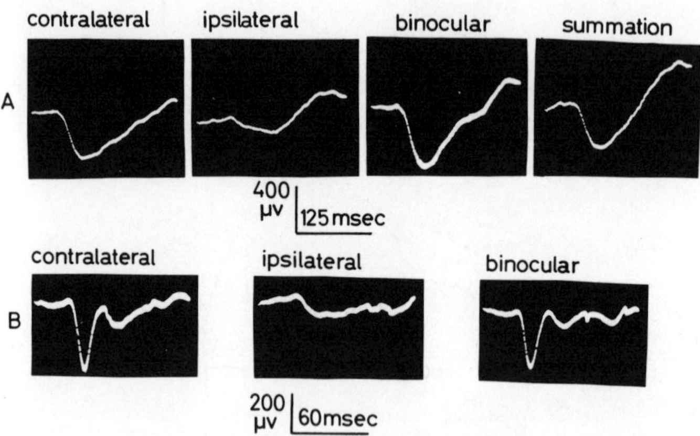


Fig. 4 VEP response of the rat to monocular and binocular stimulation. A. Recording from area 17 in the normal hemisphere of a rat visually deprived for 151 days. Fifty responses were averaged; positivity downward. B. Responses of a normal animal. Recording from area 17; positivity downward. Arithmetical summation of contralateral and ipsilateral responses. Note the large difference between contralateral and ipsilateral responses and the similarity between the amplitudes of the binocular and contralateral responses.

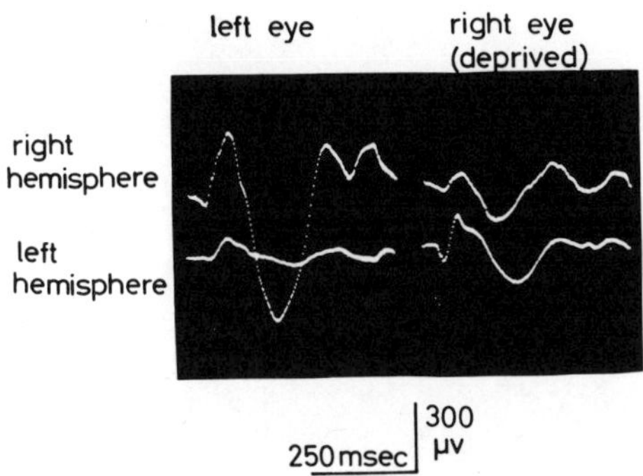


<u>Fig. 5</u> VEP of the "normal" and "deprived" cortices in a rat unilaterally deprived for 70 days. Responses to stimulation of either eye were recorded simultaneously from corresponding points of both cortices in area 17. Each trace represents an average of 50 VEP's, positivity upward. Note the large contralateral response in the "normal" cortex in comparison with the "deprived" cortex. The ipsilateral responses are similar.

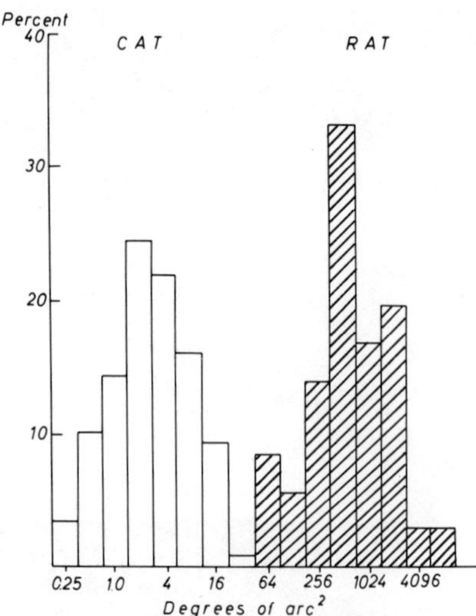


Fig. 6 Comparison between receptive field sizes of 36 neurons of the rat visual cortex and 117 neurons of the cat visual cortex (Hubel & Wiesel, 1962). Data on the cat has been pooled from simple and complex cells.

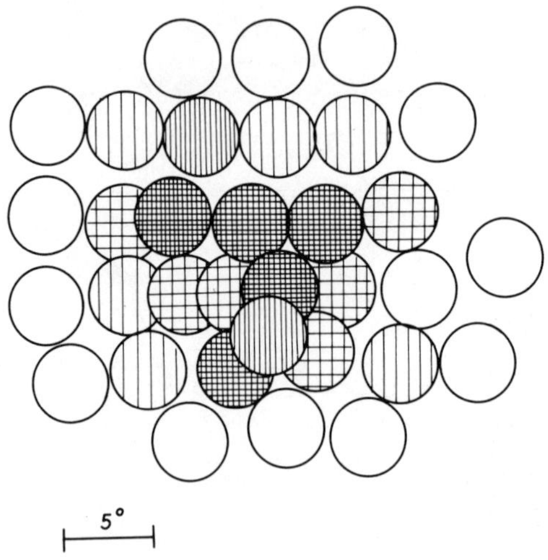


Fig. 7 Plot of a receptive field of a typical motion-selective cell to stationary spot stimuli. Stimulus intensity 1.4 ft. cd.; stimulus size 4° dia. |||| "off" responses; ╪╪╪ "on-off" responses; 0 no response. Density of lines indicate strength of response.

No difference was seen between the rate and pattern of firing of neurons during spontaneous activity in "normal" as compared to "deprived" cortices (Fig. 8).

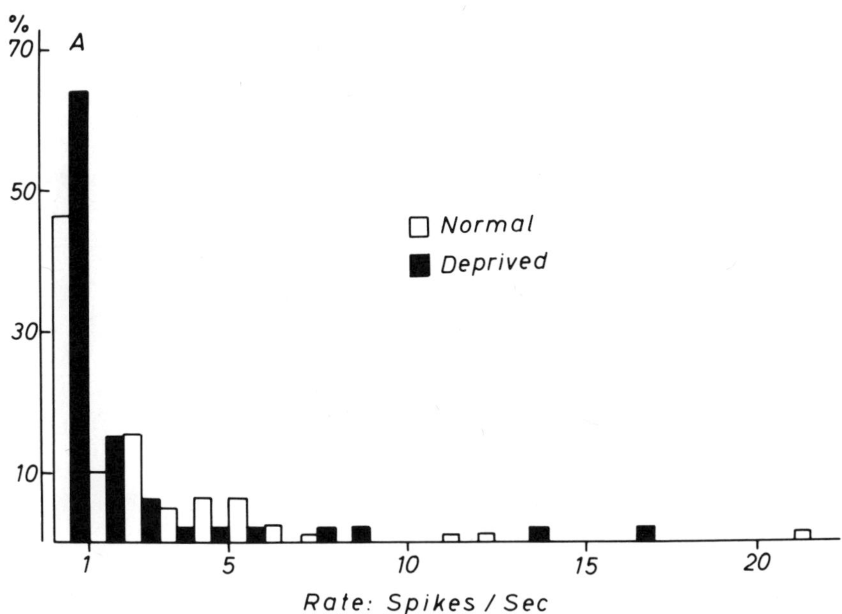


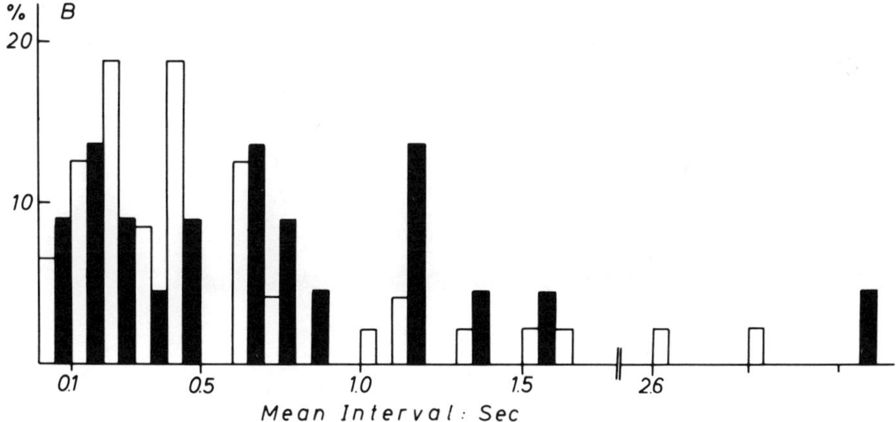


Fig. 8 Spontaneous activity of units from "normal" and "deprived" visual cortex of the rat. A. mean rate of firing (spikes/sec). B. mean interval of firing (seconds).

Units were grouped according to Chow *et al.*'s (1971) classification for neurons of the rabbit visual cortex. Motion-selective cells responded optimally to stimuli of any orientation and direction moving through their receptive field. For orientation-selective cells, the stimulus eliciting the maximal response was usually a slit of light or black bar moving in a particular orientation (Fig. 9). Stimuli of other orientations elicited weaker, if any, response. For direction-selective cells, the presence of the non-responsive direction at 180° to the optimal direction is the significant feature. The fourth group was identified as indefinite cells; their receptive field could not be mapped, although the cell responded to diffuse, punctate and/or moving stimuli in many areas of the visual field, regardless of stimulus size and orientation. From the small number

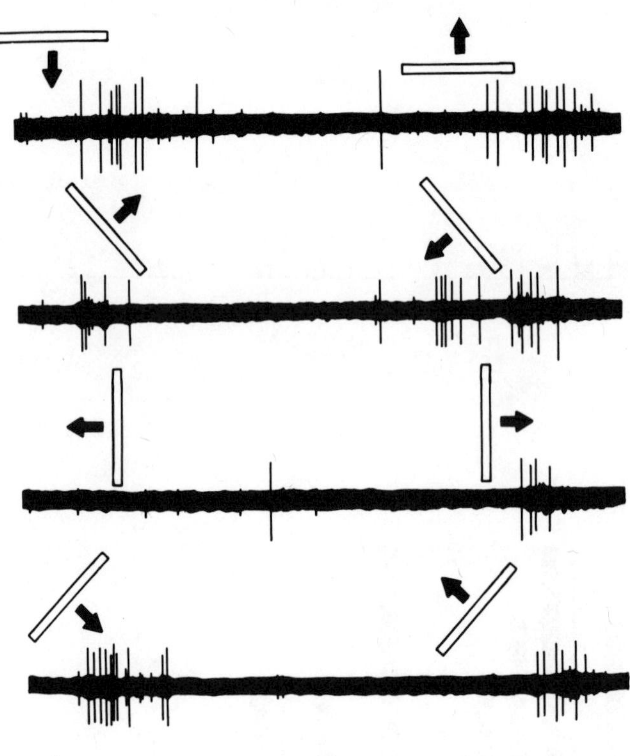

Fig. 9 Orientation selective cell of the rat visual cortex. Responses to a slit (6.9° x 1.9°) moving through a receptive field of area 6.9° x 7.2°. Average stimulus speed 17°/sec. Stimulus intensity 1.4 ft. cd. Time calibration 0.5 sec.

of cells having these receptive field properties in the "deprived" cortex we can conclude that only the level of neuronal responsiveness is influenced (Fig. 10).

If the difference in VEP between the normal and the deprived hemisphere recorded in our experiments were the result of neural degeneration, a greater change would be expected in the VEP of the "deprived" hemisphere. The VEP's obtained in our experiments were clearly demonstrable even after six months of deprivation. In comparison, enucleation of the eye in the rat after birth leads to degeneration of optic nerve fibers and of higher centers within a period of three months (Tsang, 1963). This finding is supported by Terry *et al.* (1962) who compared the effects of unilateral enucleation and deprivation in the mouse. They demonstrated extensive degeneration of the visual pathways in enucleation and no demonstrable change in deprivation. Fifkova and Hassler (1969) however have shown morphological changes in both L6B and visual cortex of pattern deprived rats.

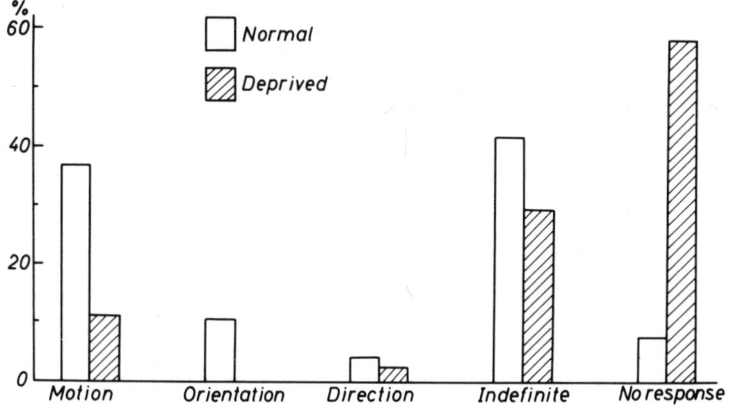


Fig. 10 Distribution of receptive field properties of 104 neurons of "normal" and 45 neurons of "deprived" cortex of 32 rats. Normal cells were pooled from the "normal" cortex of deprived rats and from normal controls.

The changes found in the deprived rat could not be correlated with behavioral findings, due to great variability in the latter. Slomin & Pasnak (1972) found visual deficits in depth perception in rats reared in the dark. However, Walk *et al.* (1957), Nealey & Edwards (1960) and Carr & McGuigan (1965), under similar experimental conditions, found no differences in depth perception of visually deprived rats. Moreover, since these experiments were carried out on light deprived rats, findings might differ for unilaterally deprived animals and even for animals which were binocularly pattern-deprived by sutures.

Our experiments have shown that in the rat visual system, due to the almost complete absence of binocular interaction, the input from the deprived and the normal eyes do not compete. Therefore, unlike in the cat (Wiesel & Hubel, 1965; Guillery, 1973), the deprivation effect is caused in the rat independently of the seeing eye. These results suggest that the rat cells have been functionally deafferentiated by the deprivation which might be due to a synaptic block at the termination of optic radiation fibers.

## REFERENCES

1. BAXTER, B.L. & RIESEN, A.H. *Science 134:*1626, 1961.
2. CARR, W.J. & MC GUIGAN, D.I. *Anim. Behav. 13:*25, 1965.
3. CHOW, K.L., MASLAND, R.H. & STEWART, D.L. *Brain Res. 33:*337. 1971.
4. CORNWELL, A.C. & SHARPLESS, S.K. *Vision Res. 8:*389, 1968.
5. CREEL, D.J. & SHERIDAN, C.L. *Psychon. Sci. 6:*89, 1966.
6. FIFKOVA, E. & HASSLER, R. *J. Comp. Neurol. 135:*167, 1969.
7. GANZ, L., FITCH, M. & SATTERBERG, J.A. *Exp. Neurol. 22:*614, 1968.
8. GUILLERY, R.W. *J. Comp. Neurol. 148:*417, 1973.
9. HAMASAKI, D.I. & FLYNN, J.T. *Arch. Ophthal. 89:*473, 1973.
10. HAMASAKI, D.I. & POLLACK, J.G. *Vision Res. 12:*835, 1972.
11. HUBEL, D.H. & WIESEL, T.N. *J. Physiol. 160:*106, 1962.
12. KRIEG, W.J.S. *J. Comp. Neurol. 84:*221, 1946a.
13. KRIEG, W.J.S. *J. Comp. Neurol. 84:*277, 1946b.
14. MONTERO, V.M., ROJAS, A. & TORREALBA, F. *Brain Res. 53:*197, 1973.
15. NADEL, L. & BURESOVA, O. *Nature 220:*914, 1968.
16. NEALEY, S.M. & EDWARDS, B.J. *J. Comp. Physiol. Psychol. 53:* 468, 1960.
17. VON NOORDEN, G.K., DOWLING, J.E. & FERGUSON, D.C. *Arch. Ophthal. 84:*206, 1970.
18. SHAW, C., YINON, U. & AUERBACH, E. *Vision Res. 14:*311, 1974.
19. SHERMAN, S.M. & STONE, J. *Brain Res. 60:*224, 1973.
20. SLOMIN, V. JR. & PASNAK, R. *Vision Res. 12:*623, 1972.
21. TERRY, R.J., ROLAND, A.L. & RACE, J. *J. Exp. Zool. 150:*165, 1962.

22. TSANG, Y. *J. Comp. Neurol.* *66:*211, 1963.
23. WALK, R.D., GIBSON, E.J. & TIGHE, T.J. *Science* *126:*80, 1957.
24. WIESEL, T.N. & HUBEL, D.H. *J. Neurophysiol.* *26:*1003, 1963.
25. WIESEL, T.N. & HUBEL, D.H. *J. Neurophysiol.* *28:*1029, 1965.
26. YINON, U. & AUERBACH, E. *Exp. Neurol.* *38:*231, 1973.
27. YINON, U., SHAW, C. & AUERBACH, E. *Exp. Neurol.* In press, 1974.

# SENSORY AND NEURONAL MECHANISMS UNDERLYING ACOUSTIC COMMUNICATION IN ORTHOPTERAN INSECTS

Franz Huber

Max Planck Institut für Verhaltensphysiologie
Abtl. Neuroethologie
Seewiesen, Federal Republic of Germany

## INTRODUCTION

In Orthoptera, intraspecific acoustic communication occurs during the period of reproduction of the adult insects and is realized by means of species-specific sound signals. These signals are generated by the males only in crickets, but by both sexes in grasshoppers. Periodic movements which produce the sound are made either with the front wings in crickets and tettigonid grasshoppers or with the hindlegs in acridid grasshoppers. Auditory organs located within the front legs in crickets and tettigonid grasshoppers or laterally within the 1st abdominal segment in acridid grasshoppers receive the acoustic information which is processed in certain parts of the CNS. The auditory input can give rise to phonokinetic behaviour in the females of crickets and grasshoppers and to acoustic responses in one of the sexes (crickets) or in both the sexes (grasshoppers).

For the last twenty years, a quite comprehensive investigation has been carried out with the following goals:

1. To describe acoustic behaviour of interest both in the field and under laboratory conditions (Alexander 1967; Busnel 1963; Markl 1972).

2. More particularly, to analyse problems concerned with:

a) the parameters of the sound signals and the structures performing them (Bailey 1970; Bailey and Broughton 1970; Bennet-Clark 1970, 1971; Busnel 1973; Dumortier 1963; Loher 1957; Michelsen and Nocke 1974; Nocke 1971).

b) the external environment through which the sound is propagated which is a background to the communication (Popov 1971a, 1972, 1974a,b; Shuvalov and Popov 1971; 1973a,b; Zhantiev and Dubrovin 1974),

c) the species-specific recognition process both at the behavioural level (Busnel 1963; v.Helversen 1972; Murphey and Zaretsky 1972; Zaretsky 1972; Popov 1974a,b) and at the level of the participating sensory and other neuronal elements (Adam 1969, 1970; Johnstone *et al.*, 1970; Kalmring 1971; Kalmring *et al.*, 1972a,b; McKay 1969, 1970; Michelsen 1966, 1968, 1971, 1972; Michelsen and Nocke 1974; Nocke 1972; Popov 1965, 1967, 1969, 1971b, 1974a; Rheinlaender *et al.*, 1972; Rheinlaender and Kalmring 1973; Rowell and McKay 1969a, b; Schwartzkopff 1973; Stout and Huber 1972; Worden and Galambos 1972; Zaretsky 1971, 1972),

d) the relationship between signal input and behavioural output, and the internal conditions on which such relationships depend (Heiligenberg 1966, 1969; Jones 1966a,b; Jones and Dambach 1973; Loher 1966; Loher and Huber 1964, 1966; Popov 1974a,b; Renner 1952),

e) the neuromuscular and neuronal mechanisms underlying sound production and associated movements (Bentley 1969a,b; Bentley and Kutsch 1966; Elsner 1967, 1968, 1970, 1973, 1974a,b,c; Elsner and Huber 1969, 1973; Ewing and Hoyle 1965; Huber 1955, 1960, 1962, 1963, 1965, 1970, 1974a,b; Josephson and Halverson 1971; Kutsch 1969; Kutsch and Huber 1970; Kutsch and Otto 1972; Möss 1971; Otto 1967, 1969, 1971),

f) the genetical and the ontogenetical basis of acoustic behaviour (Bentley 1971, 1973; Bentley and Hoy 1970; Hörmann-Heck 1957; Perdeck 1958).

Only some of these problems will be discussed in this contribution; we shall concentrate firstly on sound producing mechanisms and their neuromuscular and neuronal basis, and next on the auditory system and on sound recognition.

## ETHOGRAM

A part of the intraspecific communication system of the cricket *Gryllus campestris* L. and of the acridid grasshopper *Gomphocerippus rufus* L. is seen in Fig. 1 A,B. The diagram illustrates: a) the sequential arrangement of the behavioural events performed by the two sexes in the reproductive period; b) that different sensory systems come into play - in crickets mainly the auditory system, but also the mechanoreceptors situated on the antennae or cerci, and in grasshoppers both the auditory and the visual system. c) that

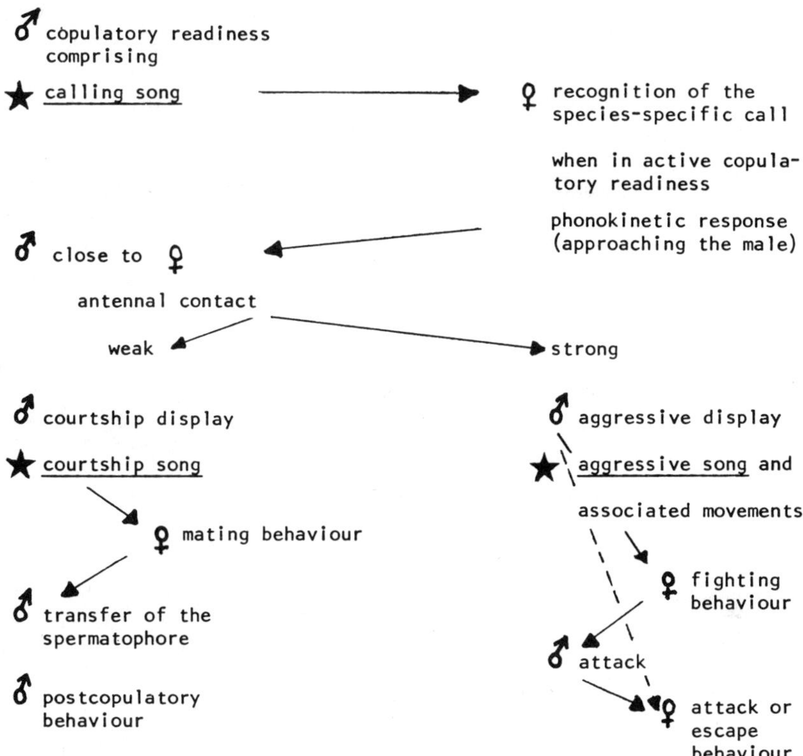


Fig. 1A Events in the sexual behaviour of male and female *Gryllus campestris* (After Huber 1974a).

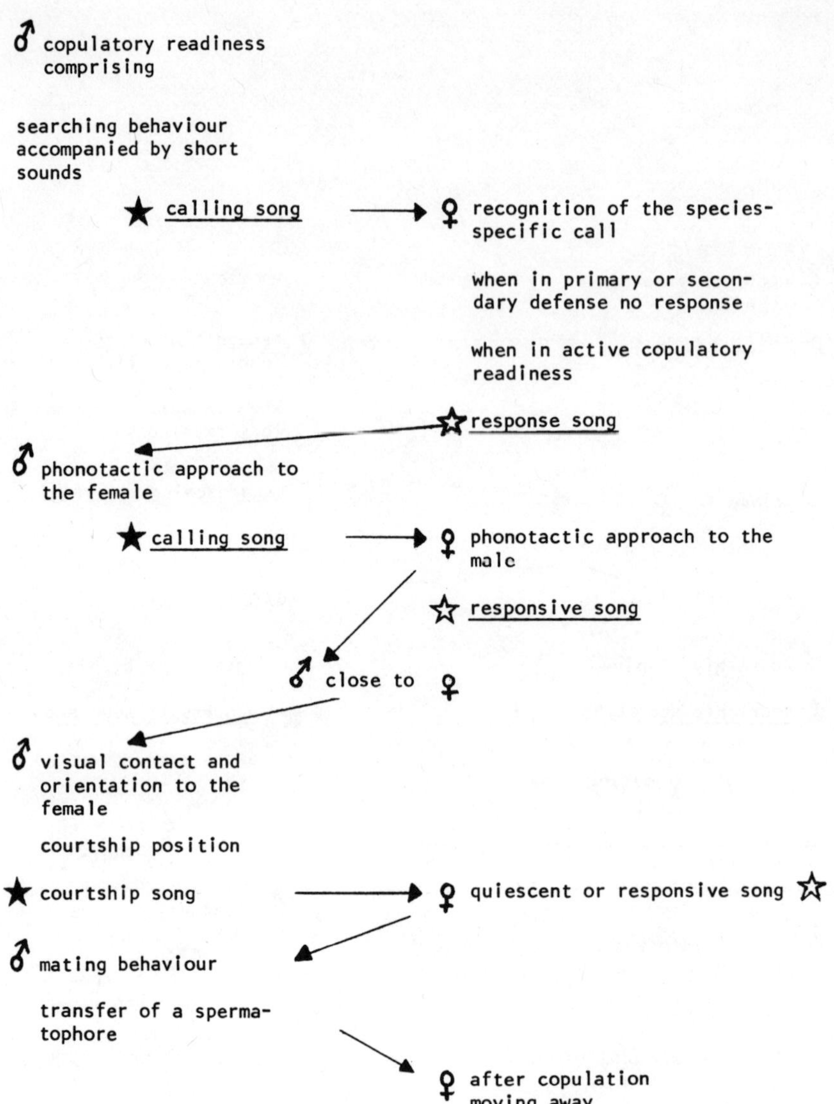


Fig. 1B Events in the sexual behaviour of male and female *Gomphocerippus rufus* (After Loher and Huber 1966).

the species produce different types of songs according to the biological situation in which they find themselves, for instance, calling, aggressive and courtship songs; and d) that the performance of some of the behavioural activities listed (phonokinesis, courtship, aggressive behaviour) depends entirely upon a preceding sensory stimulation, whilst others (e.g. calling song) apparently occur without any recognizable external stimulus, but nevertheless require certain internal conditions. For instance, in male *Gryllus campestris*, a long-lasting calling song is usually correlated with the presence of a spermatophore (Huber 1955), and the defensive behaviour or the state of active copulatory readiness in female *Gomphocerippus rufus* depends upon conditions of the endocrine system (Loher, 1966; Loher and Huber 1966).

## SOUND PRODUCTION AND THE UNDERLYING MOVEMENTS

In grasshoppers, the sound produced by hindleg stridulation is emitted within a rather broad frequency range, up to 40 kHz. Both the calling and the courtship songs are composed of short-lasting and highly damped oscillations, each caused by one impact of small pegs situated on the inner side of the hind femora against a vein located on the front wing (Fig. 2). These single oscillations are arranged as syllables and chirps, and their timing reflects an underlying temporal pattern of hindleg movements (Elsner 1970, 1974a). Hindleg movements can be recorded simultaneously with the sound through a semi-conducting element (Hall-generator) and a small magnet placed on the animal, as seen in Fig. 3. With this method it is possible to correlate the syllables with the up and down strokes of the femora.

In male crickets, the sounds produced by front wing stridulation are nearly pure tones of 4 - 5 kHz which are emitted as a result of specific resonance properties of the harp (Nocke 1971). These vibrations (Fig. 4) result from rubbing a file which is situated underneath each tegmen against a scraper located on the other wing. But unlike in grasshoppers, the sound is emitted only during wing-closure (Fig. 5) whilst wing-opening occurs soundlessly (Innenmoser 1974).

Comparing the sound signals within orthopteran species, we see that they can differ mainly with regard to two parameters - the type of the frequency components and the overall frequency range - and even more strikingly in the timing of syllables and chirps, and therefore, in the timing of the underlying leg and wing movements.

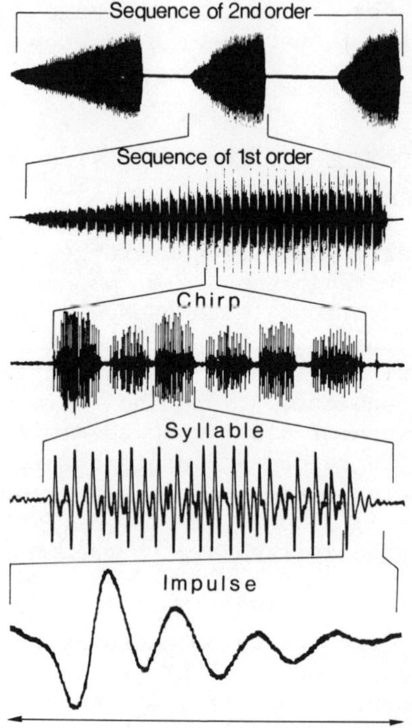


Fig. 2 Structure and terminology of a grasshopper song (*Chorthippus biguttulus*). Time marker (↔): 15 sec for the sequence of 2nd order; 2.9 sec for the sequence of 1st order; 72.5 msec for the chirp; 9.1 msec for the syllable; 0.9 msec for the impulse (= single oscillation) (After Elsner 1974a).

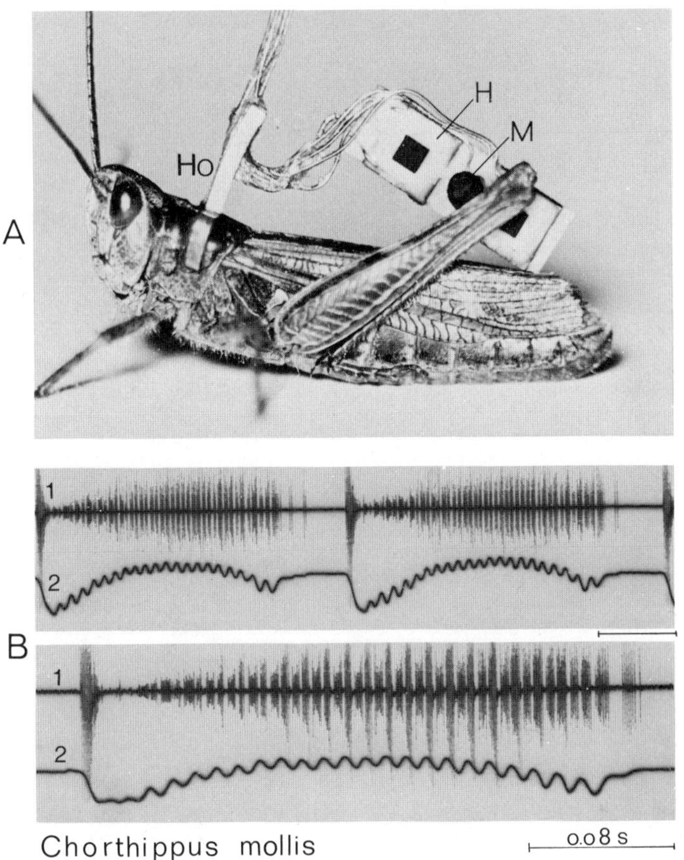


Fig. 3 *Chorthippus mollis:* A, in stridulatory position with the Hall-generator (H) fixed on a cupper holder (Ho) and placed above the abdomen approximately in the midline, and a small magnet (M) placed at the inner side of the distal part of the femur. B, simultaneous records of the sounds (1) and the voltage changes (2) in the Hall-generator. Upward deflections in (2) are correlated with upstrokes, downward deflections of the voltage are related to downward movements of the leg (After Elsner 1970).

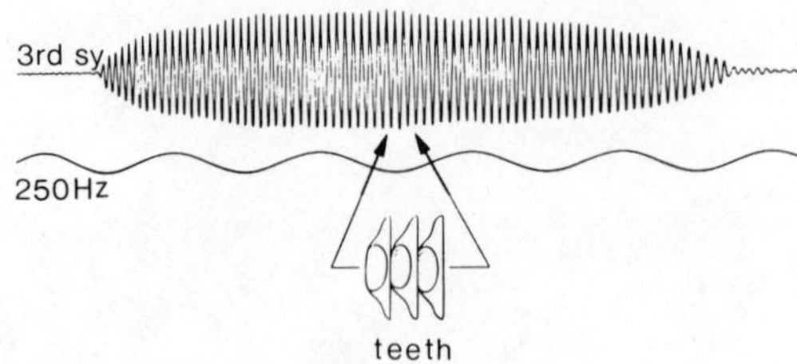


Fig. 4 *Gryllus campestris:* calling song, train of oscillations during the 3rd syllable (3rd sy) in a chirp. Time marker 250 Hz. Arrows indicate the correlation between the impact of the teeth situated on the file and the oscillations (After Huber 1970).

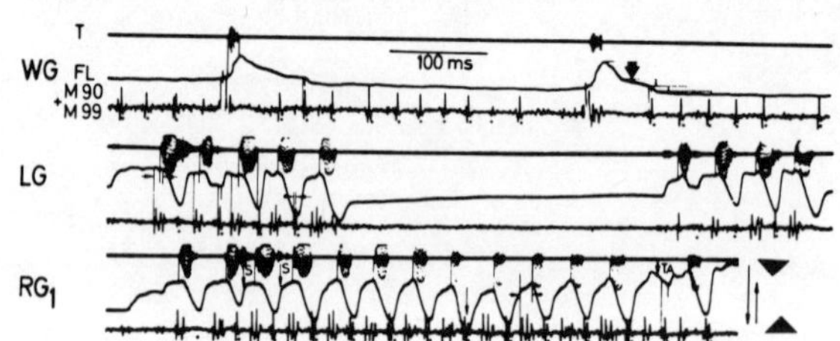


Fig. 5 *Gryllus bimaculatus:* simultaneous recordings of the songs (upper traces), the movements of the right frontwing (middle traces) and the motor activity of two stridulatory muscles (lower traces). T = sound recording; WG = courtship song; LG = calling song; $RG_1$ = part of the aggressive song; FL = wing movement registered with the Hall-generator. ▲ upward deflection indicates opening of wings, ▼ downward deflection indicates wing closure. M 90 and M 99 = remotor and subalar muscle. The electrical activity preceding wing closure is related to M 90 while activity starting with wing opening (S) is related to M 99. TA = muscle activity and wing movement with the production of sound (After Innenmoser 1974).

## NEUROMUSCULAR MACHINERY UNDERLYING SOUND PRODUCTION

In crickets, the different song patterns - calling, courtship and aggressive songs - as well as transitional stages between them are generated and timed even in the complete absence of commands from the head ganglia (Kutsch and Otto 1972), and their basic rhythm persists without any thoracic proprioceptive input (Bentley 1969b). However, this does not exclude the importance of proprioceptive feedback in the control of other song parameters and of the overall acoustic behaviour (Elsner and Huber 1969; Kutsch and Huber 1970; Möss 1971). Furthermore, in some species, input from the abdominal nerve cord is essential for the song generating system, apparently in order to produce that level of excitation which is necessary for the performance of calling and courtship displays (Huber 1955; Kutsch and Otto 1972). Till now, all our data with regard to crickets indicate a system of neurones, located within the thoracic nerve cord, which is responsible for the generation and timing of the song patterns. In the intact animal this system, however, receives input from various parts of the nervous system, mainly from the brain (Huber 1960; Otto 1971).

In grasshoppers, the songs are generated by the action of neurones which lie within the 3rd thoracic ganglion. However, unlike in crickets, stridulation disappears completely after severing the connections to the head ganglia (Loher and Huber 1966; Elsner and Huber 1969). Input from the abdominal cord is only important in the control of the female's song and of its copulatory readiness (Loher and Huber 1966; Loher 1966). The reason why grasshoppers apparently need input from rostral parts of the CNS seems to lie in the fact that stridulation is coupled with other kinds of movements taking place in anterior regions of the body (Elsner 1968) which are triggered by command neurones.

Extracellular recording of electromyograms is possible even in unrestrained and singing orthopterans (Huber 1965; Ewing and Hoyle 1965; Bentley and Kutsch 1966; Elsner 1967, 1968; Kutsch 1969). This technique allows the motoneuronal output to the various muscles to be registered during the behaviour of interest.

What we have learnt so far from this type of approach can be summarized as follows:

This technique is very useful for describing the time and phase relationships of single motor units, as well as for analysing the timing of groups of stridulatory muscles. However, the recording of electromyograms turns out to be inadequate to analyse the mechanisms of neuronal interaction at the synaptic level, for which intracellular recording techniques must be used (Bentley 1969a, b). However, it should be realized that these methods are rather difficult to apply to unrestrained animals from which we expect normal behaviour.

Despite this disadvantage, the recording of electromyograms is still a valuable tool with which to start solving the problems concerned with the neuronal and neuromuscular organization of behaviour.

## Levels of Complexity

Since stridulation involves motor units located in one muscle, then, those in groups of muscles acting as synergists or antagonists and also units in homologous groups of muscles bilaterally arranged within the corresponding segment, we have to think in terms of different levels of complexity.

On analysing the activity and time relationships of single motor units in one muscle, we found that they are recruited in a strict order (Elsner 1968; Kutsch 1969), and, as recently shown by Elsner (1974c) for different grasshopper species, they are always recruited in such a way, irrespective of the particular behaviour with which the muscle is involved. Some general rules should be mentioned.

a) Slow motor units are always activated before fast ones, possibly indicating that the former have a lower threshold as compared with the latter (Fig. 6A).

b) If the muscle contains more than one fast motor unit, the one is always recruited before the other, and not *vice versa* (Fig. 6B).

c) During performance, different degrees of synchronization among units can be achieved.

Therefore, the activation and timing of motor units at this level require a special kind of coupling between the corresponding motoneurones innervating them, one which occurs irrespective of the behaviour. The mechanism which causes such coupling cannot be worked out from recording electromyograms, but certain possible mechanisms can be proposed and checked by intracellular recordings.

In crickets, direct electric coupling was indicated by Bentley (1969a), but the timing observed could also result from direct synaptic coupling among them, and the anatomy does not contradict this hypothesis. Elepfandt (pers. comm.) stained the two fast motor neurones of the subalar muscle (Fig. 7) which is an opener in cricket stridulation. He found that their main and even finer axonal branches run close and often parallel to each other, providing a basis for direct synaptic contact. However, there is only sparce electrophysiological evidence that motoneurones excite each other directly, so

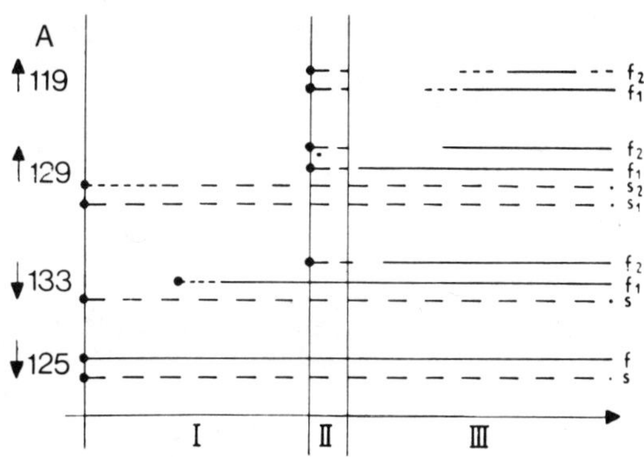


Fig. 6A *Gomphocerippus rufus:* Timing of slow (s) and of fast motor units (f) during the subroutines I, II, III in the courtship song of the male. 119 and 129 = upstroke muscles, 125 and 133 = downstroke muscles (Modified after Elsner 1968).

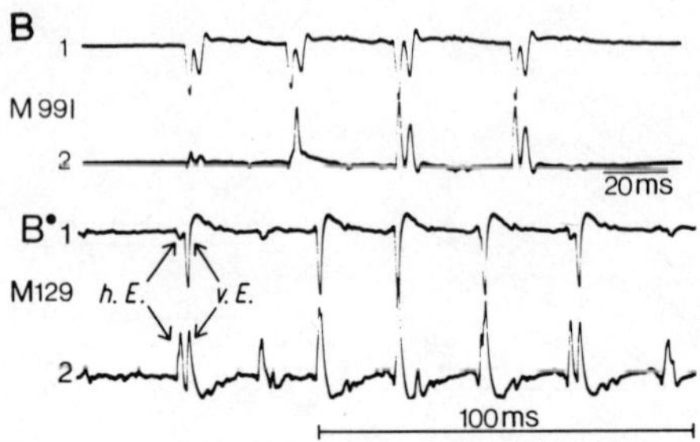


Fig. 6B *Gryllus campestris* (B) and *Gomphocerippus rufus* (B˙): timing of the two fast motor units belonging to the subalar muscles (M99 and M129 respectively). $B_1$, potentials recorded from the outer and $B_2$, from the inner part of the left muscle. In $B_1$ double firing of the 1st unit, in $B_2$, single and double firing of the 2nd unit. Initially the 1st unit precedes the 2nd, later in the chirp a nearly perfect synchrony is established (After Kutsch 1969). $B^{\cdot}_1$, potentials recorded from the anterior, and $B^{\cdot}_2$, from the posterior part of the muscle. The posterior unit (h.E.) precedes the anterior one (v.E.) during the initial and final part of the chirp, or both units become simultaneously active, and their potentials superimpose ($B^{\cdot}_2$, middle part of the chirp) (After Elsner 1967).

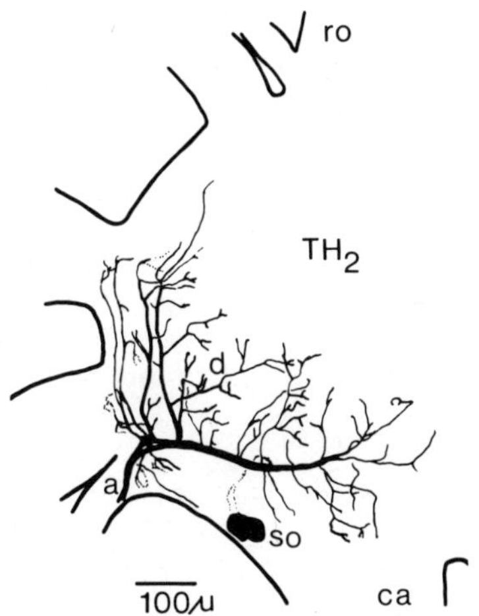


Fig. 7 *Gryllus campestris*, camera lucida drawing made from whole mount preparations of the left half of the 2nd thoracic ganglion ($TH_2$) - dorsal view - with the two fast motoneurones innervating the subalar muscle and stained with CoS. The two cell bodies (so) are located caudally in the ganglion and are attached to the main axonal branches (a) and the dendritic trees (d) by very thin processes; ro = rostrad, ca = caudad (After Elepfandt, unpubl. results).

that we also have to consider that interneuronal input and/or proprioceptive feedback may be important.

The possibility of interneuronal commands was proposed by Bentley (1969a, b) and is supported by the observation that motor units are often recruited after intervals which last much longer than a single electric or monosynaptic delay; and that they can even be activated in the absence of any other motoneuronal discharge or of proprioceptive feedback. This leads us to suppose that the animal uses a special interneuronal or motoneuronal topological arrangement for timing which appears to be rather constant for any given muscle.

At the level of groups of muscles which act during stridulation as openers and closers, or as upstroke and downstroke elements (Fig. 8), we again do not know the cellular and synaptic timing mechanisms. However, the finding that muscles can change their phase relationships rather rapidly as soon as the animal switches over to another mode of behaviour, for instance, from flight to stridulation, as seen in Fig. 9, or even when they change phase within the same behavioral activity, makes it rather unlikely that the corresponding pools of motoneurones are permanently, directly and strongly coupled. There are however, some features common to both the flight and the stridulatory pattern of crickets and grasshoppers.

a) The repetition rate at which single motor units operate in the two activities remains rather constant, indicating a basic oscillatory property.

b) The phase relationship, however, changes either gradually or abruptly, as Elsner (1968, 1974c) found when comparing different grasshopper species. There are those in which the stridulation pattern is monostable and others in which it is bistable.

If, therefore, interneurones or feedback systems are part of the timing device, it is supposed that they mainly control the phase relationships and not the repetition rate in the firing of the motoneurones.

## Asymmetry Within the System

Cricket songs in particular are known for their transitional stages which indicate the change from a calling song to a courtship song, and also from a calling song to an aggressive song and *vice versa*. The switch is usually initiated via sensory input (Huber 1955, 1960).

Considering only the change in song from calling to courtship in male crickets, and the reverse from courtship to calling, the

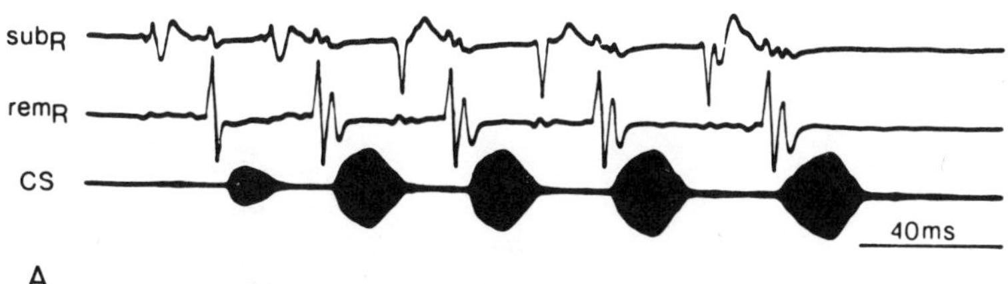


Fig. 8A *Gryllus campestris*, antagonistic recruitment of motor units in the subalar muscles ($sub_R$) and in the remotor muscles ($rem_R$) during a single calling chirp (CS). $rem_R$ shows single and double firing which precedes the syllables (closer), the subalar unit ($sub_R$) recorded here comes in at the end of each syllable (After Kutsch 1969).

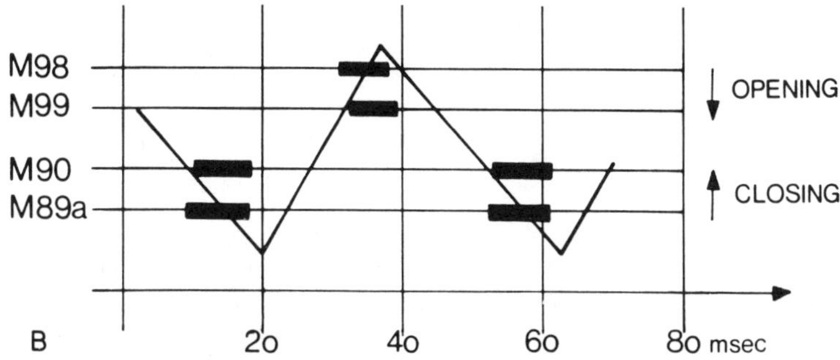


Fig. 8B *Gryllus campestris*, schematic illustration of the reciprocal action of two opener and two closure muscles during a one and a half wing beat cycle. Note the synchrony of the synergists (After Huber 1974b).

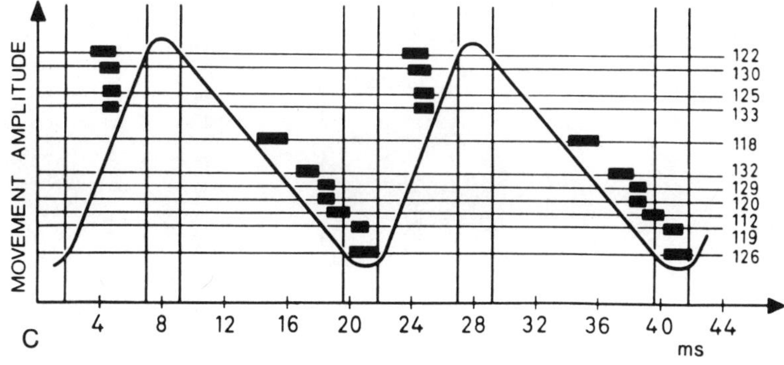


Fig. 8C *Gomphocerippus rufus*, illustration of the recruitment of stridulatory muscles during two up- and downstrokes in the courtship song. The downstroke muscles are smaller in number and far better synchronized than the upstroke group (After Elsner 1968).

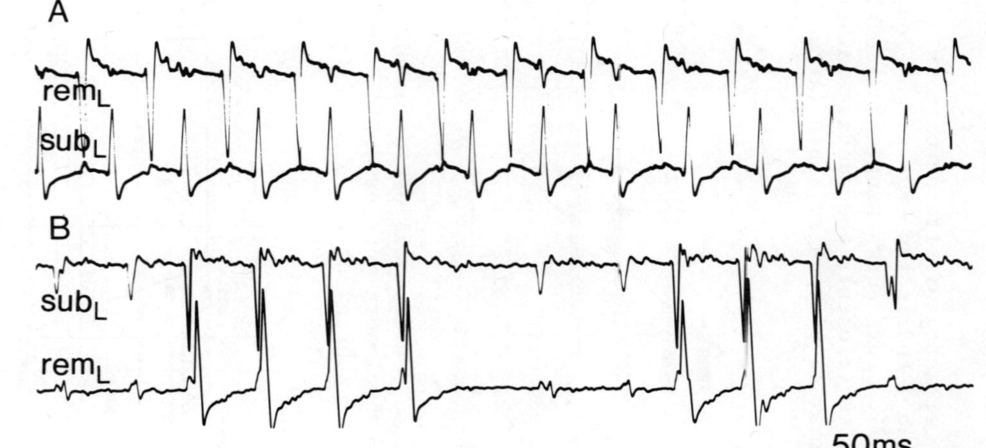


Fig. 9 *Gomphocerippus rufus*, motor activity of the remotor ($rem_L$) and the subalar muscle ($sub_L$) during flight (A) and stridulation (B). Note the antagonistic action of the two muscles in flight, and their synchronous recruitment in stridulation. The two motor units fire at very similar repetition rates in both behavioural events but with a distinct phase shift in flight (After Elsner 1968).

following features have been noted (Innenmoser 1974, Weber 1974).

a) If the switch takes place suddenly, a pause is usually found between the two patterns, indicating that some time is needed for the system to operate.

b) Electromyograms recorded from unrestrained and singing males show that the motoneurones involved also undergo a change in their timing, and this occurs earlier than the change in sounds which are recorded simultaneously. This means that parts of the neuromuscular machinery start to switch over before the change is seen in the sound pattern. As shown in Fig. 10, the motor units of different muscles do not switch simultaneously. The change from calling to courtship activity is already indicated during the last calling chirps preceding courtship by a burst of activity of the subalar muscle which was found to be characteristic of the courtship song, whilst the antagonist, namely the remotor muscle, still discharges according to the pattern of the calling song. On the other hand, if the animal switches back, the remotor sometimes indicates the change first, and the subalar continues to stay in the courtship pattern.

Altogether, these data lead to the conclusion that the courtship song is initiated by interneuronal input, preferably acting on the opener motoneurones (see also Bentley 1969b), whereas the calling song when developing from a courtship pattern, is first indicated at the neuromuscular level by a change in activity of the closer motoneurones. This means that for both activities not only different interneuronal-motoneuronal relationships are needed, but also that they come into play out of phase with each other.

## Features of the Song Generating System

Several years ago, we formulated the hypothesis that in cricket stridulation at least two oscillating mechanisms are present. One was thought to set the syllable rate at a frequency of 30 Hz, this being modulated by a second system controlling the chirp rate at about 4 - 5 Hz, and in multiples of the syllable interval (Kutsch 1969; Kutsch and Otto 1972; Otto 1971). The hypothesis was based on three findings:

a) While often in the calling song single chirps are missing, nevertheless the chirp rate is unaltered (Fig. 11A).

b) In brain-stimulated males as well as in normal animals which started to call spontaneously, the chirp intervals were found with multiples of the final interval (Fig. 11B).

c) In both cases the 'syllable oscillator' remained unaffected.

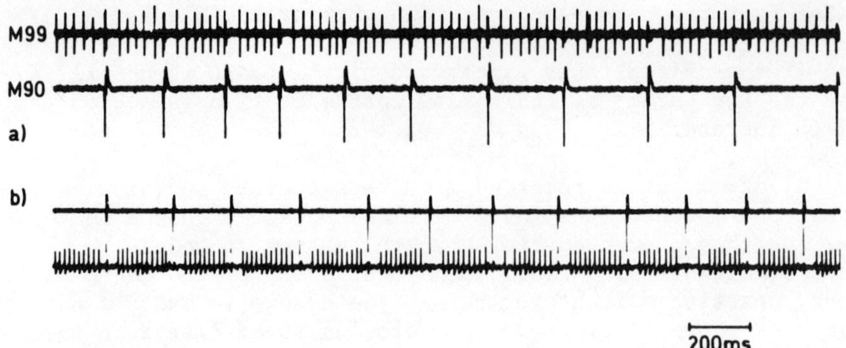


Fig. 10A *Gryllus campestris*, motor activity recorded during the final part of a longer lasting courtship song (Aa) where the male had no contact with the female, and during a courtship song (Ab) with the male in contact with the female. M99, subalar motor units, M90, several remotor motor units superimposed. Note the more or less tonic firing of M99, which is briefly interrupted when the M90 comes in (After Weber 1974).

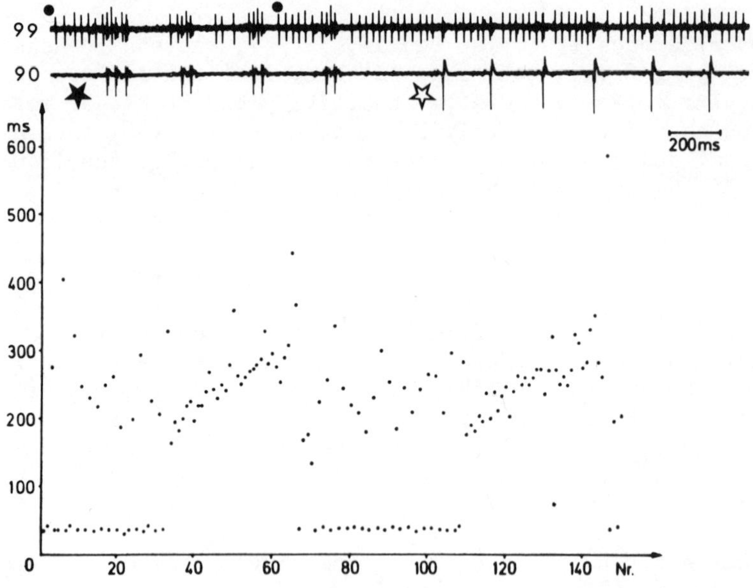


Fig. 10B *Gryllus campestris*, transition from calling (★) to courtship song (☆). Upper part of the figure, motor activity recorded from the subalar (99) and the remotor muscle (90). The subalar starts firing in bursts ( ● ) already at the final part of the calling song which is marked by the three- and the two-syllabic pattern of the remotor muscle. Lower part of the figure, sequential interval histogram of syllable and chirp intervals (After Weber 1974).

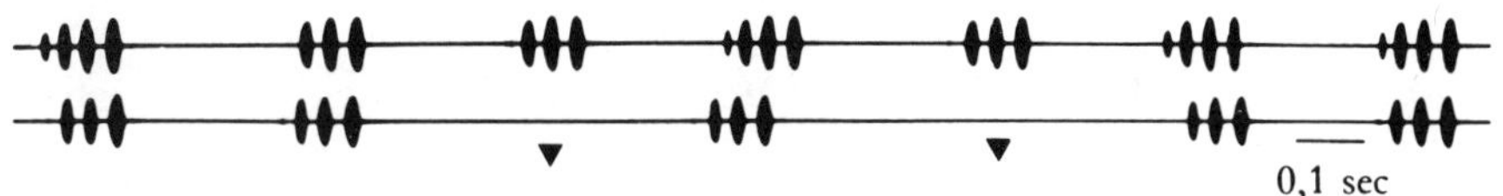


Fig. 11A *Gryllus campestris*, calling song (continuous record) with two chirps missing ( ▼ ) but with no change in the chirp rate. (After Kutsch 1969).

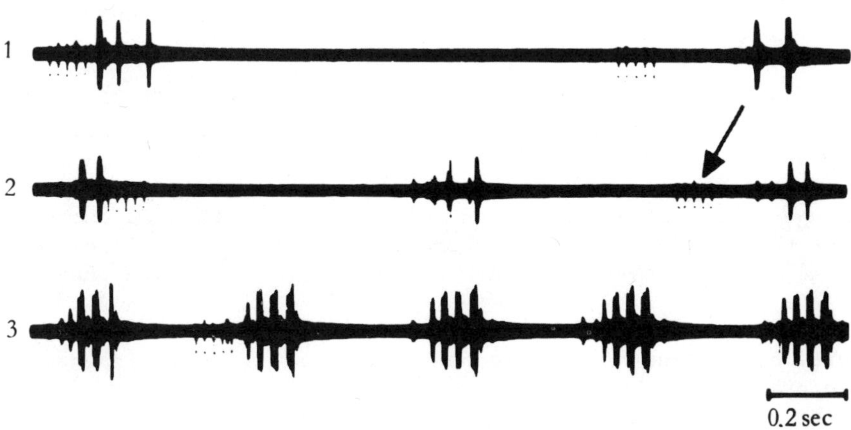


Fig. 11B *Gryllus campestris*, sound pattern similar to the calling song elicited through brain stimulation with stimulus bursts (arrow) of 5 square waves each at intervals of 800 msec. Note that the chirps in the traces 1 and 2 are grouped in multiples of the final interval (3) (After Otto 1971).

By a quantitative analysis of either the intervals between syllables and chirps, or the intervals between correspondent muscle potentials, Innenmoser (1974) and Weber (1974) have elucidated certain features of the song-generating system in more detail.

As shown in Fig. 12, the joint interval histograms for the calling song indicate strongly that the syllable intervals remain extraordinarily constant, despite the variation in the chirp intervals. The very small variation of the syllable intervals has a gaussian distribution, with a standard deviation of about 5% from the mean value of 40 msec. This deviation is several times smaller than the duration of a single epsp in the motoneurones, which could mean that it is caused by subthreshold random fluctuations of an underlying synaptic process.

If in the calling song, the syllable intervals would vary independently of each other, one should expect that the sum of all intervals in a chirp would vary much more than in each single class because of the superimposed variations. However, this is not the case. Therefore, it turns out that each single syllable is triggered and timed independently of the variation occurring in the preceding one, and this leads one to suppose that common interneurones are involved.

Considering the time relationships between consecutive synergistically and antagonistically operating motoneurones in stridulation, Innenmoser (1974) found that the subalar preceding the remotor interval is the most constant time parameter and is independent of the change in the syllable period (Fig. 13). In other words: subalar motoneurones and remotor motoneurones appear to be latency-locked, whilst all other intervals change with the period and are phase-locked.

A plausible hypothesis could be that stridulation is mainly triggered by command neurones connected primarily to the opener motoneurones (see also Bentley 1969b). The trigger input would then start the syllable oscillator in these neurones, for instance, by depolarizing them for a certain amount of time and initiating an inbuilt oscillation. Due to latency-locking, the timing of the antagonist could be achieved, and the observed coupling would be based on the mechanism which guarantees this type of coupling between openers and closers.

The chirp intervals vary much more, and only they are influenced by external stimuli, as shown in Fig. 14, where acoustic stimuli, when presented at the right time within the interchirp intervals, delay the next chirp and reset the cycle (Jones 1966a,b; Jones and Dambach 1973). Joint interval histograms of the chirp intervals (Fig. 12) demonstrate clearly their limitation to shorter values, which means that a male cricket cannot increase the chirp rate above

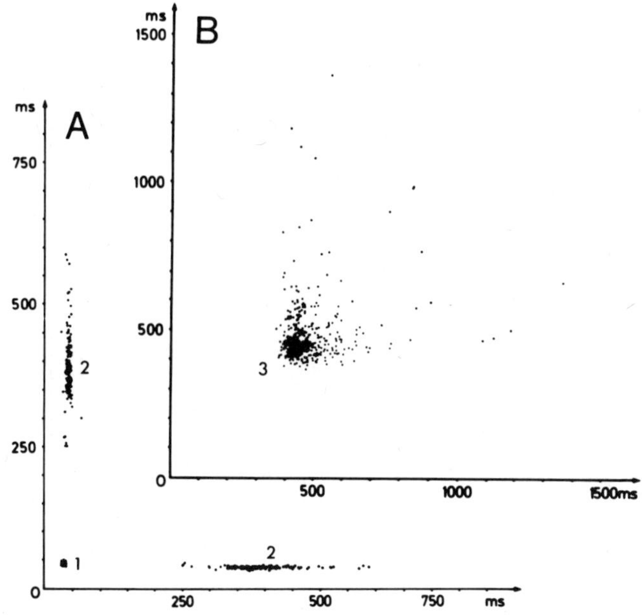


Fig. 12 *Gryllus campestris*, A, joint interval histogram of 400 chirps, plotted from recordings of the corresponding motor activity of the remotor muscle 30 minutes after onset of the calling song. 1, highly constant syllable intervals, 2, variation of the chirp intervals. B, joint interval histogram of 400 interchirp intervals (V in C) plotted from recordings of the corresponding motor activity of the remotor muscle 20 minutes after onset of the calling song. Note the sharp demarkation towards shorter intervals (3) and the normal distribution of longer intervals.

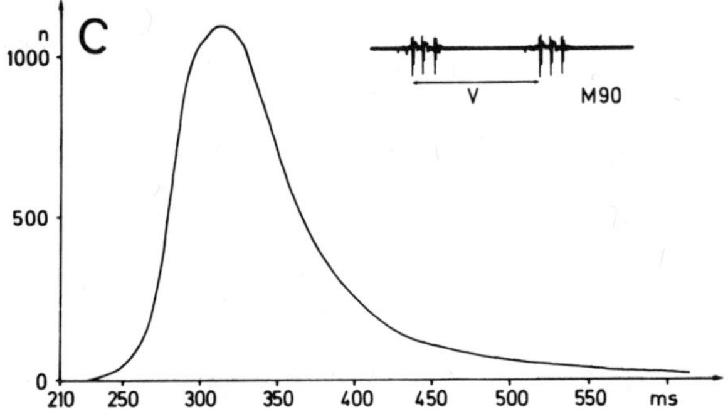


Fig. 12C *Gryllus campestris*, distribution of interchirp intervals of three-syllabic chirps (upper right corner) during the initial part of the calling song (After Weber 1974).

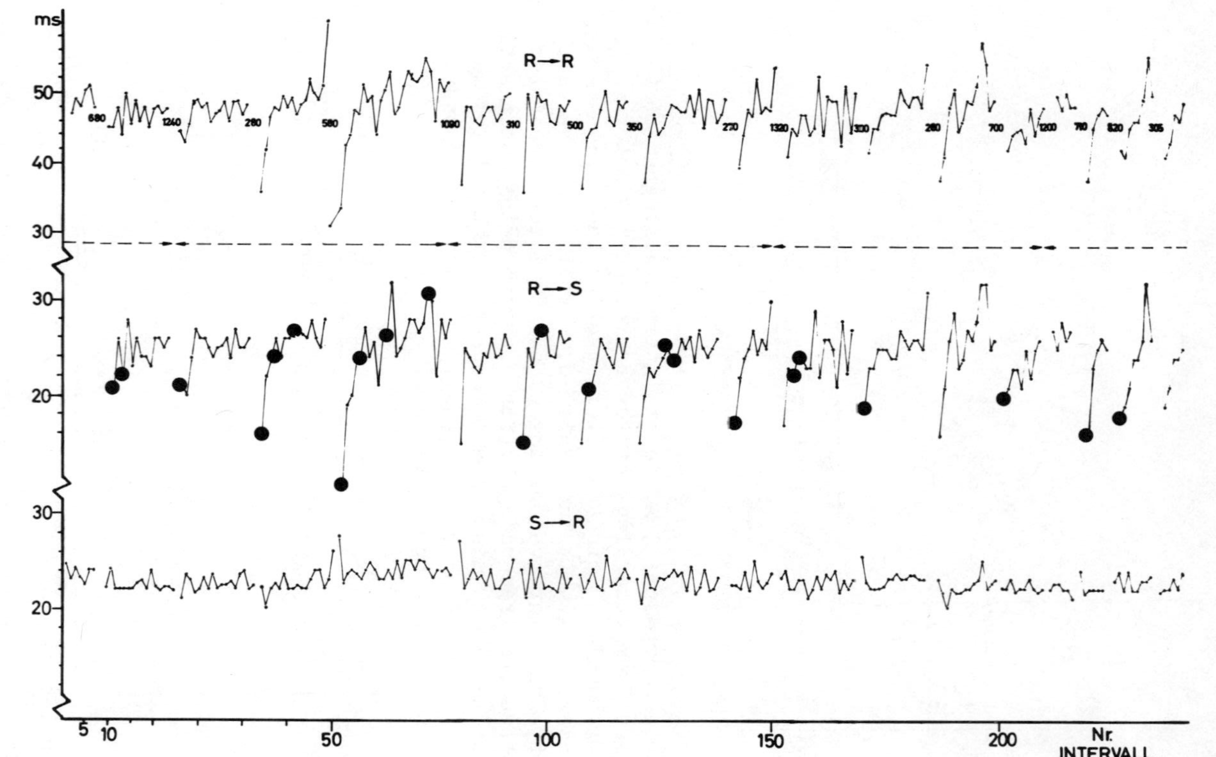


Fig. 13 *Gryllus bimaculatus*, sequential histograms of the remotor-remotor (R-R), remotor-subalar (R-S) and subalar-remotor (S-R) intervals of 18 consecutive chirps of the aggressive song. Numbers in (R-R) show the duration of chirp intervals in msec; dotted line with arrows indicates aggressive chirps which follow closely; (●) intervals with no sound production. (After Innenmoser 1974).

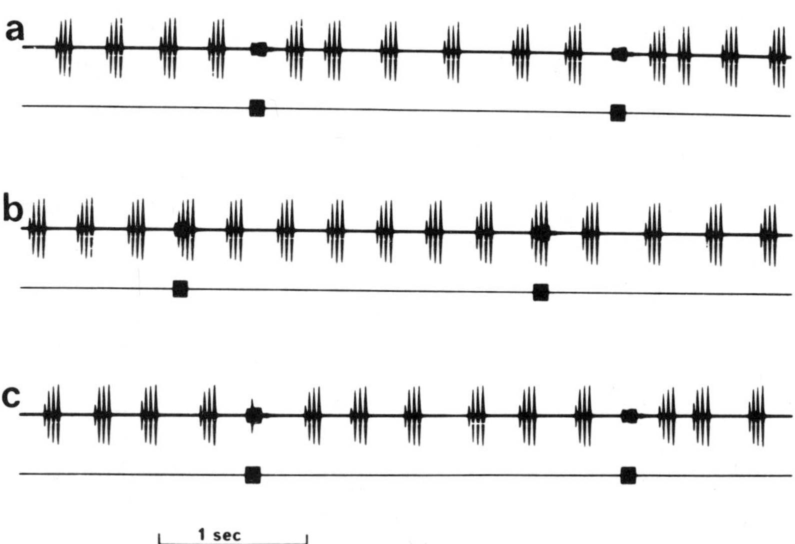


Fig. 14A *Gryllus campestris*, effect of artificial sound signals (■) (100 msec, 5 kHz, 80 dB) on the stridulation of an intact male. Upper traces in a, b, c = signals plus chirps; lower traces = signals only.

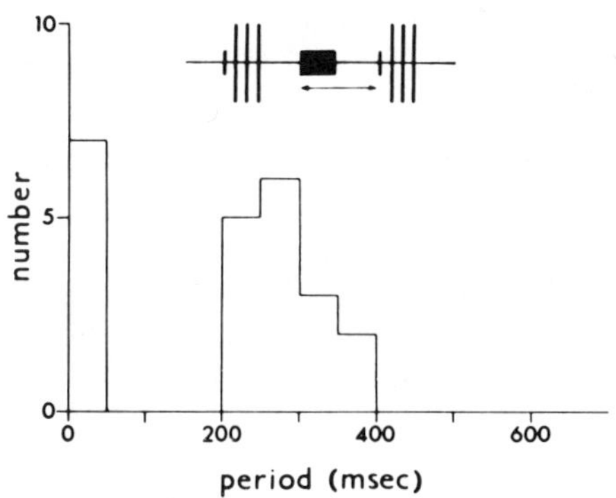


Fig. 14B *Gryllus campestris*, distribution of signal to chirp period during the experiment demonstrated in A (After Jones & Dambach 1973).

4 - 5 Hz. But Fig. 12 also indicates that the longer chirp intervals are randomly distributed, which is, so far, the best evidence we have that these intervals can no longer be considered as 'multiples' of some faster running oscillating process, for instance, the syllable generator.

Our recent quantitative analysis gives little support to the idea that the mechanisms generating the chirp rate determine the syllable rate, and *vice versa*. Both appear to be independent processes based on two quite separate neuronal machineries.

## SPECIES-SPECIFIC SOUND RECOGNITION

One of the most important questions arising out of our consideration of acoustic communication in orthopteran insects deals with the structures and mechanisms responsible for the species-specific sound recognition.

A comparative study of the time and spectral characteristics in a variety of calling songs of different cricket species, and also of different types of songs within one species, shows that these signals as a rule lack frequency modulation. However, they can easily be distinguished by the number of time parameters which potentially can be used by the perceiving system (Popov 1971a, b, 1973, 1974a, b). In grasshoppers, pulse frequency modulation is thought to be another parameter (Elsner 1974a).

To date, there seems to be no unique parameter by which a certain song can be discriminated, and this points to sound-processing nervous machineries which deal with more than one parameter of the signal at the same time (Adam 1969; Kalmring 1971; Popov 1974a; Stout and Huber 1972; Zaretsky 1972; Zhantiev and Tshukanov 1972a, b).

### Behavioural Experiments on Sound Recognition

The elucidation of the quantitative features of the time parameters in cricket songs, both under different external conditions - temperatuer, light cycle, vibratory or tactile stimuli, etc. - and in different internal conditions relating to the animal has been due to the work of A.V. Popov based on comparative field studies. His work leads to the conclusion that only a few parameters are highly stable and independent of external and internal factors. Stable are the syllable rate and the chirp duration; variable were found to be the chirp rate, sound intensity, syllable duration and the syllable amplitude envelope (Popov 1974a, b). In grasshoppers, extensive investigations of this kind are still lacking.

In crickets, phonokinesis by the female is the only behavioural response which can be used to determine the sound parameters important in intraspecific recognition. As shown by Zaretsky (1972), the female of *Scapsipedus marginatus* is attracted by the conspecific syllable pattern or by artificial acoustic dummies which simulate the natural conspecific song. However, it is not important whether the pattern is played back with the normal sound frequency of approximately 5 kHz or with another frequency within the auditory range of the animal. General locomotion of the female can also be elicited with non-specific acoustic stimuli (arousal effect) but the conspecific input is required for successful phonokinesis (Table I).

A phonokinetically responding female is only able to approach the sound source if both hearing organs remain intact. With one destroyed, the female starts to circle to the side of the intact organ (Fig. 15) and never reaches the 'male'. Similar experiments with female *Gryllus campestris* in the field (Klopffleisch 1973) confirm Zaretsky's findings (Fig. 16).

Since females with only one ear intact can be stimulated to phonokinesis, the auditory information picked up with one tympanal organ seems to be sufficient only for species-specific recognition. Popov (1973, 1974a, b) studied sound recognition in *Gryllus campestris* and *Gryllus bimaculatus* by presenting sound models and natural songs in a maze where the female had either no choice to compare because only one signal was presented or it could compare between two different signals which were emitted in competition. The results can be summarized as follows:

a) Rough models such as continuous tones of 4.5 kHz, or a series of sound pulses (syllables) with a carrier frequency of 4.5 kHz but with different chirp rates and chirp durations, as well as unpulsed chirps, stimulated the female, when these were presented alone.

b) However, when these model sounds were emitted simultaneously and in competition with the conspecific call or with closely matching artificial acoustic dummies, the females clearly preferred the conspecific song or its mimic dummy.

c) In the case of choice between two conspecific calling songs, the female in the maze always chose the one with the higher intensity or the higher chirp rate.

At least in these two species, the process of recognition must be based on the evaluation of only a few most stable parameters in the calling song: namely, syllable period and chirp duration. This was confirmed by further studies (Popov 1974b). Females of *Gryllus bicmaculatus* respond phonokinetically in a maze if the call is constructed of chirps each containing at least 4 but not more than 10

TABLE I

A. ASSOCIATION BETWEEN SPECIFICITY OF THE CALLING SONG AND SOUND LOCATING ABILITY IN KINETICALLY RESPONDING FEMALES *SCAPSIPEDUS MARGINATUS* (ZARETSKY 1972)

| Song type | Success | Failure | Total | $\chi^2$ | P |
|---|---|---|---|---|---|
| *Scapsipedus marginatus* calling song | 45 | 15 | 60 | 17 | 0.001 |
| Sympatric species calling song | 5 | 18 | 23 | | |

B. ASSOCIATION BETWEEN SPECIFICITY OF THE CALLING SONG AND PHONO-KINESIS OF FEMALES *SCAPSIPEDUS MARGINATUS* (ZARETSKY 1972)

| Song type | Kinesis | No response | Total | $\chi^2$ | P |
|---|---|---|---|---|---|
| *Scapsipedus marginatus* calling song | 60 | 8 | 68 | 15.8 | 0.001 |
| Sympatric species calling song | 23 | 21 | 44 | | |

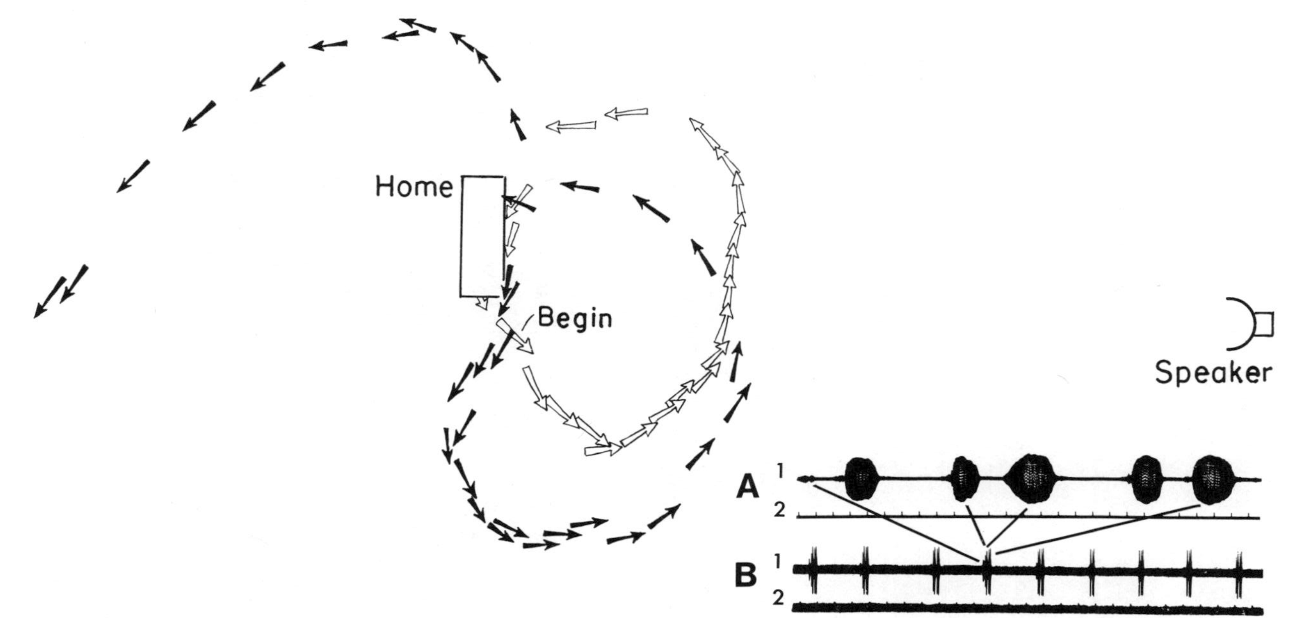


Fig. 15 *Scapsipedus marginatus*, path-indicated by arrows - of a female with the right tympanal organ destroyed when stimulated with the natural call (A1, B1) or with artificial calls matching the natural song. A2 - time marker 10 msec, B2 - time marker 0.5 sec, A1 - single chirp, B1 - series of chirps. Two successive circus movements are shown. The initial movement is indicated by open arrows (After Murphey and Zaretsky 1972; Zaretsky 1972).

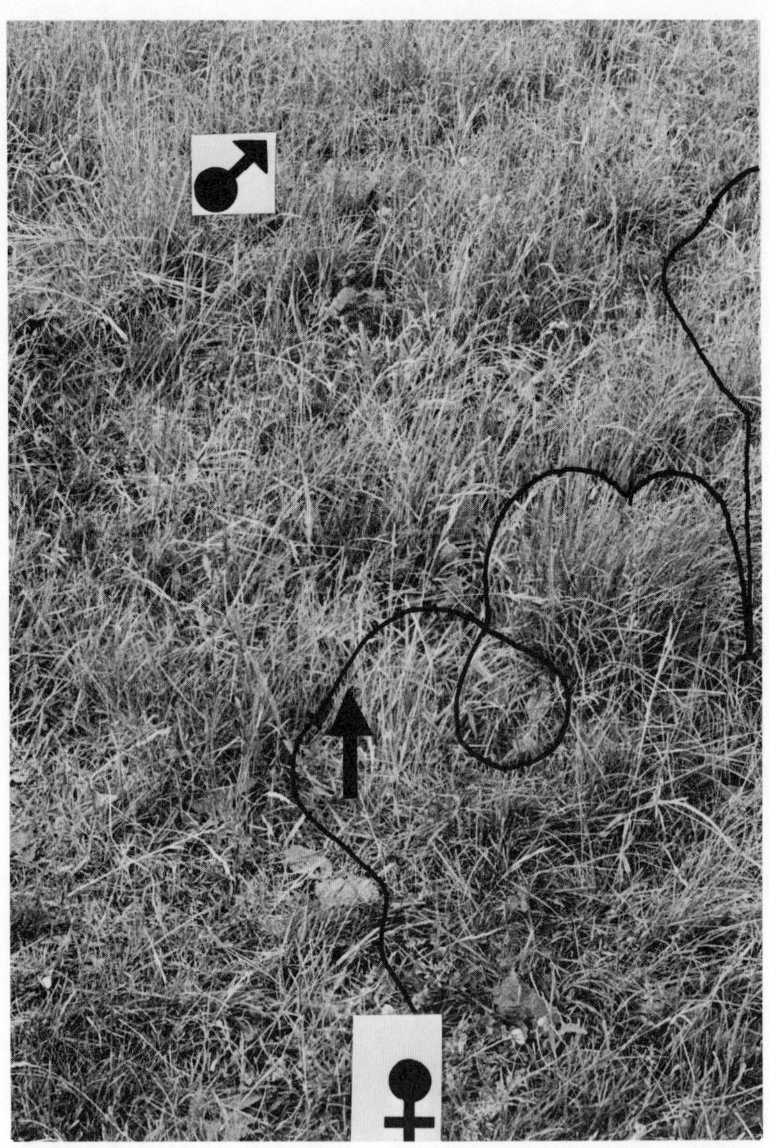

Fig. 16 *Gryllus campestris*, path in the field of a female (♀) (arrow) with the left tympanal organ removed stimulated by the calling song of a male situated at the upper left corner (♂) approximately 2 meters away (After Klopffleisch 1973).

syllables, whereas a continuous trill is ineffective (Fig. 17). Within these limits, models with the same syllable period which followed the rule n > 3 but < 10, when presented simultaneously with the natural call of 4 syllables/chirp, were each equally effective. On the other hand, females of *Gryllus campestris* are more specific in their demands. This could be shown for *G. bimaculatus* and *G. campestris* which live sympatrically in Azerbaijan. Non-sympatric males of *G. campestris* usually produce chirps composed of 4 syllables each and so also do those of *G. bimaculatus*. Fig. 17 indicates that the probability of the female's response in *G. campestris* (P%) is tuned to chirps with 4 syllables. The Azerbaijanian subspecies, however, differs. Here, male *G. campestris* never increase the number of syllables in one chirp above 3, while the males of *G. bimaculatus* never reduce the syllable number per chirp below 4. Discrimination, therefore, is apparently based on chirp duration.

In acridid grasshoppers, sounds are produced with the two hindleg apparatuses; we know that syllables are generated during both the up- and the downstroke, and that animals stridulating with only one hindleg exhibit a more refined temporal pattern (Fig. 18) than those stridulating with two legs because of their being partly out of phase (Loher and Huber 1964, 1966; Elsner and Huber 1969; Elsner 1974a).

Here, the question arises whether the female recognizes the conspecific song by taking into account the information generated in the more refined pattern produced by one leg, despite the biological noise generated by the partly out-of-phase action of the other leg; or whether it deals with the features of the overall amplitude modulation in the songs produced with the two legs. Since females are equally well attracted to one leg- and to two leg-singers, both patterns seem to be effective. But we are still faced with the question of which are the important parameters.

The work of v.Helversen (1972) provides reliable evidence that females of *Chorthippus biguttulus* in the state of active copulatory readiness respond to the male's song acoustically, but do not process the information contained in the pattern of single up- and downstrokes produced by each leg. Instead, they seem to evaluate a combination of two closely related parameters: the chirp duration (equivalent to a series of up- and downstrokes) and the interchirp interval (i.e. the pause between consecutive chirps). As shown in Fig. 18, the female responds to several chirp-pause combinations and the correlation is such that longer chirp durations are combined with longer pauses and *vice versa*. Her response range lies within the chirp-pause combinations that the males usually exhibit in the natural habitat.

*Chorthippus biguttulus* at least seems to possess certain features of the overall amplitude-modulation still present in the

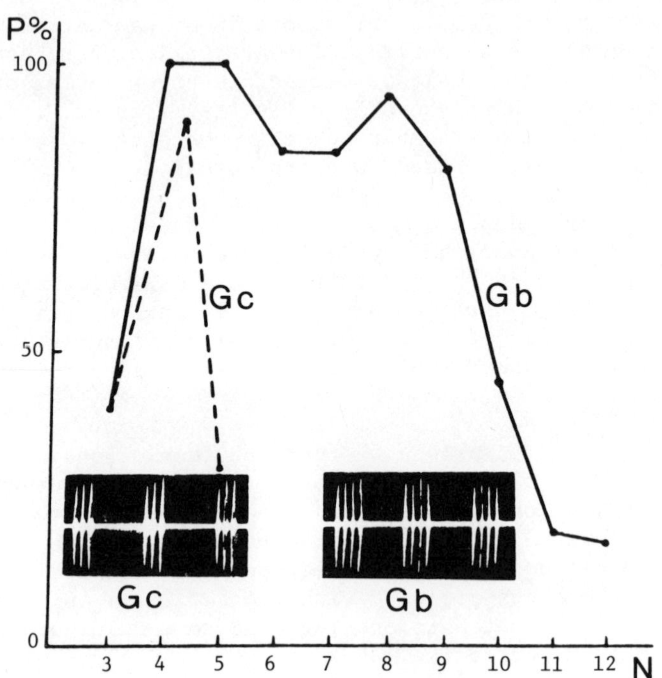


Fig. 17 *Gryllus campestris* (Gc) and *Gryllus bimaculatus* (Gb), probability (P%) of the female's positive phonokinesis as a function of the number of syllables in the chirps (N) of the male's calling song. Solid curve (*Gryllus bimaculatus*) is tuned to chirps containing 4 - 10 syllables each; dotted curve (*Gryllus campestris*) is tuned to 4 syllabic chirps. The calling song was matched by a sound model with a syllable rate of 28 Hz, and chirp rate of 2.3 Hz and a syllable duration of 24 msec. (After Popov 1974a).

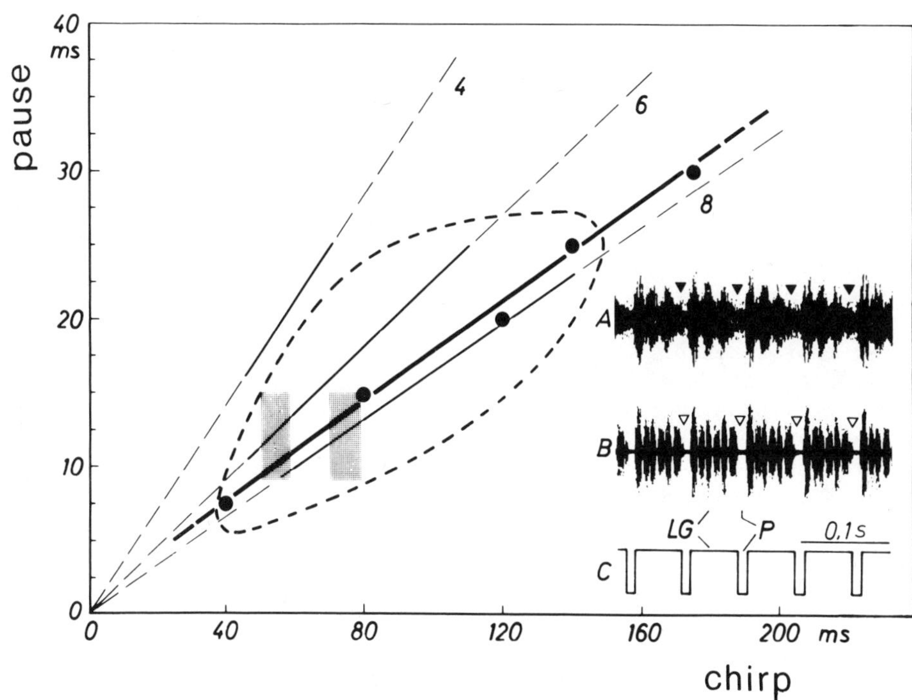


Fig. 18 *Chorthippus biguttulus*, A chirps of the male's song produced with the two hindlegs where the pause is missing between successive chirps ( ▼ ); B, chirps produced with one hindleg only - clear separation of up- and downstrokes, with a pause between consecutive chirps ( ▽ ); C, diagram of the artificial sound pattern produced by a noise generator. LG = chirp, P = pause. The sign ● in the main figure indicates the maximal response of the female in terms of response songs to the sound dummies (C) as a function of different chirp-duration pause-duration combinations. The dotted line encircles an area of chirp-pause-combinations to which the females responded once per stimulus presentation. Shaded rectangles show the variation of the song pattern in terms of chirp-pause combinations in conspecific males at 35°C, the test temperature. The dotted straight lines (numbered 4, 6 and 8) characterize the average chirp-pause combinations of the songs, and the unbroken lines in between characterize those in the temperature range of 24 - 38°C. The numbers 4,6, and 8 refer to songs with chirps which contain 4,6 and 8 up- and downstrokes respectively (Modified from v. Helversen 1972).

song produced with the two hindlegs. However, due to the phase shift between the two legs there is no real pause (Fig. 18) which separates consecutive chirps; instead, the sound intensity in this part of the song is merely reduced (Elsner 1974a). Thus if the female uses chirp-pause combinations it must discriminate rather small intensity changes of the order of 5 - 8 dB.

## Signal Processing Within the Auditory Pathway in Crickets

The auditory system of crickets consists of two hearing organs located within the proximal part of the tibiae in the front legs, each exposing two tympanal membranes to the environment. A set of 40 - 50 primary sensory neurones arranged in a row form the *crista acustica* (Michel 1973), which is considered to be that part of the complex tibial sensory system reacting to airborne sound. The crista is in close contact with tracheal membranes which also partly form the outer tympanal membranes. The fibres of the primary auditory neurones form the auditory nerve which enters the 1st thoracic ganglion as part of the main leg nerve (Nocke 1972, Rehbein 1973, Eibl 1974). Within the ganglion, the fibres diverge slightly and branch ipsilaterally where they end in the so-called 'acoustic neuropile' (Fig. 19). This neuropile region is bilaterally and symmetrically arranged and no decussations were found between the two ganglionic halves (Eibl 1974). It is here that the sensory neurones synapse with 2nd order auditory fibres.

a) Coding in the hearing organs. A complete knowledge of how different sound parameters are processed by hearing organs must encompass that gained from studies on the mechanical properties of the tympanal membranes (see Michelsen 1971; Michelsen and Nocke 1974; Johnstone *et al.* 1970), as well as the features of single auditory neurones, such as their response to different frequency components, their coding of sound intensity, their degree of adaptation, and their ability to code temporal parameters of the songs (Nocke 1972; Zhantiev and Tshukanov 1972a, b). If we consider only the auditory neurones, it is seen that recordings from the whole auditory nerve and from single primary neurones give the following results. The ears of *Gryllus campestris* are most sensitive to and tuned to those parts in the sound spectrum which are emitted at the highest intensity (Fig. 20), and the threshold curve matches the sound spectrogram virtually precisely. Therefore, crickets are able to discriminate at least between the lower (4 - 5 kHz) and the higher part (12 - 16 kHz) in their sound spectrum. This discrimination is achieved by two populations of auditory sensory neurones (Fig. 21) which are specifically tuned to either the lower part (NF-cells) or to the higher part (HF-cells) of the spectrum. The HF-cells cease to discharge when the smaller tympanum is destroyed (Nocke 1972). Similar results were obtained in *G. bimaculatus* by Zhantiev and Tshukanov (1972a, b).

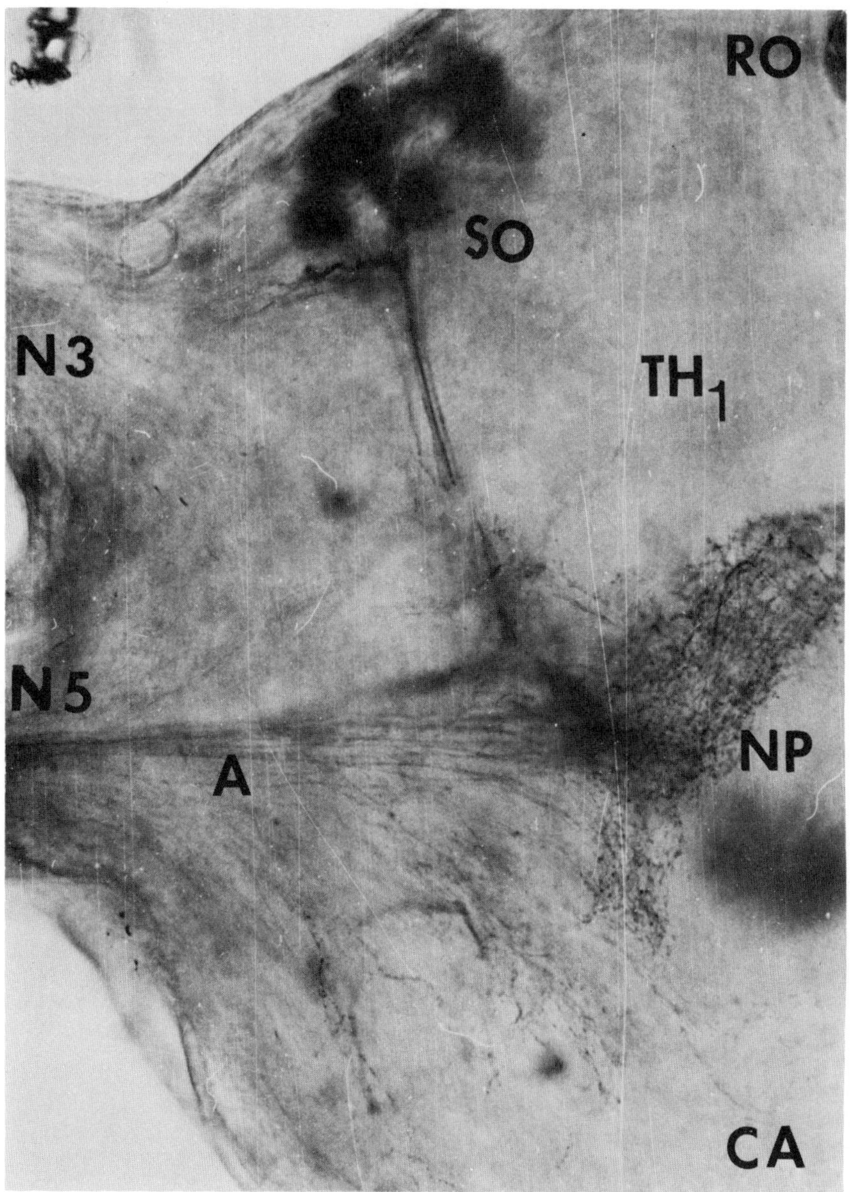


Fig. 19 *Gryllus campestris*, left half of the 1st thoracic ganglion ($TH_1$), dorsal view, stained with CoS to demonstrate the entrance of the axons from primary sensory auditory fibres (A) through nerve 5 (N5) and the acoustic neuropile (NP). SO = somata of some motoneurones innervating leg mescles, RO = rostrad, CA = caudad, N3 = nerve three (After Eibl 1974).

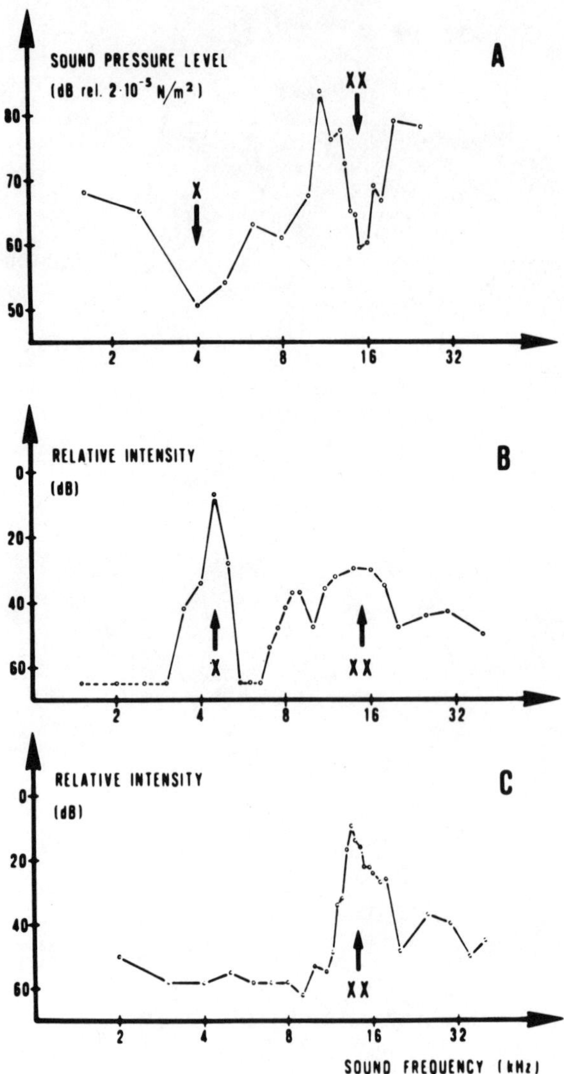


Fig. 20 *Gryllus campestris*, comparison of the hearing threshold curve (A) with the sound spectrograms of the calling (B) and the courtship song (C). X and XX with arrows mark the agreement of the hearing threshold optima with the corresponding maxima of the song spectrum (After Nocke 1972).

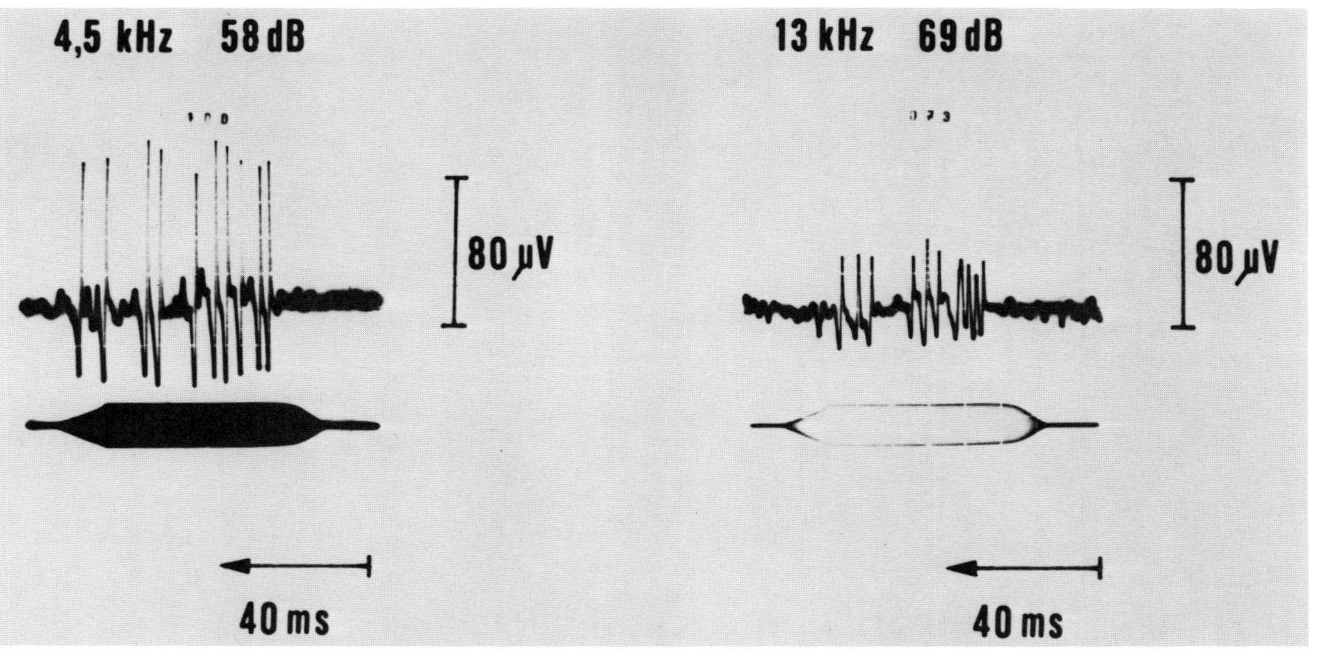


Fig. 21 *Gryllus campestris*, single unit activity of primary auditory neurones recorded extracellularly from the auditory nerve to demonstrate at least two populations of sense cells, one sensitive and tuned to the lower frequency part (4.5 kHz) and the other sensitive and tuned to the 3rd harmonic (13 kHz) in the sound spectrum (After Nocke unpubl.).

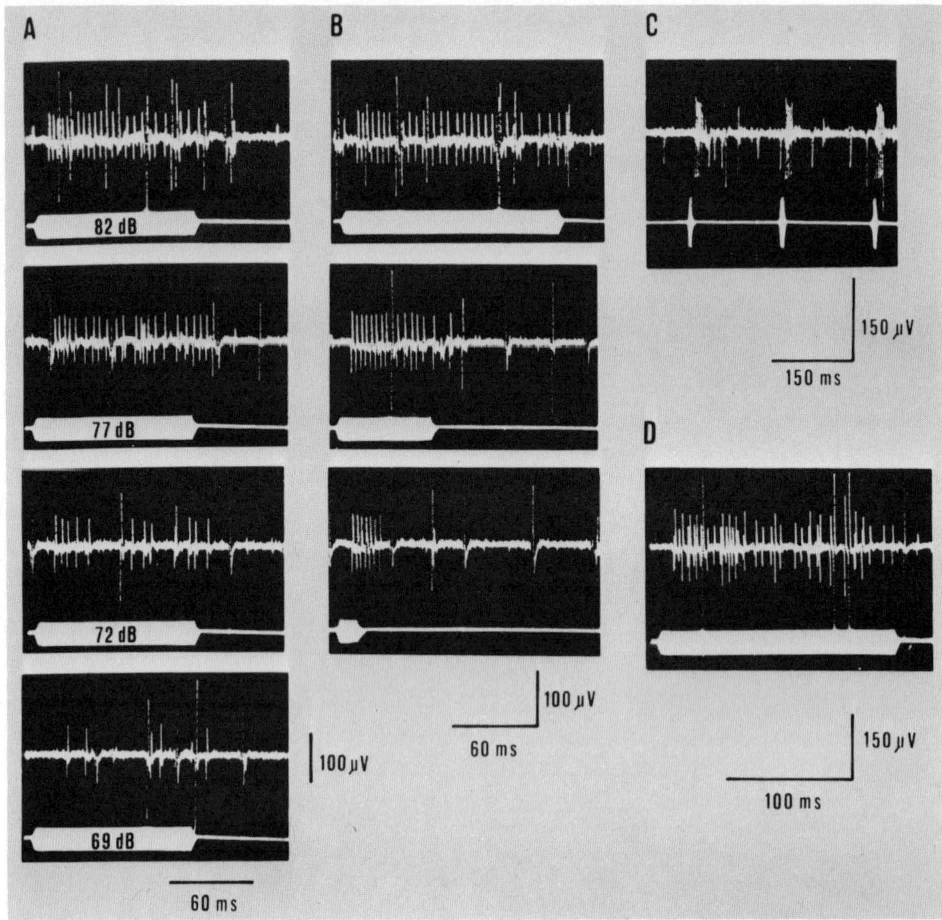


Fig. 22 *Gryllus campestris*, some coding qualities of the high frequency unit (see Fig. 21). A, response to a 13.5 kHz stimulus of different intensities (69, 72, 77, 82 dB); B, response to the same intensity but to different sound durations (22, 70, 157 msec); C, each 14 kHz/75dB/15 msec stimulus is answered by 3 - 4 spikes; D, a 13.5 kHz/70dB/200 msec stimulus is answered by 2 high frequency units. Note that in all recordings an acoustically non-correlated background activity is present and marked by large spikes (After Nocke 1972).

As in the hearing organs of many other animals, the sound intensity in the cricket ear is coded in a non-linear way. The CNS reads out sound intensity by processing the interspike intervals, e.g. the time relationships of incoming signals.

The duration of a sound signal and its temporal pattern are coded by the duration of related spike trains and train patterns, because so far no primary sensory neurones have been found to discharge phasically. But, as seen in Fig. 22, there is no evidence in crickets that the sensory neurones are specifically tuned to the time parameters exhibited in the conspecific songs (Nocke 1972). This could explain why females respond with arousal on listening to sound of sympatric species (Zaretsky 1972; Popov 1974a, b).

b) Coding in the 2nd order auditory neurones. Within the auditory neuropile, the primary sensory neurones converge, apparently in different combinations, on to a relatively small number of 2nd order neurones. There is also evidence that some 2nd order elements are T-shaped so that they conduct impulses up to the head ganglia and simultaneously down to the motor centres in the 2nd thoracic ganglion.

Electrophysiological recordings from 2nd order fibres have been obtained successfully in restrained as well as in unrestrained animals. Some respond with a rather short delay of about 8 - 10 msec whilst others start to discharge after some 15 - 25 msec (Popov 1967, 1969, 1971, 1974a, b; Zaretsky 1972; Zhantiev and Tshukanov 1972a, b). Furthermore, we know that male crickets with the two tympanal organs destroyed sing normally. Thus auditory feedback is not necessary to start stridulation nor to sustain it. However, feedback could be used to control the excitatory state of the motor centres and so to influence the chirp rate.

Out of a variety of 2nd order auditory neurones so far studied in different cricket species, some were found to respond phasically to the onset of sound stimulation, and code the timing of the syllables, while others discharged tonically as long as the stimulus was present. Units which adapted quickly could be separated from others which showed no sign of adaptation or habituation. Since we are mainly interested in the processing of the conspecific calling songs, we concentrated on non-habituating units. This is justified from a behavioural point of view because females need longer-lasting calling songs to be attracted and guided to the male (Murphey and Zaretsky 1972).

With a technique utilizing plastic suction electrodes to record extracellularly the responses of 2nd order auditory neurones from the neck connectives (Stout 1971), we found single unit activity which was clearly related to a calling song played to the animal (Fig. 23). Two units are of special interest and they were encountered

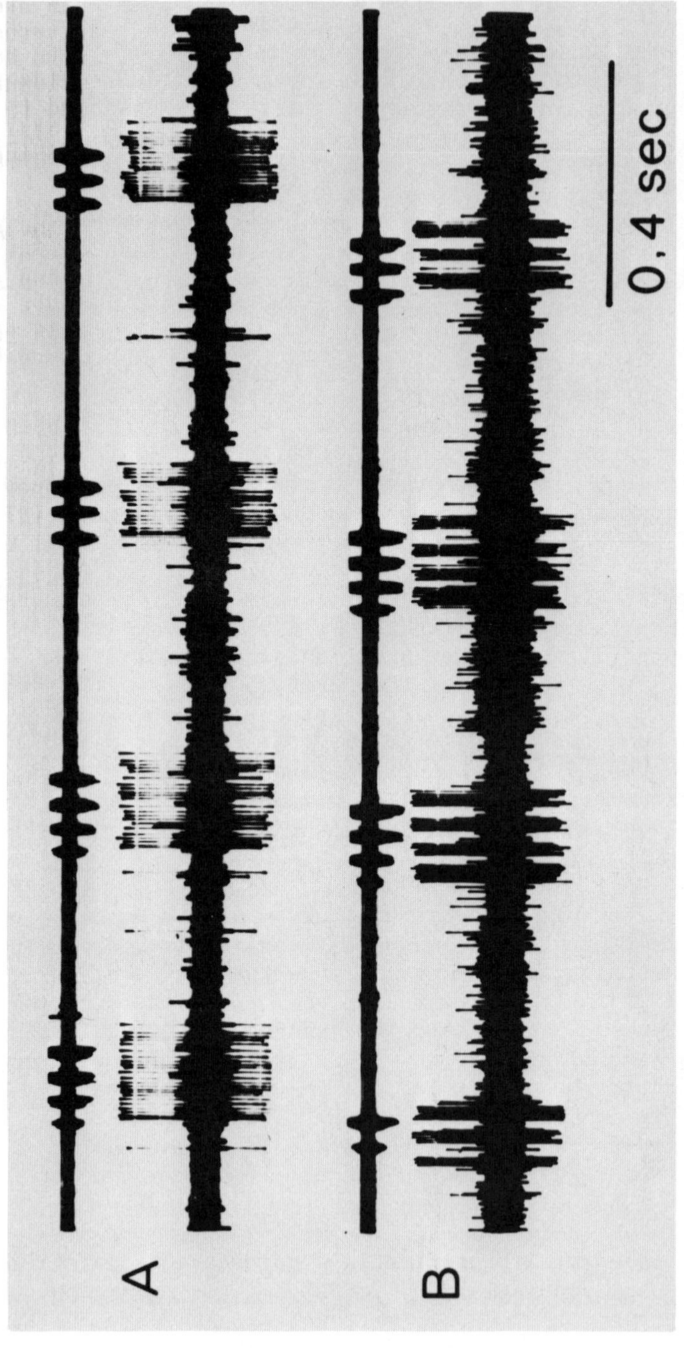


Fig. 23 *Gryllus campestris*, responses of two auditory interneurones picked up at the level of the left neck connective (lower trace) in a female during playback of the conspecific calling song of the male (upper trace). A, signals the chirp rate and chirp duration of the natural call, and B, codes, in addition, syllable sequences within single chirps (After Stout and Huber 1972).

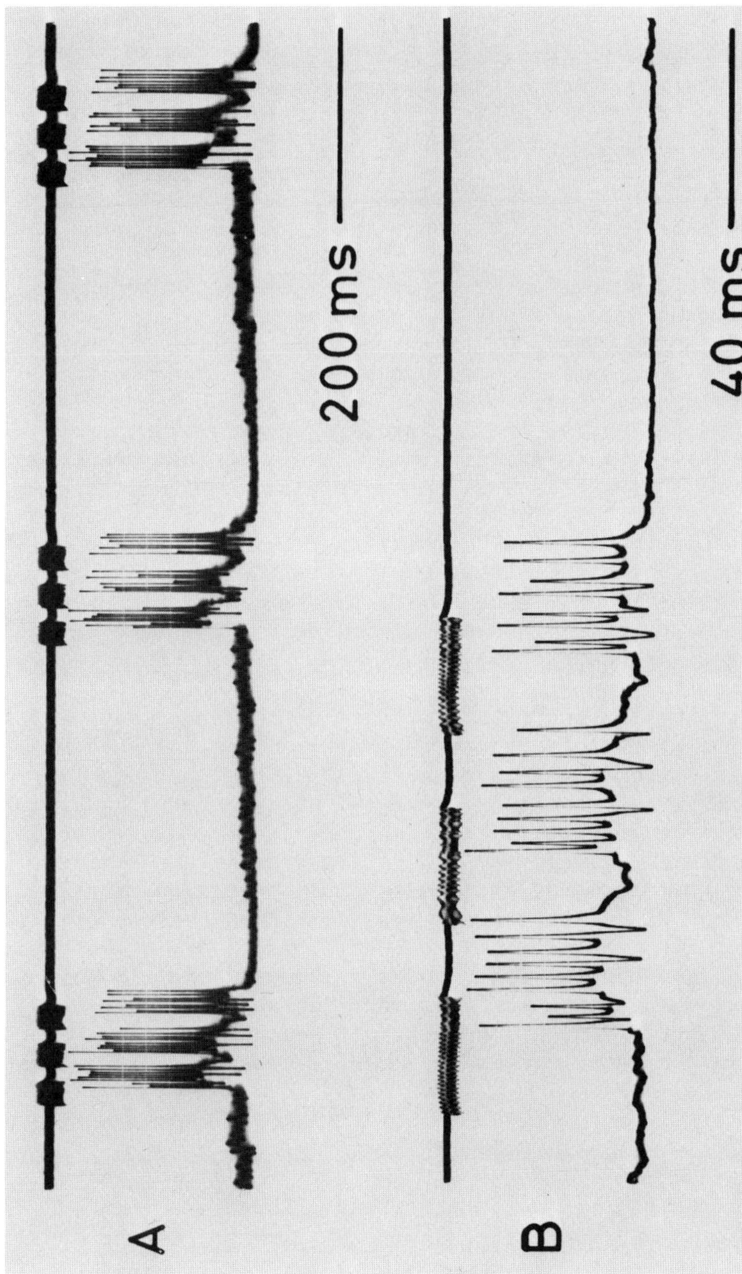


Fig. 24 *Acheta domesticus*, responses of a pulse coding auditory interneurone recorded from the neuropile of the 1st thoracic ganglion with micropipettes. A, three chirps of an artificial calling song (upper trace) and correlated responses (lower trace); B, single chirp at higher speed and related response. The base line shows little bumps which result from subthreshold synaptic activity, the depolarization of the membrane during the stimulus and the related spike train (After Stout, unpubl. results).

in each connective both in females and males. One when stimulated with the natural calling song gave responses which matched chirp rate and chirp duration (chirp coding unit), while the other matched the syllable rate and the syllable duration (pulse coding unit). That we are dealing with two separate units has recently been demonstrated by Stout (pers. comm.) who has computerized our data. Stout was also able to penetrate the prothoracic neuropile of *Acheta domesticus* and to record the pulse coding unit, apparently intracellularly. As indicated in Fig. 24, sound pulses depolarize the membrane and give rise to a train of spikes, correlated with each single pulse, which cease suddenly before the next pulse starts.

Here we may ask a number of questions, for example: Are these units specifically tuned to the natural and conspecific song pattern, or are they merely a link in the neuronal network dealing with species-specific sound recognition? All our recent data lead to the conclusion that pulse-and chirp-coding units within the thoracic nerve cord cannot be considered as the 'species-specific-filters' which the ethologists need to explain their results. This means we have to search for other candidates. We have also some indication that these units respond equally well in females which are in a non-receptive state as in those in the state of active copulatory readiness. In other words, the well known changes in the behaviour of female crickets which show no response, or escape behaviour, or even phonokinesis, to the conspecific sound signal cannot be based on the auditory machinery mentioned so far.

c) Conclusions. From our recent results it appears that species-specific song recognition in orthopteran insects is established by the cooperation of neurones within a multineuronal network distributed within the CNS (thoracic nerve cord and head ganglia), in which the participating members have certain features in common. Through connections at different levels and interactions among the single neurones, a new system property evolves which is tuned toward the processing of essential parameters and parameter combinations by which species-specific recognition is characterized. It is doubtful whether we shall find 'complex feature detecting neurones' in our animals; we rather favor the hypothesis that the whole network has some still unknown optimizing properties. To search for those and subsequently to investigate them is an immediate goal of our research.

## ACKNOWLEDGEMENTS

I am greatly indebted to my former group of students at the University of Cologne and to foreign scientists who joined our laboratory; without their work and enthusiasm this chapter would never have been written.

## REFERENCES


1. ADAM, L.J. *Z. vergl. Physiol.* *63:*227, 1969.
2. ADAM, L.J. *Verh. Dtsch. Zool. Ges. Köln*, 245, 1970.
3. ALEXANDER, R.D. *Ann. Rev. Entomol.* *12:*495, 1967.
4. BAILEY, W.J. *J. Exp. Biol.* *52:*495, 1970.
5. BAILEY, W.J. & BROUGHTON, W.B. *J. Exp. Biol.* *52:*507, 1970.
6. BENNET-CLARK, H.C. *J. Exp. Biol.* *52:*619, 1970.
7. BENNET-CLARK, H.C. *Nature* *234:*255, 1971.
8. BENTLEY, D.R. *J. Insect Physiol.* *15:*677, 1969a.
9. BENTLEY, D.R. *Z. vergl. Physiol.* *62:*267, 1969b.
10. BENTLEY, D.R. *Science* *174:*1139, 1971.
11. BENTLEY, D.R. In: Developmental Neurobiology of Arthropods. D. Young, editor. Cambridge University Press, p. 147 (1973).
12. BENTLEY, D.R. & KUTSCH, W. *J. Exp. Biol.* *45:*151 (1966).
13. BENTLEY, D.R. & HOY, R.R. *Science* *170:*1409, 1970.
14. BUSNEL, R.G. Acoustic Behaviour of Animals. Elsevier Publ. Comp. Amsterdam (1963).
15. DUMORTIER, B. In: Acoustic Behaviour of Animals. R.G. Busnel, editor. Elsevier Publ. Comp., Amsterdam, pp. 277, 346, 583, (1963).
16. EIBL, E. *Staatsarbeit der Universität zu Köln* (1974).
17. ELSNER, N. *Zool. Anz. 31, Suppl. Bd.* 592, 1967.
18. ELSNER, N. *Z. vergl. Physiol.* *60:*308, 1968.
19. ELSNER, N. *Z. vergl. Physiol.* *68:*417, 1970.
20. ELSNER, N. In: Symp. Neurobiology of Invertebranes, Tihany 1971, p. 261 (1973).
21. ELSNER, N. *J. Comp. Physiol.* *88:*67, 1974a.
22. ELSNER, N. *J. Comp. Physiol.* *89:*227, 1974b.
23. ELSNER, N. *J. Comp. Physiol.* In press. 1974c.
24. ELSNER, N. & HUBER, F. *Z. vergl. Physiol.* *65:*389, 1969.
25. ELSNER, N. & HUBER, F. *Fortschr. Zoologie* *22:*1, 1973.
26. EWING, A. & HOYLE, G. *J. Exp. Biol.* *43:*139, 1965.
27. HEILIGENBERG, W. *Z. vergl. Physiol.* *53:*114, 1966.
28. HEILIGENBERG, W. *Z. vergl. Physiol.* *65:*70, 1969.
29. HELVERSEN, D. VON *J. Comp. Physiol.* *81:*381, 1972.
30. HÖRMANN-HECK, S. VON *Z. Tierpsychol.* *14:*137, 1957.
31. HUBER, F. *Z. Tierpsychol.* *12:*12, 1955.
32. HUBER, F. *Z. vergl. Physiol.* *44:*60, 1960.
33. HUBER, F. *Evolution* *14:*429, 1962.
34. HUBER, F. In: Acoustic Behaviour of Animals. R.G. Bushnel, editor. Elsevier Publ. Comp., Amsterdam, p. 440 (1963).
35. HUBER, F. *Naturw. Rundschau* *18:*143, 1965.
36. HUBER, F. Rheinisch-Westf. Akad. Wiss., Westdeutscher Verlag Opladen, p. 41 (1970).
37. HUBER, F. Symposium of the Institute of Biology *21:*61, Chapt. 4, Blackwell Scientific Publ. Oxford (1974a).
38. HUBER, F. In: Simple Nervous Systems, D.R. Newth, editor, Chapt. 10, p. 381. E. Arnold, London (1974b).

39. INNENMOSER, J. *Dissertation Universität zu Köln* (1974).
40. JOHNSTONE, J.R., SAUNDERS, J.C. & JOHNSTONE, B.M. *Nature 227:*625 (1970).
41. JONES, M.D.R. *J. Exp. Biol. 45:*15, 1966a.
42. JONES, M.D.R. *J. Exp. Biol. 45:*31, 1966b.
43. JONES, M.D.R. & DAMBACH, M. *J. Comp. Physiol. 87:*89, 1973.
44. JOSEPHSON, R.K. & HALVERSON, R.C. *Biol. Bull. 141:*413, 1971.
45. KALMRING, K. *Z. vergl. Physiol. 72:*95, 1971.
46. KALMRING, K., RHEINLAENDER, J. & REHBEIN, H. *Z. vergl. Physiol. 76:*314, 1972.
47. KALMRING, K., RHEINLAENDER, J. & RÖMER, H. *J. Comp. Physiol. 80:*325, 1972.
48. KLOPFFLEISCH, K. *Staatsarbeit Universität zu Köln* (1973).
49. KUTSCH, W. *Z. vergl. Physiol. 63:*335, 1969.
50. KUTSCH, W. & HUBER, F. *Z. vergl. Physiol. 67:*140, 1970.
51. KUTSCH, W. & OTTO, D. *J. Comp. Physiol. 81:*115, 1972.
52. LOHER, W. *Z. vergl. Physiol. 39:*313, 1957.
53. LOHER, W. *Z. vergl. Physiol. 53:*277, 1966.
54. LOHER, W. & HUBER, F. *J. Insect Physiol. 10:*13, 1964.
55. LOHER, W. & HUBER, F. *Symp. Soc. Exp. Biol. 20:*381, 1966.
56. MARKL, H. *J. Ornith. 113:*91, 1972.
57. MC KAY, J.M. *J. Exp. Biol. 51:*787, 1969.
58. MC KAY, J.M. *J. Exp. Biol. 53:*137, 1970.
59. MICHEL, K. *Dissertation Universität Mainz* (1973).
60. MICHELSEN, A.A. *J. Insect Physiol. 12:*1119, 1966.
61. MICHELSEN, A.A. *Nature 220:*585, 1968.
62. MICHELSEN, A.A. *Z. vergl. Physiol. 71:*49, 1971.
63. MICHELSEN, A.A. In: Handbook of Sensory Physiology, Vol. V, Auditory Systems, Springer Verlag (In press, 1974).
64. MICHELSEN, A.A. & NOCKE, H. *Adv. Ins. Physiol. 10:*247, 1974.
65. MÖSS, D. *Z. vergl. Physiol. 73:*53, 1971.
66. MURPHEY, R.K. & ZARETSKY, M.D. *J. Exp. Biol. 56:*335, 1972.
67. NOCKE, H. *Z. vergl. Physiol. 74:*272, 1971.
68. NOCKE, H. *J. Comp. Physiol. 80:*141, 1972.
69. OTTO, D. *Zool. Anz. 31. Suppl. Bd.* 585, 1967.
70. OTTO, D. *Zool. Anz. 33. Suppl. Bd.* 472, 1969.
71. OTTO, D. *Z. vergl. Physiol. 74:*227, 1971.
72. PERDECK, A.C. *Behaviour 12:*1, 1958.
73. POPOV, A.V. *J. Evol. Biochem. Physiol. 1:*239, 1965.
74. POPOV, A.V. In: Evolutionary Neurophysiology and Neurochemistry, E.M. Kreps, Editor. Leningrad:Nauka p. 54 (1967).
75. POPOV, A.V. In: Modern Problems of Structure and Function of the Nervous System in Insects. Leningrad:Nauka p. 182 (1969).
76. POPOV, A.V. In: Sensory Processes at the Neuronal and Behavioural Level. New York, Academic Press, p. 301 (1971a).
77. POPOV, A.V. *Jurnal Evol'uzionnoj Biochimii i Fiziologii 7:* 87, 1971b.
78. POPOV, A.V. *Entomol. Obozr. 57:*17, 1972.

79. POPOV, A.V. *Jurnal Evol'uzionnoj Biochimii i Fiziologii* *9:* 265, 1973.
80. POPOV, A.V. In: Symposium on Mechanoreception. J. Schwartzkopff, editor. (In press, 1974).
81. POPOV, A.V. *Rev. Entomol. URSS* (In press, 1974).
82. REHBEIN, H.G. *Verh. Dtsch. Zool. Ges. Mainz* *184:*1973.
83. RENNER, M. *Z. Tierpsychol.* *9:*122, 1952.
84. RHEINLAENDER, J., KALMRING, K. & RÖMER, H. *J. Comp. Physiol.* *77:*208, 1972.
85. RHEINLAENDER, J. & KALMRING, K. *J. Comp. Physiol.* *85:*361, 1973.
86. ROWELL, C.H.F. & MC KAY, J.M. *J. Exp. Biol.* *51:*231, 1969a.
87. ROWELL, C.H.F. & MC KAY, J.M. *J. Exp. Biol.* *51:*247, 1969b.
88. SCHWARTZKOPFF, J. *Nova Acta Leopoldina 37/2:*223, 1973.
89. SHUVALOV, V.F. & POPOV, A.V. *Jurnal Evol'uzionnoj Biochimii i Fiziologii* *7:*612, 1971.
90. SHUVALOV, V.F. & POPOV, A.V. *Jurnal Evol'uzionnoj Biochimii i Fiziologii* *9:*177, 1973a.
91. SHUVALOV, V.F. & POPOV, A.V. *Zool. J.* *52:*1179, 1973b.
92. STOUT, J.F. *Z. vergl. Physiol.* *74:*26, 1971.
93. STOUT, J.F. & HUBER, F. *Z. vergl. Physiol.* *76:*302, 1972.
94. WEBER, T. *Dissertation Universität zu Köln* (1974).
95. WORDEN, F.G. & GALAMBOS, R. *Neurosciences Res. Progr. Bull.* *10:* 1972.
96. ZARETSKY, M.D. *Nature* *229:*195, 1971.
97. ZARETSKY, M.D. *J. Comp. Physiol.* *79:*153, 1972.
98. ZHANTIEV, D.R. *Zool. Zh.* *50:*507, 1971.
99. ZHANTIEV, D.R. & TSHUKANOV, V.S. *Vestn. Mosk. Univ., Ser. VI,* *2:*3, 1972a.
100. ZHANTIEV, D.R. & TSHUKANOV, V.S. *Zool. Zh.* *51:*983, 1972b.
101. ZHANTIEV, D.R. & DUBROVIN, N.N. *Zool. Zh.* *53:*345, 1974.

# NEURAL TRANSACTIONS DURING ACOUSTIC STIMULATION OF NOCTUID MOTHS

K.D. Roeder
Department of Biology
Tufts University
Medford, Mass., U.S.A.

## INTRODUCTION

Moths of several families have acoustic organs capable of detecting the echolocation cries made by insectivorous bats. The afferent nerve responses of these auditory organs have been studied as follows: the thoracic tympanic organs of noctuid moths (Roeder and Treat, 1957, Roeder, 1964, 1966a, 1974); the abdominal tympanic organs of geometrids (Roeder, 1974), and the cephalic palp-pilifer organs of choerocampine sphingids (Roeder and Treat, 1970, Roeder, 1972). In the case of the noctuid tympanic organ, the fine structure of the receptor region has been described by Ghiradella (1971), and the biophysics of acoustic transduction is being investigated by Adams (1971, 1972 and in press).

In noctuid moths, two types of avoidance behavior are elicited when the tympanic organs are excited by bat cries or by bat-simulating ultrasonic pulse patterns. Observations in the field (Roeder, 1962) revealed that moths tend to turn and fly directly away from a faint or distant source of ultrasonic pulses, while they loop and dive in an apparently random and non-directional pattern when the sounds reaching them are intense. These two behavioral patterns were confirmed in the laboratory (Roeder, 1967) using moths mounted in stationary flight whose tendency to turn on exposure to ultrasonic pulses was measured by means of a differential anemometer.

The noctuid tympanic organ contains two acoustic sense cells, designated A1 and A2. The A1 sense cell alone responds with a proportional train of spikes when exposed to sound intensity levels equivalent to those that elicit turning-away behavior in intact moths. Sense cell A2 begins to respond proportionally at a sound intensity level 20-30 dB higher, at which point the A1 response reaches saturation (Roeder, 1974). This finding suggests that excitation of A1 alone in both ears may release turning-away from a distant and unalerted predator while excitation of A1 and A2 simultaneously may elicit the non-directional diving, looping and falling observed when the predator is nearby and in a position to track the moth by means of its echo (Roeder, 1966a).

One might expect behavior having such apparent survival value as the turning-away response to be automatic and invariant under natural conditions. Yet the anemometer studies carried out in the laboratory with restrained moths showed that the incidence of turning-away attempts was often erratic (Roeder, 1967). Some specimens would constantly attempt to turn away from the side at which the sound pulses were directed on one occasion and then not at all when examined a few hours later. Other specimens would make erratic turning attempts even in the absence of acoustic stimulation, or would respond only in a fragmentary fashion. Still others would fly steadily and make no response to acoustic stimulation. It must be presumed that the unpredictability of this behavior is due in part both to the restraint needed and to the fact that an unknown number of field conditions could not be replicated in the laboratory. This leads to the conclusion that the mechanism mediating acoustic input and motor output to the alar muscles (controlling the wings' differential angle of attack and hence steering during flight) is subject to modulation by other inputs. In other words, a neural control akin to attention is included in the behavioral mechanism of bat avoidance.

Various investigations have sought to elucidate the interneuronal connections between the sensory input of A1 and the alar motor nerves. The mechanism appears to be limited to the pterothoracic ganglion (the partially fused meso- and metathoracic ganglia of the wing-bearing segments). These neuronal connections remain to be worked out, but various forms of integration of the incoming A1 spike train have been described in 2nd- and 3rd-order interneurons belonging to the thoracic neuropil (Roeder, 1966b, Paul, in press). Procion-yellow injection of the A1 axon has revealed that the central terminations of A1 branch widely, but only ipsilaterally, within the meso-and metathoracic ganglia (Paul, 1973), from which region also arise the alar motor nerves. The projection of the A1 axon into the prothoracic ganglion, where its arborizations terminate in the posterior ipsilateral segment, may provide the link to the ascending acoustic interneurons discussed below.

Treat (1956) showed that the direct component of the mechanism concerned in changes in the pattern of wing movement is contained within the thoracic ganglia. He recorded behavioral responses from headless moths in stationary flight when they were exposed to bursts of ultrasound. These responses of decapitated moths lacked the sustained character of turning-away behavior observed in intact moths, and mostly took the form of brief twitches or perturbations of the rhythmically flapping wings. This suggests that the ganglia in the head exert a facilitating control over the thoracic system in sustaining steered flight.

This suggestion requires neurophysiological support through a demonstration that 1) axons of interneurons excited by the A1 spike train ascend through the prothoracic ganglion and cervical connectives to the brain, and 2) that neurons in the brain are activated by these units and in their turn transmit spike patterns that descend to the thoracic center so as to exert a sustaining or facilitative (regenerative) control over the local system. The possibility also exists that these facilitative (regenerative) pathways are complemented by acoustically-activated descending pathways that have an inhibitory (degenerative) modulating control over the local system.

The following account describes a preliminary neurophysiological search for these postulated ascending and descending signals and for the forms of neural integration that they might exhibit.

## MATERIAL AND METHODS

In most of the experiments we employed specimens of *Prodenia eridania* Cramer which were obtained as pupae during the winter months. In summer, a variety of other noctuids were collected at night in a u.v. trap and used the following day. No significant species differences were noted in acoustic sensitivity or neuronal performance.

Methods for mounting the moths, insertion of insulated steel microelectrodes in the neuropil, generation of ultrasonic stimulus pulses and registration of the results have been fully described in the publications cited above. Methods special to this study will be described where they become relevant. Diagrams of the two exposures of the nervous system are shown in Fig. 1.

## RESULTS

### Ascending Spike Signals

While probing the thoracic neuropil for acoustically activated spike signals, it was previously noted that a complex of acoustic units ascends the nerve cord through the prothoracic ganglion and cervical connectives (Roeder, 1966b). Subsequently, stimulus-

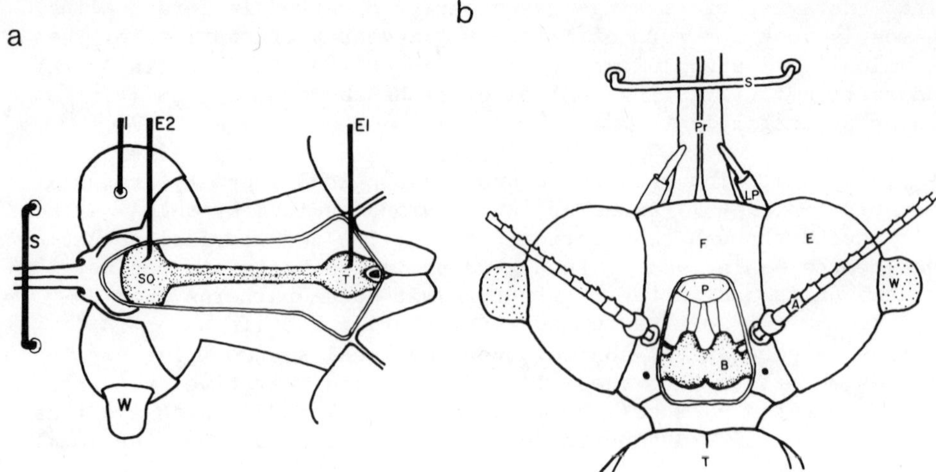


Fig. 1 a) Diagram of the exposure used in two-electrode penetrations of the ventral nerve cord. E1 and E2, recording electrodes: I, indifferent electrode; S, small staple immobilizing the proboscis; SO, subesophageal ganglion; T1, prothoracic ganglion; W, wax post affixed to the compound eye in order to stabilize the head. b) Exposure of the protocerebral ganglia used in probing the brain neuropil. B, protocerebral ganglia; E, compound eye; F, frons which has been partly dissected away together with part of the vertex; LP, labial palp; P, pharyngeal pump visible through opening in frons; Pr, proboscis; S, staple; T, tergum; W, wax post stabilizing the head.

synchronized spike trains were recorded from an electrode in the neuropil of the lateroventral quadrant of the protocerebral ganglia and these were studied in some detail (Roeder, 1969a, 1969b, 1970, 1973). These spike trains last for about the duration of the acoustic stimulus pulse and generally show a latency of 8-15 msec with respect to the onset of the acoustic stimulus, depending on its intensity.

My interest centered on these protocerebral spike responses, which resemble repeaters (1966b), because although they show only minor temporal transformation of the afferent spike trains originating in the tympanic organs, they possess three properties indicating integration of the acoustic inputs. The first property is that if these brain responses (to 1/sec stimuli) are observed and followed for several hours at low acoustic intensities, the spike trains may show (in about 20% of cases) curious lapses in acoustic responsiveness. Lapses commonly begin about one hour after the preparation has remained otherwise undisturbed and was kept in dim light or darkness (Fig. 2a). The spike response fails, commonly abruptly but sometimes gradually, and remains absent for periods ranging from a few seconds to an hour. There may be a number of lapses before the preparation finally responds in a stable fashion. In a few cases, lapses seem to be precipitated by illumination and terminated by strong acoustic stimuli (Roeder, 1969a, 1970). The second property indicating acoustic integration is that one of the units contributing to the spike train is sometimes responsive at low sound intensities but becomes suppressed at high intensities, suggesting an inhibitory action by sense cell A2. The third indication of acoustic integration is a complex of two or three repeater units recorded from the right protocerebral ganglion, which is excited for instance, by stimulus pulses directed at either the right or the left tympanic organ, but is generally slightly more sensitive (by about 4 dB) to sounds directed at the right side of the moth. When sounds are directed at both tympanic organs, sensitivity of the protocerebral response is greater than with monaural stimulation (Roeder, 1973). The slight ipsilateral bias of the protocerebral response cannot be due alone to the considerable directional properties of the tympanic organs (Payne *et al.*, 1965), for if the brain response is studied after destruction of one tympanic organ the unilateral bias in favor of the intact side is much greater (10-15 dB or more). This was inadvertantly checked in summer when using species of *Leucania*. A considerable asymmetry in acoustic responsiveness was encountered in two or three specimens, irrespective of the side of the brain under the electrode. A subsequent check of these specimens revealed that one tympanic sensillum had been destroyed by the gamasine mite, *Dicrocheles phalaenodectes* (Treat, 1954).

These three properties indicate integration of afferent signals not only from the ipsilateral A1 and A2 sense cells but also of those from both the right and left tympanic organs. This at first led me to conclude that the spike trains originated in higher-order interneurons in the brain and that these signals might possibly be descending the nerve cord (Roeder, 1969a, 1969b, 1970). Present evidence indicates that this is not the case and that these spike responses detected in the brain with a latency of 8-15 msec represent activity in the cerebral terminations of ascending fibers.

Evidence for this conclusion was obtained by probing the neuropil with two electrodes - one in the prothoracic ganglion and the other in the subesophageal ganglion. The electrode arrangement is shown in Fig. 1A. When the electrode in one ganglion encountered

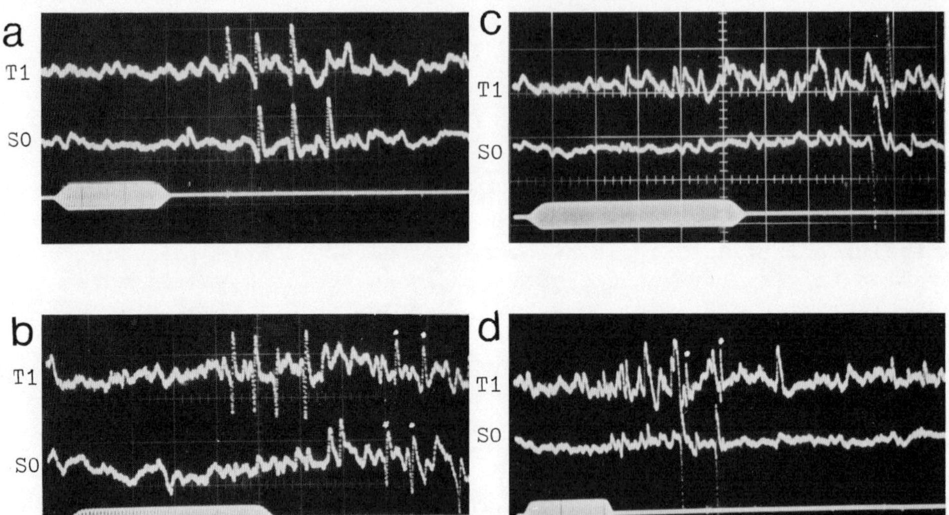


Fig. 2 *Prodenia eridania*. Acoustic responses recorded simultaneously at a subesophageal electrode (SO) and prothoracic electrode (T1). a) ascending train of 3 repeater spikes registered at both electrodes. b) ascending train of 4 repeater spikes in the T1 channel and 2 descending spikes (marked by dots) registered at both electrodes. c) single large descending spike registered in both channels. d) the same preparation as c), two descending spikes registered in each channel. Stimulus pulses (lower traces) were 45 kHz and 5 msec in duration in a); 10 msec in duration in b), c) and d). Total sweep length, 20 msec in a), b) and c); 40 msec in d).

repeater spikes in response to acoustic stimulation (1/sec) the neuropil of the other ganglion (or in some cases the cervical connectives) was searched with the second electrode for slightly phase-shifted spikes time-locked to the first spike sequence.

This method was used in 90 experiments, a few of which were successful in locating the same unit under both electrodes. In each case, repeater spikes in the 8-15 msec latency time-frame arrived first at the prothoracic (T1) electrode (Fig. 2A). The conduction velocity of these spikes is 1.3 to 1.5 meters/sec through the cervical connectives.

The latency of these signals as well as their form and response characteristics suggest that they most probably belong to the same units previously reported (Roeder, 1969a, 1969b, 1970) from the protocerebral ganglia. Additional evidence supporting the identity of these ascending signals with 8-15 msec brain responses was supplied by the incidental observation that lapses sometimes occurred in the ascending acoustic responses when registered in the prothoracic ganglion or cervical connectives (Fig. 3C and D). These findings indicate that a considerable amount of integration takes place in the pterothoracic ganglion.

## Descending Acoustic Signals

Having established the conduction direction of the spike train in the 8-15 msec latency time-frame generated by acoustic stimulation, it became feasible to seek the signals postulated above as originating in the brain and descending the nerve cord to modulate and sustain the flight-steering mechanisms of the pterothoracic ganglion.

Such descending signals might be expected to make their appearance in the nerve cord with latencies longer than 15 msec; also, they might be expected to show a completely different pattern of spikes from the stimulus-bracketed repeater trains, as well as an even greater lability than that indicated by the ascending repeaters' lapses in responsiveness. These expected instabilities might be expected to compound with still others suggested by the observation (Roeder, 1967) that intact moths mounted and in stationary flight show great lability in their turning-away behavior, for the situation of a moth completely immobilized for electrode insertion and subjected to surgical insult is undoubtedly even more 'unnatural'. For these reasons, the current search for descending spike signals is being carried on with the expectation of only a small percentage of successful experiments.

First, it was necessary to demonstrate that signals correlated in some fashion with the acoustic stimuli do in fact descend the

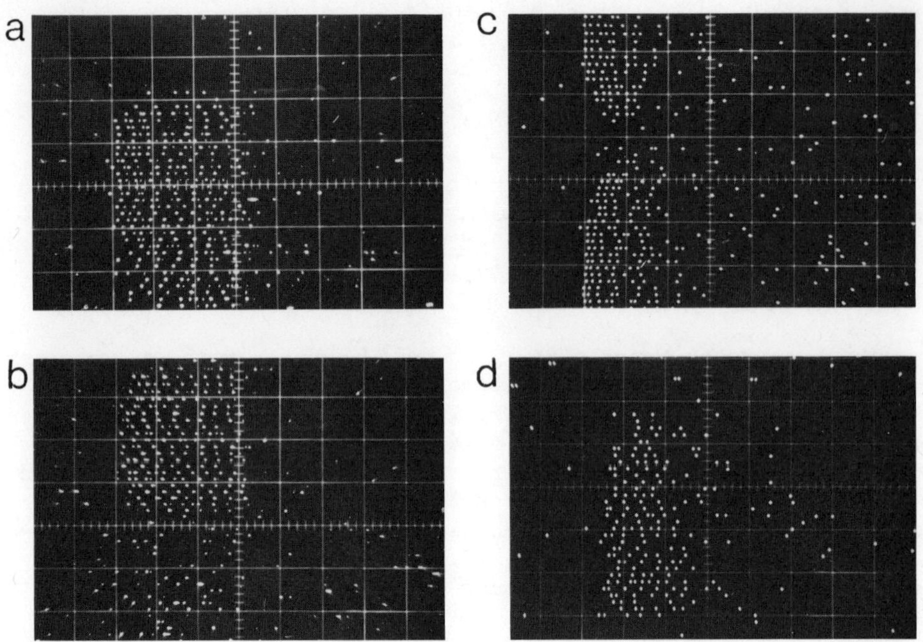


Fig. 3 *Prodenia eridania*. Lapses of acoustic responsiveness in the nervous system. a) and b) continuous record of the responses of a repeater unit in the protocerebral ganglion. Total vertical time-span covered by the two frames is about 2 minutes. 45 kHz pulses 15 msec in duration were delivered continuously at 1/sec (interval between lines of dots). Sweep time-scale, 5 msec/division. c) lapse in a repeater unit located in the prothoracic ganglion. d) lapse in a unit located in the cervical connectives. Time and stimulus parameters the same as in a) and b).

nerve cord from the brain to the thoracic centers. It was possible to accomplish this in 2 out of the 90 experiments described above. In the experiment illustrated in Fig. 2B, the T1 electrode (upper trace) registered a train of 4 ascending repeater spikes in response to the acoustic stimulus (lower trace). The subesophageal electrode (SO, center trace) was apparently not placed so as to record this ascending train, but instead registered a pair of spikes (dots over), the first at about 15 msec. A similar pair of spikes also appears on the upper (T1) trace but is slightly displaced, indicating later arrival at the prothoracic ganglion. This temporal displacement corresponds to slightly more than 1 msec. In the second successful experiment (Fig. 2C and D) neither electrode registered distinct ascending responses to the stimulus, but a single large spike appears at 15-16 msec on the SO (center) trace. This is followed after a small delay by a corresponding single spike on the T1 (upper) trace. Fig. 2D is from the same experiment on a contracted time base. Here, two time-locked spikes appear, the first in the SO channel at a latency of 19 msec, closely followed by a corresponding pair in the T1 channel.

Presented only with these single traces, it might be thought that the timing of the SO-T1 spikes occurred by chance, or might be unrelated to acoustic stimulation. These possibilities were negated in the second successful experiment, where the system remained stable for about one hour and permitted the registration of a large number of stimulus-triggered sweeps as well as dot patterns. In this case fortunately, the background spike activity on the subesophageal channel was low compared with the acoustically-triggered spikes. This made it possible to allow the large SO spikes, rather than the stimulus, to trigger the oscillograph sweep at a high (0.1 msec/division) writing rate. From this it was demonstrated that the T1 spike invariably followed the SO spike with a constant delay of 0.8 msec. This measurement indicated a conduction velocity in the descending unit of 2.2 meter/sec. The descending spikes were found to follow the stimulus at a repetition rate of 1/sec, but, unlike the ascending repeaters, the descending response failed rapidly at slightly higher stimulus repetition rates. This descending response consisted of one and occasionally two spikes, a signal similar to that of a pulse-marker (Roeder, 1966b), particularly one of the labile type recently discovered by Paul (in press).

## Candidate Descending Signals from the Brain

There can be no doubt about the conduction direction of the signals described in the preceeding section. This is not the case with spikes detected in the protocerebral neuropil because morphological considerations preclude the placing of two electrodes, one in the brain and the other in the ventral nerve cord, without causing extensive surgical destruction. Since the extent of such damage would seem to reduce still further the chances of detecting labile acoustic responses in the brain, a two-electrode preparation has so far not been attempted. Thus, in the following experiments I employed single-electrode penetrations of the protocerebral neuropil. The method of preparation (Fig. 1 B) has been described previously (Roeder, 1969a). However, unlike in the earlier work, the present series is being investigated with the knowledge that the spike trains generated 8 to 15 msec after the stimulus belong to ascending pathways. Therefore, the search for candidate descending signals possibly modulating the thoracic mechanisms of turning-away behavior could be concentrated on later signals. The present series consists of 77 preparations.

As previously reported, spike responses correlated in some degree with acoustic stimulation were detected only in the lateroventral regions of the protocerebral neuropil, although other regions were routinely probed. In all successful preparations, the ascending trains of spikes in two or three units were detected 8-15 msec after the onset of the stimulus pulses (Fig. 4 A). In addition, three types of acoustically correlated spike responses have been detected so far at greater latencies.

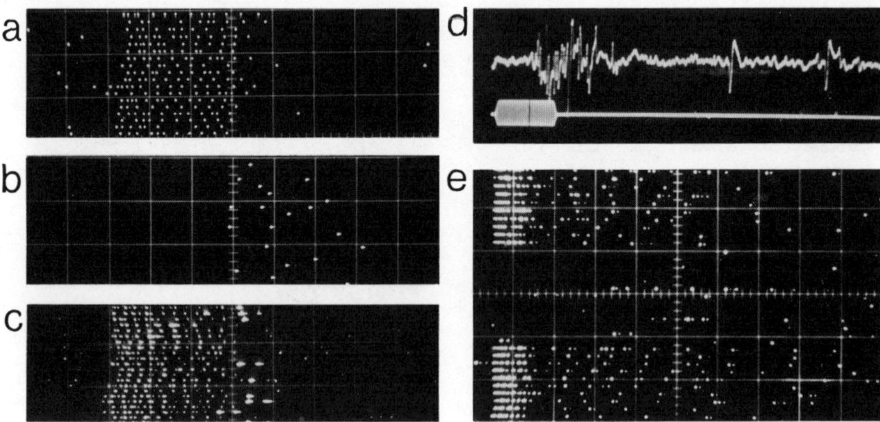


Fig. 4 *Prodenia eridania*. The response of units in the protocerebral neuropil to ultrasonic pulses delivered 1/sec (interval between lines of dots). a) typical ascending repeater trains in response to low-intensity pulses (42.6 kHz, 15 msec duration). b) the same preparation as a); the electrode tip was displaced slightly so that it failed to register the repeater responses and detected only a pulse-marker spike. c) another preparation; owing to the greater spike height (larger dots) of the pulse-marker both response types can be distinguished. d) single sweep showing a diffuse repeater volley followed after a delay by the first two spikes of an afterdischarge unit. The stimulus (lower trace) is 10 msec in duration. e) the same responses as in d) presented as dot patterns and on a contracted time base (20 msec/division). Stimuli were delivered 1/sec (interval between lines of dots). The repeater responses appear at the left of each line and are followed by the afterdischarges. The stimulus was switched off for about 14 seconds in the center section of the frame. The horizontal time scale in a), b) and c) is 5 msec/division; in e) 20 msec/division.

The signal in this category that was most frequently encountered (12 preparations) was a labile pulse-marker (Paul, in press) or phasic spike that appeared singly or occasionally in groups of two or three, 18 to 40 msec after the stimulus. The example in Fig. 4B was registered soon after the recording of 4A. A slight displacement of the electrode tip caused it to lose contact with the repeaters and register in their place one or more well-spaced spikes with a latency of 24 to 40 msec. A similar response is shown in 4C, the pulse-marker spikes being in this case larger than and thus clearly distinct from, the repeater trains. A third example is shown in Fig. 5A and B, the isolation of the late phasic spike in B being accomplished in this case by passing the taped signal through a spike-height analyser. Units of this type tend to fail, leaving only the repeater train, and rarely respond to each stimulus at stimulus repetition rates much above 1/sec. It seems likely that these labile pulse-marker responses are identical with the spikes demonstrated in the preceeding section to descend the nerve cord.

Less often encountered was a unit that begins to generate spikes only 40-50 msec after the acoustic stimulus (Fig. 4D) and continues to do so for 150 to 200 msec. This prolonged afterdischarge is better appreciated in the dot pattern recorded on a time base of 20 msec/division (Fig. 4E). In the upper part of this frame, each acoustic pulse elicits a repeater train, seen as a partially overlapping row of dots to the left of each line. The afterdischarge is spread out as a row of dots over the rest of the line. The 1/sec acoustic stimulus was switched off at a time corresponding to the middle of the frame, and it is clearly shown that the afterdischarge follows acoustic stimulation. The significance of this afterdischarge response wil be discussed later.

A third type of protocerebral response is inhibitory. This has been encountered only once in the present series. However, the unit remained sufficiently stable that it was possible to make a fairly complete study of its response characteristics. In the absence of acoustic stimulation this unit showed a tonic discharge of spikes that fluctuated between about 15 and 25/sec (upper part of Fig. 5D). When the moth was exposed to acoustic stimuli (1/sec) of an intensity only just sufficient to evoke a repeater train (short dot patterns at extreme left of frame) the tonic spikes were suppressed for 150 to 200 msec (Fig. 5C and D). An increase of 5 dB suppressed the spikes for about 400 msec, while a +15 dB stimulus caused suppression lasting as much as 600 msec after the stimulus pulse (Fig. 5E). When the repetition rate of the acoustic pulses was increased to 10/sec and delivered at moderate intensity for a period of 20 sec, the spikes of this unit remained almost completely absent throughout the period. Stimulation at a repetition rate of 1/sec at a moderate intensity for 14 sec revealed that the inhibited tonic unit adapted over this period; the duration of suppression following each stimulus

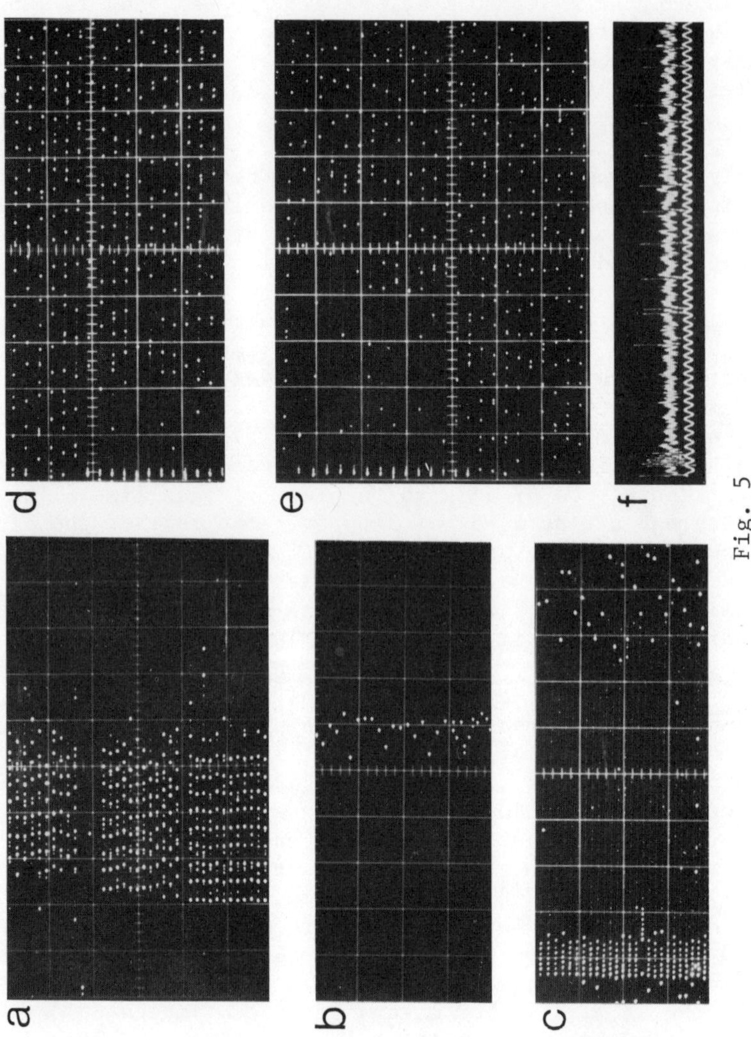


Fig. 5

<u>Fig. 5</u>

*Prodenia eridania*. All recordings made from a single brain preparation. Stimulus pulses were 45.3 kHz and 15 msec duration.

a) ascending repeater trains at near-threshold stimulus intensity (upper segment), at intensities of +5 dB (center segment), +15 dB (lower segment).

b) pulse-marker responses differentiated by means of a spike height analyser from part of the same recording.

c) the electrode moved slightly, when it began to register the inhibited unit. Dot pattern (20 msec/division) showing repeater responses (left column) and period of suppression of unit at low stimulus intensity. A few spikes of the inhibited unit appear just before and just after the repeater trains.

d) the same, horizontal time scale 100 msec/division. Repeater trains now appear as a vertical column of short lines to the extreme left. In the upper part of the frame the acoustic stimuli were too weak either to elicit repeater trains or to interrupt the tonic discharge of the inhibited unit. Stimulus was increased by 5 dB near the center of the frame causing repeater trains and inhibition of the tonic discharge.

e) the same; stimulus intensity increased to +15 dB and continued at 1/sec for 14 seconds. Inhibition of the tonic unit shows adaptation over this period.

f) a single response of the repeaters (left) followed by inhibition of the tonic unit. One tonic spike falls just ahead of the repeater train. Time line; 0.1 Hz.

dropped from 600 msec at the beginning to 200 msec at the end (Fig. 5E).

The low frequency (15-25/sec) of spikes in the tonic discharge prevented any determination of the latency of inhibition. A conventional spike trace of one response is shown in Fig. 5F. The repeater train is shown at the left of the trace; it is just preceded by one spike of the inhibited unit, which then drops out, only to return. The preparation in which this inhibited unit was encountered was also remarkable in yielding at a slightly different site in the neuropil a pulse-marker response of the type discussed above (Fig. 5B) as well as a typical ascending train of repeater spikes (Fig. 5A). All these units were encountered by making minute displacements of the electrode tip through a single hole pierced in the tough sheath enclosing the left protocerebral ganglion. The exceptional productivity of this preparation may have derived from the minimal mechanical and osmotic damage to the neuropil resulting from this single penetration of the sheath. In this case, as in the majority of preparations, no saline was added since the insect's hemolymph kept the brain adequately irrigated.

## SUMMARY AND DISCUSSION

The two-electrode experiments provide definite evidence that a short train of repeater spikes in response to each brief acoustic stimulus ascends the nerve cord and cervical connectives, arriving in the protocerebral ganglion with a latency of 8 to 15 msec, depending on stimulus intensity. Evidence is also strong that this signal, usually transmitted by two or three fibers, is identical with that recorded from the noctuid brain and described previously (Roeder, 1969a, 1969b, 1970, 1973). This conclusion is further supported by observations that the lapses in responsiveness described in these earlier papers were also occasionally present in the repeater units detected in the cervical connectives or prothoracic ganglion (Fig. 2C and D).

A review of behavioral evidence indicates that the brain both modulates and sustains the thoracic interneuronal system that couples the afferent signals from the A1 and A2 tympanic sense cells to the motor innervation of the alar muscles responsible for steering during flight. The ascending train of repeater spikes seems to constitute the ascending limb of this regulatory system. This signal already shows evidence of considerable integration, both of the A1 with A2 responses in each tympanic nerve (Roeder, 1969b) and of the A1 responses generated in the right with those from the left tympanic organ (Roeder, 1973). In addition, this ascending repeater signal shows evidence of lability in the form of the unexplained lapses in acoustic responsiveness (Roeder, 1969a, 1970).

This evidence of instability in the ascending signal forecasts a low order of success in the search for still higher-order nerve responses to acoustic stimulation that might possibly be candidates for the descending signals postulated to modulate and sustain turning-away behavior. This low order of success is likely to compound with what may be called malfunction of the behavioral mechanism due to removal of the moths from field conditions, the physical restraint required by the experimental situation, and the surgical damage incurred on exposing the ganglia and probing the neuropil. Indeed, out of 77 experiments performed in the present series only 14 yielded candidate descending signals of interest.

The majority of these successful experiments revealed a phasic response at a latency of up to 40 msec. The two-electrode experiments showed this response to be descending. The response pattern usually consisted of one but occasionally of two or three spikes. The failure of this response to follow stimulus frequencies much above 1/sec suggests a similarity to the labile pulse-marker encountered by Paul (in press) in the pterothoracic ganglion. The response characteristics of these labile phasic units do not reveal their role in connection with the neuronal mechanism responsible for avoidance behavior in the presence of bat cries, which are emitted at about 10/sec by a cruising bat. This matter is discussed by Paul (in press).

Two other response patterns were detected but only once apiece in the present series. However, since their signals remained stable for a period sufficient to permit measurement of some of their properties they have been described in some detail. In view of the long odds against registering such signals the fact that it has been possible to define them at all is grounds for some degree of gratification.

Of particular significance in the behavioral context is the unit that responded to a stimulus pulse with a latency of about 40 msec and then continued to afterdischarge for 150-200 msec. Presumably, this unit would have fired steadily during stimulation at a repetition rate of 10/sec, but unfortunately this was not tested. This stimulus repetition rate would have approximated the ultrasonic pulse pattern of a cruising bat. If such an afterdischarge can be shown to descend the nerve cord it might well serve to potentiate and sustain the turning-away behavior shown in flight by a moth in the presence of faint ultrasonic pulses.

The second unit in this category showed sustained activity that was inhibited for hundreds of milliseconds following reception of a faint and brief ultrasonic pulse. Although its response mode is reversed, the inhibited unit could well complement the afterdischarge unit and belong to the same modulation system. However, unlike the afterdischarge unit, which fired only for about 200 msec after the stimulus, the inhibited unit remained inactive for as long as 600 msec. The behavior of the inhibited unit was observed in response to 10/sec acoustic stimulation, which caused it to remain almost completely 'silent' during a stimulation period of 14 seconds.

In seeking behavioral correlates to the performance of the inhibited unit, it can be noted that many free-flying moths cease flapping their wings and drop to the ground when they encounter intense ultrasonic stimuli (Roeder, 1962). This suggests the possibility that the inhibited tonic unit may serve to sustain the thoracic 'flight oscillators' (Wilson, 1961). However, in the experiment reported above the unit in question was suppressed for 200-300 msec by the faintest of pulses capable of generating a response in the ascending repeaters (Fig. 5D). Since moths tend to fly with greater vigor when turning away from an ultrasonic source (Roeder, 1967) such behavior would contraindicate a flight-sustaining role for the inhibited unit. Further speculation is unprofitable until the performance of these and possibly other units can be confirmed and extended.

## ACKNOWLEDGEMENTS

This work was supported by Research Grant 00947 and by a Research Career Award from the National Institutes of Health. Dr. Asher E. Treat read the manuscript and offered many valuable suggestions. Pupae of *Prodenia eridania* were supplied regularly during the winter months by Dr. Samuel Ristich of the Boyce Thompson Institute for Plant Research, Yonkers, New York.

## REFERENCES

1. ADAMS, W.B. *J. Gen. Physiol.* *58:*562, 1971.
2. ADAMS, W.B. *J. Exper. Biol.* *57:*297, 1972.
3. GHIRADELLA, H. *J. Morphol.* *134:*21, 1971.
4. PAUL, D.H. *J. Insect Physiol.* *19:*1785, 1973.
5. PAYNE, R.S., ROEDER, K.D. & WALLMANN, J. *J. Exper. Biol.* *44:*17, 1966.
6. ROEDER, K.D. *Animal Behaviour* *10:*300, 1962.
7. ROEDER, K.D. *J. Insect Physiol.* *10:*529, 1964.
8. ROEDER, K.D. *J. Insect Physiol.* *12:*843, 1966a.
9. ROEDER, K.D. *J. Insect Physiol.* *12:*1227, 1966b.
10. ROEDER, K.D. *J. Insect Physiol.* *13:*873, 1967.
11. ROEDER, K.D. *J. Insect Physiol.* *15:*825, 1969a.
12. ROEDER, K.D. *J. Insect Physiol.* *15:*1713, 1969b.
13. ROEDER, K.D. *Amer. Scientist* *58:*378, 1970.
14. ROEDER, K.D. *J. Insect Physiol.* *18:*1249, 1972.
15. ROEDER, K.D. *J. Insect Physiol.* *19:*1591, 1973.
16. ROEDER, K.D. *J. Insect Physiol.* *20:*55, 1974.
17. ROEDER, K.D. & TREAT, A.E. *J. Exper. Zool.* *134:*127, 1957.
18. ROEDER, K.D. & TREAT, A.E. *J. Insect Physiol.* *16:*1069, 1970.
19. TREAT, A.E. *J. Parasitol.* *40:*619, 1954.
20. TREAT, A.E. *Ann. Entomol. Soc. Amer.* *48:*272, 1955.
21. WILSON, D.M. *J. Exper. Biol.* *38:*471, 1961.

# SPECULATIONS ON A NEURAL SUBSTRATE FOR IMMEDIATE MEMORY

Moshe Abeles, Yaakov Assaff, Yehezkel Gottlieb, Yehiel Hodis and Eilon Vaadia
Department of Physiology
Hebrew University - Hadassah Medical School
Jerusalem, Israel

## INTRODUCTION

We carry with us a fairly detailed memory of the immediate past. In the course of time, a huge bulk of information passes through this memory, but only a fraction remains available for long periods. It is generally accepted that the memory of the near past is carried by the electric activity of the cerebral nerve cells. This assumption is based mainly on two arguments: (a) It is hard to conceive of any mechanism whereby stored information could be continuously modified to encompass an endless spectrum of variations except by electrical activity. (b) Any major disturbance of the electrical activity of the brain (such as electro-shock, hypoglycemic shock or concussion) disrupts the memory of events preceding the disturbance.

Psychophysical studies of memory show that there are a multitude of different processes that could be called "memory" (Iversen, 1973; Warrington & Weiskrantz, 1973). Short term memory is usually studied by asking the subject to recite a list of digits or nonsense syllables. There is good indirect evidence that this memory is carried by internal rehearsal of the digits. The amount of information that can be carried by such a mechanism is limited, and it might well be that this mechanism of short term memory is associated with our verbal ability. Internal verbal rehearsing would be expected to be of little use in lower animals.

Another type of short term memory is that whereby we capture a momentary sensory input and stretch it for a few hundreds of milliseconds. For instance, if we see a page with several rows each containing four or so letters, for a short period, we cannot recite the entire text. We have exceeded our short term memory capacity. However, if we are asked within a second after the disappearance of the page to recite one particular line, we can remember the entire line. This type of memory is called sometimes sensory register. In the present paper we would like to suggest a neural mechanism for this sensory register.

Since the description of closed loops of neurons by Lorente de Nó (1949), it is believed that the memory of the immediate past is carried by reverberating activity in closed loops. Hebb (1949) suggested that activity in such loops might switch among several alternating paths, using a more complicated cell assembly than a simple loop; but in both cases, we expect to see some degree of rhythmicity in the activity of the cells carrying this process.

In single unit recording, however, one sees rhythmic activity mainly when the animal is anesthetized with barbiturate or when it is drowsy, but very seldom in unanesthetized animals. Cortical cells tend to fire in synchrony when the EEG shows large alpha waves, but this type of activity is absent in the aroused state when the cells are supposed to have their reverberating activity.

In our studies, we have computed autocorrelation functions for the firing of 314 cells in unanesthetized cats treated with muscle relaxants. Except for 6 cells, which fired in synchrony with respiration, all others showed no trace of rhythmicity. In another study, one of us (Gottlieb, 1971) showed that in the same preparation cells could be made to fire rhythmically by administration of small doses of barbiturate to the animal. Furthermore, under the circumstances, cells which are close together fire in synchrony with each other and with the local alpha wave. In summary, we have very little evidence for reverberating cell activity as a carrier of sensory information in the alert animal.

Even if we do not consider reverberation as the carrying mechanism for immediate memory, it is hard to understand how the sensory information is retained immediately after the cessation of the stimulus, since most of the cortical cells only show transient responses (Abeles & Goldstein, 1972; Gerstein & Kiang, 1972; Goldstein *et al.*, 1968). In figure 1, we see responses of a single unit (from the primary auditory cortex of the unanesthetized cat) to tone bursts of different intensities. Except near threshold, when the cell responds throughout the duration of the stimulus, the responses are transient. With all intensities there is no activity that can carry information about the stimulus for hundreds of milliseconds after its cessation.

We shall now examine some more (indirect) experimental observations and suggest a mechanism to explain how the brain is able to maintain the electrical activity aroused by a stimulus for several hundreds of milliseconds after its cessation.

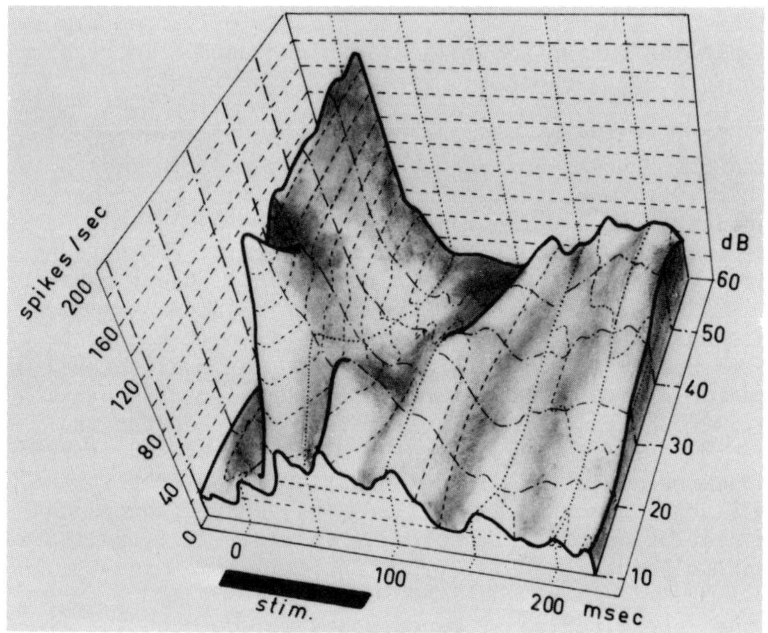


Fig. 1 Responses of a single auditory unit to tone bursts. Three dimensional graphs describing the response of a single unit from AI of the cat to tone pips of 26.7 kHz. The vertical axis shows the firing rate of the unit. Time is represented on the horizontal axis. The tone was turned on between time 0 and time 100. The depth axis shows the tone intensity in dB SPL.

## SINGLE UNIT RECORDING

We have carried out experiments designed to understand what is happening when one employs the technique of single unit recording. The main purpose was to resolve the discrepancy between the number of units recorded when an electrode passes through the cortex and the expected number. Physiologists assume that one can record an extracellular spike at distances up to 100 μ from the nerve cell generating it. If so, one would expect to record from around 2000 nerve cells (assuming a cell density of 40,000 per $mm^3$), during one electrode pass from the surface to the white matter. However, when the experiment is actually done, one records only from six to sixty units, depending on the recording technique used. To resolve this discrepancy we carried out two series of experiments.

In the first series, one of us (Vaadia, 1971) advanced an electrode into the cortex in fixed steps of 100 μ. After each such step, all the activity recorded was analyzed. Using a very concise method of representing nerve spike waveforms that we had developed (Abeles, 1974), we were able to observe that the shape of spikes tended to change at a certain depth in the cortex. This change could best be described as follows: at the first recording sites one sees generally only small spikes of moderate to long duration (2 msecs. or slightly longer); at deeper sites there appear also narrower spikes (about 1.5 msec duration). Upon reconstruction of the electrode tracks we found that the narrower spikes always appeared upon penetration of layer III. In three experiments, a lesion was made when the first narrow spikes appeared. Histological examination revealed that the lesion was in all three cases at layer III. This change corresponds to the large concentration of stellate cells in layer III (and IV) which are almost entirely absent in layer II (Sholl, 1956).

In the second series of experiments we advanced the electrode through the cortex in 2 μ steps. After each move, all nerve cell activity was recorded for 30 seconds and then another step was made. All identifiable spikes were analyzed for variations in shape and firing statistics as the electrode advanced. Again, we could define two types of cells. In the first type, the spike size first increased, reached a clear cut maximum and then decreased (Fig. 2A). This cell type had stable statistics both with regard to the average firing rate and to the autocorrelation function of the firing (Fig. 3A). The other type showed a tendency to only small size variations along large distances and non-stationarity in its firing patterns (Figs. 2B and 3B). Cells of the first type were distributed throughout layers II and VI and had broader spike shapes, whereas cells of the second type were found more in layers III and IV and had narrower spike shapes.

It should be stressed that the examples of Figures 2 and 3 represent the extremes of a continuous spectrum. Of course, we cannot

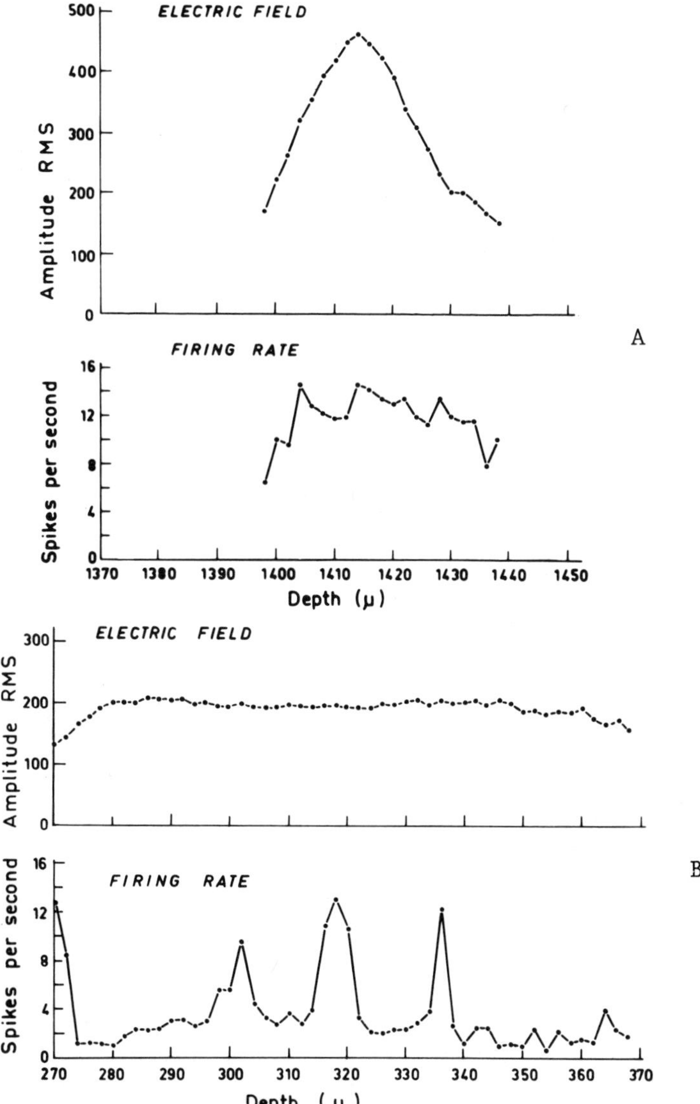


Fig. 2 Extracellular field and firing rate of two cells as a function of electrode position in the cortex. The abscissae represent the position of the recording electrode below the surface of the cortex. A recording was taken every 2 μ. The ordinate for the electric field is the amplitude of the spike in arbitrary units. The background noise did not permit us to carry out measurements when the size of the spike was below 100 - 150 units. The firing rate was computed by counting the spikes for 30 seconds at each point. A) Typical cell exhibiting a stationary firing rate. B) Cell with flat field showing a non-stationary firing rate.

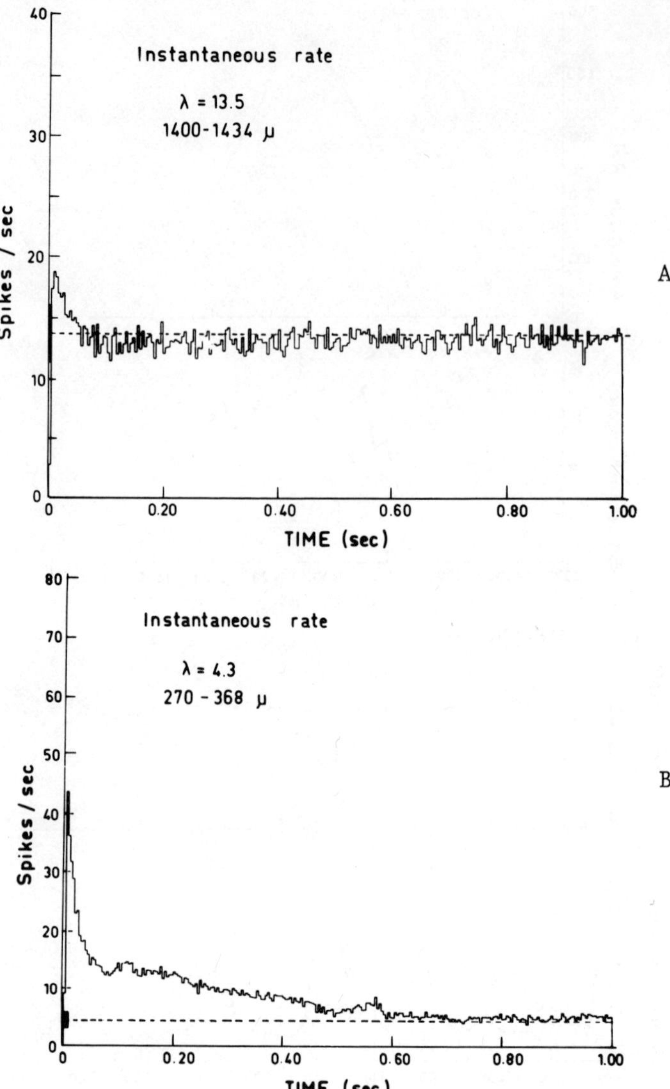


Fig. 3 Autocorrelation functions for the two cells of Figure 2. The abscissae represent the time after a spike occurred. The rate of firing is shown as the ordinate. If the process had a pure Poisson distribution, the curve would appear flat at the level of the broken line. The black bar near the ordinate gives the 1% confidence level for a Poisson process. A) Except for a slight tendency for bursting (shown by the hump in the first 50 msec) the process follows the statistics of a Poisson distribution. B) In the non stationary cell, high firing levels tend to be maintained for about half a second.

expect to find really sharp differences in cortical cell properties if we remember that histological examination reveals all types of intermediate cells between the typical pyramidal and typical stellate cell and, functionally, any spike activity of one cell would be reflected through its synaptic connections onto other cells. Nevertheless, we feel that we can talk about prototypes of cells just as one can talk about prototypes of personality despite the existence of a continuous range of intermediate variations.

## DISCUSSION

We are trying to find explanations for the following findings: stellate cells are concentrated in cortical layers III and IV. Some of the cells in these layers have a broad extracellular electric field in which the spike amplitude is almost constant. These cells tend to have non-stationary firing characteristics. Stellate cells are characterized by their spherical dendritic fields and many have axons distributed only within the limits of their dendritic field - for example, cells 24 and 25 in Fig. 4. During the development of an action potential in such cells, one expects to find an approximately constant current density in the volume embraced by the axonal branches; thus, the extracellular spike is expected to show an approximately constant amplitude throughout this volume. The size of this extracellular field is about 100 μ (Fig. 2B), in agreement with the histological data.

The non stationarity of the firing patterns of these cells may be explained in two alternative ways. Either they are part of some positive feedback loop, which tends to maintain high levels of activity for prolonged periods, or some of the transmitters acting on these cells act for long durations. The hypothesis of reverberations in a closed loop would be an example of a positive feedback mechanism, but, as pointed out earlier, the lack of any periodicity in the autocorrelation functions seems to exclude this possibility. Only if there were many positive feedback loops, each with a different cycle time, could we expect to see some kind of positive feedback without a trace of rhythmicity. The simplest mechanism of this sort could be generated by connecting the axons of the stellate cell, so that they re-excite their own dendrites; but so far we have no histological evidence for such an arrangement in stellate cells.

Whatever may be the mechanism of the non-stationarity, it exists, and we would like to explore its functional significance.

The afferent fibers to the cortex terminate mainly in layers IV and III; this was confirmed recently by Sousa-Pinto (1973) for AI, the patch of the cat cortex on which we have been experimenting. These layers contain a high concentration of stellate cells with

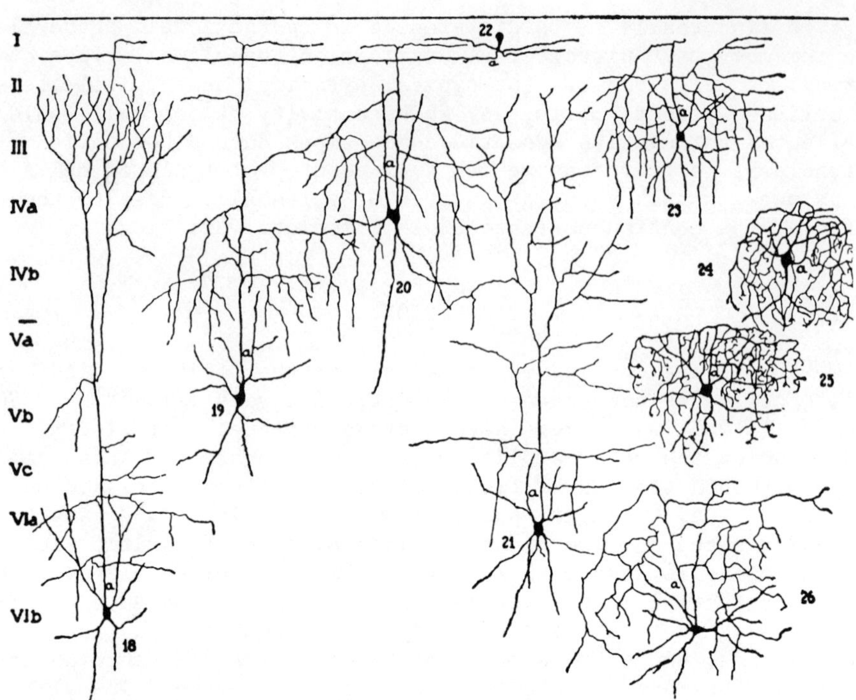


Fig. 4 Three main types of cells with intracortical axons. (From Lorente de Nó, 1949).

limited dendritic fields and axonal distribution. Furthermore, these cells are capable of maintaining a high level of activity for several hundreds of milliseconds and are thus perfectly placed for storing the incoming information. We assume that each of these cells, when activated, will have a response such as shown in Fig. 5. Detailed information on the nature of the stimulus is conveyed to the cortex by the "place code", i.e., by which of the afferent fibers is active. This information may then be stored by the prolonged activity of these stellates, the stellate cells thus serving as a sensory register.

Each of these stellate cells covers a cortical area of about 7500 $\mu^2$. The primary auditory cortex of the cat has an area of about 1 $cm^2$ (on each side), providing space for 13,000 non-overlapping storage elements. This value is within an order of magnitude of 50,000 myelinated auditory fibres in the eighth nerve (Gacek & Rasmussen, 1961). Similarly, the area of the striate cortex in man is about 30 $cm^2$, which would contain about 500,000 independent storage elements, again, a number close to the one million myelinated axons passing through the optic nerve (Polyak, 1957).

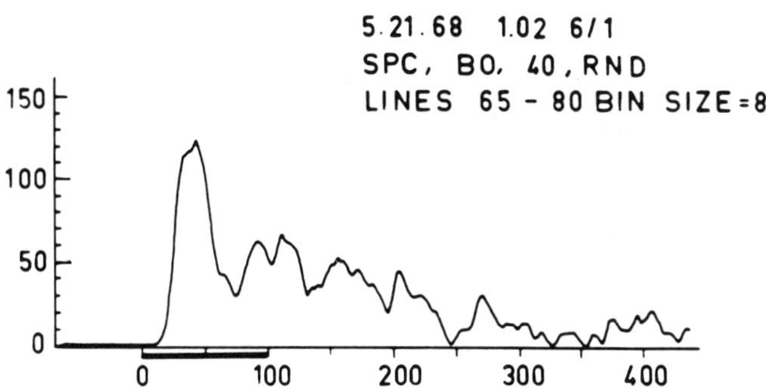


Fig. 5 Prolonged response. Post-stimulus (PST) histogram for a single unit in AI of the cat. A tone of about 4.5 kHz was turned on between times 0 and 100 msec (From Abeles & Goldstein, 1972).

It is extremely rare to find prolonged responses, such as shown in Fig. 5, in anesthetized animals or those treated with muscle-relaxants. It might well be that these responses are inhibited unless the animal is attentive. In the non-attentive state, we are able to see the effect of the direct input from the incoming afferent fibers to the pyramidal cell. Only when the storage cells are not inhibited can we see the prolonged response and only then is the cortex given enough time to process the incoming information. The suggestion that the storage is mediated through a transmitter with prolonged action is especially attractive in this context because it explains how we can notice a stimulus after its cessation. When our attention is drawn to a stimulus, the stellates of the appropriate sensory cortex are disinhibited; even if this occurs after the stimulus has stopped, the residual transmitter will reactivate the stellates in a special pattern corresponding to the previous afferent input.

Although these suggestions are highly speculative, they appear to fit much of the available data. Our group is now actively engaged in direct neurophysiological examination of short-term memory in unrestrained, unanesthetized animals.

## ACKNOWLEDGEMENT

The authors are indebted to Miss V. Horn for her devoted help throughout the experiments and to Mr. S. Ben-Yonah for preparing the figures. This research is supported in part by grant 015.9361 from the Israel Commission for Basic Research.

## REFERENCES


1. ABELES, M. A Journey Into the Brain. In: Proceedings of the International Symposium on Signal Analysis and Pattern Recognition in Biomedical Engineering. Technion, Israel. In press, 1974.
2. ABELES, M. & GOLDSTEIN, M.H. JR. *Brain Res.* *42:*337, 1972.
3. GACEK, R.R. & RASMUSSEN, G.L. *Anat. Rec.* *139:*455, 1961.
4. GERSTEIN, G.L. & KIANG, N.Y-S. *Exp. Neurol.* *10:*1, 1964.
5. GOLDSTEIN, M.H. JR., HALL, J.L. & BUTTERFIELD, B.O. *J. Acoust. Soc. Amer.* *43:*444, 1968.
6. GOTTLIEB, Y. Recording the activity of neuron pairs and of slow waves in the cortex of the cat. M.Sc. thesis submitted to the Hebrew University, 1971 (In Hebrew).
7. HEBB, D.O. The Organization of Behaviour. John Wiley & Sons, Inc., p. 60, 1949.
8. IVERSEN, S.D. Brain lesions and memory in animals. In: The Physiological Basis of Memory. (J.A. Deutsch, ed.) Academic Press, p. 305, 1973.
9. LORENTE DE NÓ, R. Cerebral cortex: architecutre, intracortical connections, motor projections. In: Physiology of the Nervous System, 3rd ed. (Fulton, J.F., ed.) Oxford University Press, p. 288, 1949.
10. POLYAK, S. The vertebrate visual system. University of Chicago Press, p. 300, 1957.
11. SHOLL, D.A. The organization of the cerebral cortex. John Wiley & Sons, Inc., 1956.
12. SOUSA-PINTO, A. *Adv. Anat. Embriol. & Cell Biol.* *48, Fasc.2:* 1, 1973.
13. VAADIA, E. Detection and identification of action potentials in the cat cortex. M.Sc. thesis submitted to the Hebrew University, 1971 (In Hebrew).
14. WARRINGTON, E.K. & WEISKRANTZ, L. An analysis of short term and long term memory defects in man. In: The physiological basis of memory (J.A. Deutsch, ed.). Academic Press, p. 365, 1973.

# ELECTROPHYSIOLOGICAL AND PSYCHOPHYSICAL CORRELATIONS IN THE AUDITORY SYSTEM OF MAN

H. Sohmer and H. Pratt*
Department of Physiology
Hebrew University-Hadassah Medical School
Jerusalem, Israel

## INTRODUCTION

When studying the relation between sensory physiology and behaviour, one is usually interested in the application of such studies to man; obviously, however, it is difficult to conduct studies directly on human subjects. This has led many workers to try to correlate single sensory nerve fiber activity in *animals* with discriminative ability in *human* subjects, or in the same species of animals, by conditioning experiments. Today, it is possible to study some electrophysiological bases of auditory behaviour directly in alert humans using non-traumatic techniques which permit the recording of gross electrical responses to sound stimuli of most parts of the auditory pathway - the auditory nerve (compound cochlear action potential), the brain stem auditory nuclei and the cerebral cortex. [This technique was originally designed to serve as an objective clinical test in cases of uncertain hearing diagnosis (Sohmer & Feinmesser, 1967) and is called electrocochleography (Sohmer *et al.*, 1972)]. At the same time, behavioural responses to the same stimuli can be elicited from the same subject, so that electrophysiological-behavioural correlations are feasible.

We present here some preliminary results of two projects in which these recording techniques were used in attempts to make such correlations.

The first of these involves measurement of the temporary subjective threshold elevation, called Temporary Threshold Shift (TTS)

*Partially supported by a stipend from the Center for the Study and Management of the Environment of the Hebrew University.

which follows exposure to intense sound stimuli. The second is concerned with a search for possible correlations between the dependence of the subjective estimate of the loudness of a click and of the electrophysiological responses of the auditory system to click stimuli, upon the intensity of that click, both in the same subject.

## METHODS

The responses from nerve and brain to click stimuli presented by earphones were recorded as the potential differences between a clip electrode on the ear lobe and a disc electrode on the vertex of the scalp. Due to a low signal-to-noise ratio, the recorded activity had to be filtered, amplified and summed by an average response computer. Further details of the technique have been reported (Sohmer *et al.*, 1972). The subject under investigation was reclining comfortably on a bed so that he was able to report, simultaneously with the electrical recordings, subjective evaluations of the same stimulus to which his nerve and brain were responding, such as threshold and loudness estimation. A schematic sketch of the arrangement is shown in Fig. 1.

The effects of noise exposure on the subjective and electrophysiological responses were studied in 10 subjects. Three sets of control, pre-exposure, recordings were made of the responses of the auditory nerve and brain-stem auditory nuclei (electrocochleography) to 50 dB SL click stimuli (i.e. 50 dB above the previously determined threshold of the particular subject). These click levels did not cause contraction of the middle ear muscles. This was followed immediately by 15 minutes exposure to 90 dB SL white noise (noise with a very broad frequency spectrum). After ten minutes of this exposure, the white noise was turned off and the electrocochleographic responses to 50 dB SL click stimuli were again recorded (each such recording took less than a minute, being the average response to 512 clicks, presented at the rate of 10 per second). The white noise was then turned on again for 5 minutes in order to complete the 15 minutes' exposure. Upon completion of this period of white noise, electrocochleographic recordings were made every few minutes. Interspersed with such recordings, the subjective threshold of the subject for hearing the click was determined. This post-exposure threshold compared with the pre-exposure one gave the actual threshold shift (TTS) of the subject. These recordings and determinations were continued until pre-exposure values were approached. The amplitude of the electrocochleographic responses and the subjective TTS could then be plotted as a function of time before, during and after the noise exposure.

In the second series of experiments, the electrocochleographic and evoked cortical responses to different intensity click stimuli were determined. At the completion of each recording at each

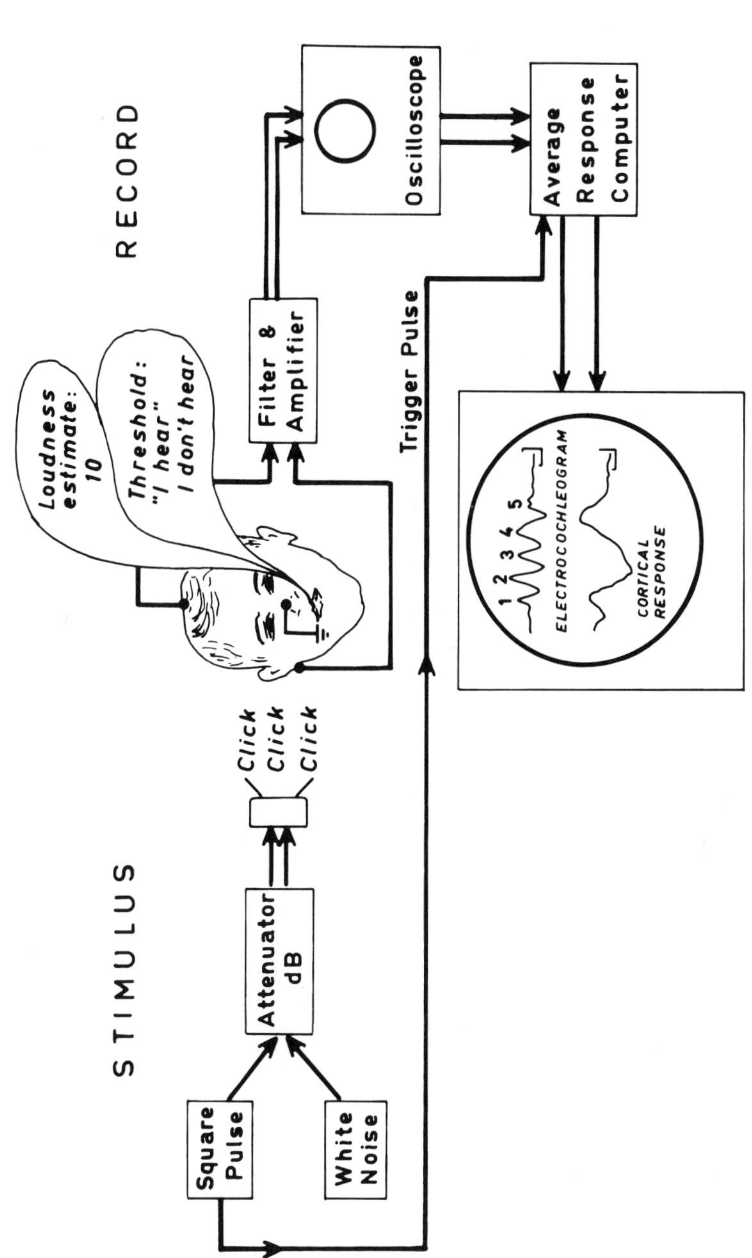


Fig. 1 Schema of the stimulus and recording system. Typical normal electrocochleographic and cortical responses to click stimuli are depicted, including the ability of the subject to give a simultaneous, subjective evaluation of the stimulus such as apparent loudness or threshold. Note the 5 electrocochleographic waves as indicated.

intensity, the subject was asked to assign a numerical value to the loudness of that click, a value which bore a simple arithmetic relationship with the apparent loudness of a standard reference click intensity presented now and then during the experiment (Stevens, 1956). The amplitudes of the electrical responses of the subject and his estimation of the loudness of the clicks could then be plotted as a function of the intensity of the clicks.

## RESULTS AND DISCUSSION

### TTS

Exposure to intense sound stimuli is followed by a temporary threshold shift, its degree and duration being functions of the intensity and duration of the noise exposure (Okada, *et al.*, 1972). Is this behavioural decrement accompanied by a neural decrement? Figure 2, data recorded from a typical subject, shows that the TTS is accompanied by a definite depression of the amplitude of the compound cochlear action potential (the first wave of the five seen). The latency of the action potential was increased. The amplitude and the latency gradually returned to control values as the TTS also decreased. Little correlation was seen between the TTS and the later recorded waves which represent neural activity of the brain-stem auditory nuclei (Lev & Sohmer, 1972; Sohmer, *et al.*, 1973). A more detailed account of these observations is presented elsewhere (Sohmer & Pratt, 1974).

These results indicate that the subjective TTS is a peripheral phenomenon, already apparent in the depression of the amplitude of the response of the first order sensory neurons, and therefore the noise exposure may influence either the primary auditory nerve fibers or an even more peripheral site.

Since relaxation of the middle ear muscles is very rapid following the cessation of an intense sound stimulus (Hung and Dallos, 1972), it is not likely that residual muscular activity contributes to the subjective threshold shift and neural decrement of TTS. This was verified by means of impedance measurements which showed that there is no apparent muscular activity after the noise exposures and with the durations used in this study. Therefore, another type of conductive loss may be responsible for the increased latency of the compound cochlear action potential.

It would be worthwhile in the future to record, in addition, the cochlear microphonic potential (the non-neural receptor potential of the cochlea) in these subjects in order to clarify the possible effects of the noise on the more peripheral receptor apparatus.

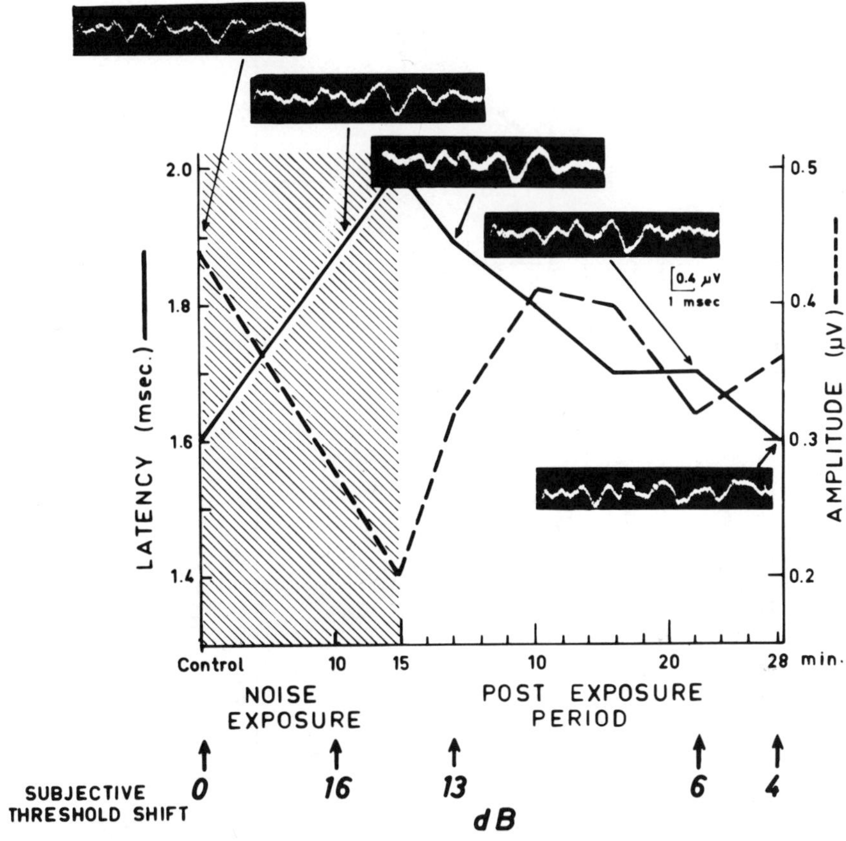


Fig. 2 Electrocochleographic responses during noise-induced temporary threshold shift. The amplitude and latency of the cochlear action potential (first wave) are plotted as a function of time before, during and after the noise exposure. The actual subjective threshold shift is also indicated.

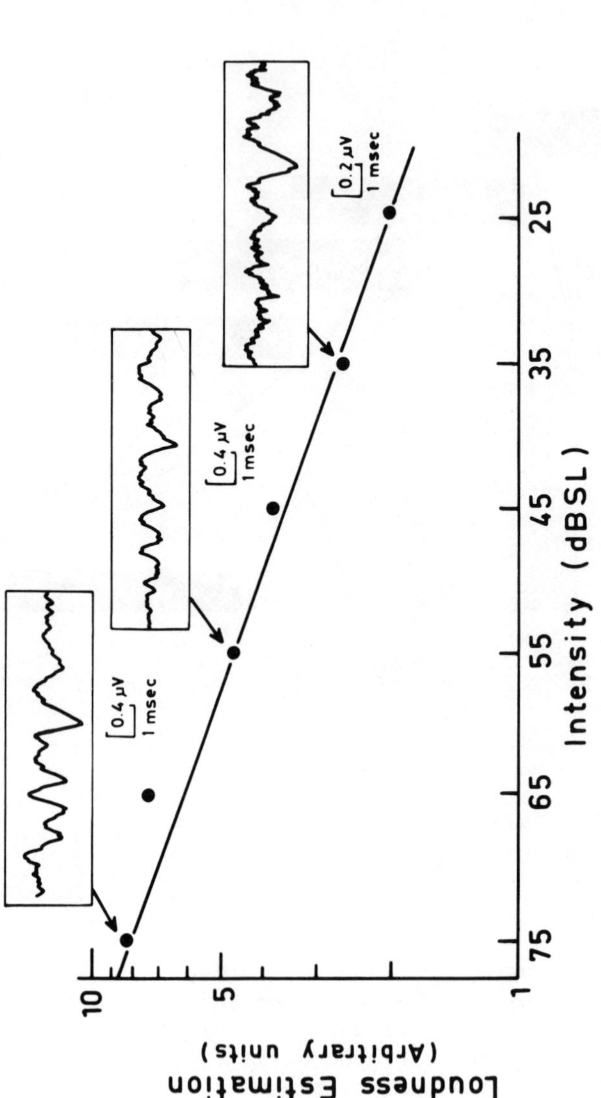


Fig. 3 Plot of the apparent subjective loudness of a click as a function of click intensity reported by a subject, together with some of the electrocochleographic responses to the same click in the same subject (insets).

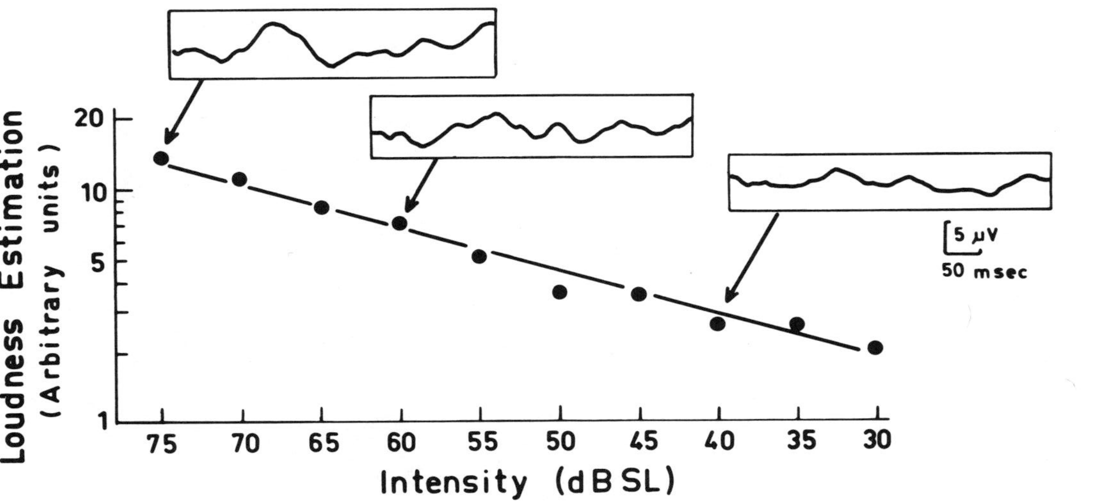


Fig. 4 Plot of the apparent subjective loudness of a click as a fraction of click intensity as reported by a subject, together with some of the cortical responses to the same clicks in the same subject (insets).

## Loudness

In Figure 3, we present a graph of the dependence of loudness estimation on click intensity with corresponding electrocochleographic responses to the same click in the same subject. Figure 4 shows a similar loudness function with corresponding evoked cortical responses. The amplitudes of the compound cochlear action potentials and of the evoked cortical response, and of course the subjective loudness, decrease with decreasing click intensity. Thus the cochlear nerve may "code" click intensity in the form of the amplitude of the compound response of the cochlear nerve, which in turn is a function of the number of synchronously-firing primary auditory nerve fibers activated by that stimulus.

These are only two examples of how the non-traumatic recording of electrophysiological responses of many levels of the auditory pathway can be used to further our understanding of the correlation between sensory physiology and sensory behaviour.

## REFERENCES

1. HUNG, I.J. & DALLOS, P. *J. Acoust. Soc. Am. 52:*1168, 1972.
2. LEV, A. & SOHMER, H. *Arch. Klin. exp. Ohr.-, Nas.-u Kehlk.-Heilk. 201:*79, 1972.
3. OKADA, A., MIYAKE, H., YAMAMURA, K. & MINAMI, M. *J. Acoust. Soc. Am. 51:*1240, 1972.
4. SOHMER, H. & FEINMESSER, M. *Ann. Otol. (St. Louis) 76:*427, 1967.
5. SOHMER, H., FEINMESSER, M., BAUBERGER-TELL, L., LEV, A. & DAVID, S. *Ann. Otol. (St. Louis) 81:*72, 1972.
6. SOHMER, H., FEINMESSER, M. & SZABO, G. *Electroenceph. Clin. Neurophysiol. 34:*761, 1973.
7. SOHMER, H., PRATT, H. *Audiology.* In press, 1974.
8. STEVENS, S.S. *Am. J. Psychol. 69:*1, 1956.

# INSECT MECHANORECEPTOR MECHANISMS

M.J. Rice
Department of Entomology
University of Queensland
Queensland, Australia

## INTRODUCTION

The study of insect mechanoreceptors has a long history. The most obvious peripheral sense organs are of course the numerous cuticular hairs with which the bodies and appendages of most insects bristle; these were named sensilla by Haeckel who also decided that the associated peripheral sense cells are derived from the epidermis. Demoll, von Rath and others classified the numerous variety of sensilla and inferred their functions from general observations on the insects' behaviour and on the structure and topography of the sensilla. By these means it was determined that setiform sensilla could monitor touch and indicate the flexion of joints; that campaniform sensilla could register bending of the cuticle; that the curiously modified setiform sensilla of *Nepa* served as static organs under water; that tympanal organs were auditory receptors and that chordotonal sensilla were responsive to movements and vibrations of the parts of the body (Historical Review by Wigglesworth, 1973). Other sensory cells associated with flexible joints and flexible areas of the body wall were described by Retzius (1890) and Zarwarzin (1912). These were thought to be involved in general mechanical and possibly thermal senses (Snodgrass, 1926). Thus, fifty years ago much of the fundamental information on insect mechanoreceptors was known or inferred. From about 1925, the emphasis shifted toward the experimental study of the role of mechanoreceptive input in the timing and regulation of muscular contractions and the resultant behavioural patterns. Changes in the patterns of muscular co-ordination were brought about by selective sectioning of nerves. It was concluded that although there was a fixed pattern of nervous organisation responsible for the sequential timing of muscular contractions, afferent nervous input was still very important in enabling an animal to display its remarkable adaptability to a wide range of normal as well as unusual circumstances (Review by Pringle, 1961). In short, it has been determined that mechanoreceptor inputs can trigger and modulate behavioural patterns but that they do not normally generate the patterns.

The whole study of insect mechanoreceptors was placed in an entirely new plane by the application of modern electrophysiological techniques (Pringle, 1938 a,b,c) and high resolution electronmicroscopical techniques (Gray, 1960). These two methods have yielded an enormous amount of fundamentally new and exciting information, much of which has yet to be fully processed and correlated with the fund of detail provided by the early workers in this field. Parts of the new material have been reviewed by different authorities in recent years (Pringle, 1961; Schwartzkopff, 1964; Bullock and Horridge, 1965; Finlayson, 1968; Howse, 1968; Thurm, 1968). Certain aspects of the origin and function of mechanoreceptors and of their role in behavioural mechanisms have not been dealt with and it is the particular purpose of the present short review to point out three such topics which are in need of closer examination. These are:

(a) the significance of the multiplicity of insect mechanoreceptor types and the possibility of a diverse origin for the two classes of neurons involved in mechanoreception.

(b) the probability that a highly adaptable bend-stretch mechanism forms the basis for mechanotransduction in most or all of the range of mechanoreceptors in insects.

(c) the manner in which a series of structurally and physiologically differentiated mechanoreceptors can operate to provide a sequential release of the successive components of a complete and complex behavioural act.

These three topics are certainly diverse, and even if all the necessary data were available, would be impossible to deal with in depth in such a short exposition as the present one. However, all three are fundamental to our comprehension of mechanoreceptor physiology in its deepest sense and deserve more attention than they are drawing from most workers in this field. The contemporary scene is one where masses of electrophysiological and ultrastructural data from a wide range of insects are accumulated each year, with little concern for the significance of the data in the context of mechanoreceptor mechanisms as a whole. At this juncture, a more broadly based approach is increasingly desirable not only for its intrinsic value but because it provides feedback that enables greater insight for the interpretation of new and particular data. An understanding of the evolutionary and developmental origins of the diversity of mechanosensitive sense organs provides the background against which their present diversity of form and function and their implication in behavioural processes can be better understood. In the same way, comprehension of the transduction mechanism is fundamental to the meaningful interpretation of the vast volume of new physiological and fine structural information that is printed each year. Finally, the analysis of individual mechanoreceptor form and function in relation to a complex behavioural act - feeding in the tsetse fly - is taken to illustrate the use which an insect makes of the specialised structural and physiological parameters of its range of mechanoreceptors.

## A BEHAVIOURAL AND DEVELOPMENTAL INTERPRETATION OF INSECT MECHANORECEPTOR DIVERSITY

The most simple and significant classification of insect mechanosensitive neurones is that of Zarwarzin (1912), who simply divided them into Types I and II. Type I neurones are always associated with some part of the cuticle and they are easily distinguished by their main morphological characteristic: a single sensory projection. Type II neurones are not associated with cuticular structures and invariably have more than one sensory projection. Finlayson (1968) has updated Zarwarzin's terminology by referring to the two types of neurones as uniterminal and multiterminal respectively. From the comparative physiological viewpoint, it is of interest to note that Type II mechanoreceptors of insects are analogous to the diffuse receptive area class of vertebrate mechanoreceptors whilst the Type I's are analagous to vertebrate punctile receptive area receptors. There seems to be strong selective pressure on an animal to differentiate and specialise two distinct channels to separately convey punctile and diffuse mechanosensitive information into the C.N.S. As in vertebrates, too, there is a tendency for the punctile Type I receptors to be rapidly adapting and the diffuse Type II receptors to be slowly adapting, though this relationship does not invariably apply.

Type I neurons innervate a very wide range of cuticle-derived sensilla, showing a truly remarkable variety of shapes and sizes. Basically, all of these structures can be reduced to three main types: TRICHOID, CAMPANIFORM and CHORDOTONAL. Although there are a number of exceptions, these three mechanoreceptor types can respectively be associated with the detection of TOUCH, STRESS and VIBRATION. On structural grounds, it would appear that the original sensillum was trichoid and that by reduction of the hair shaft to a small plate the campaniform condition was arrived at. Further

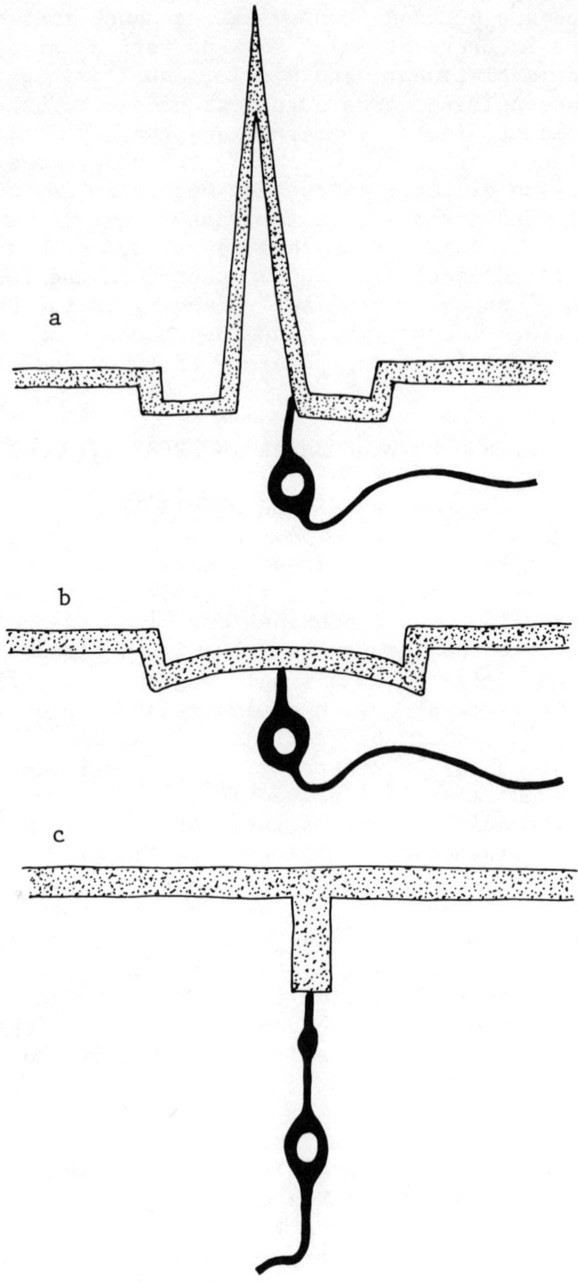


Fig 1 Hypothetical relationship between insect sensilla. a. trichoid; b. campaniform; c. chordotonal.

migration along the same axis would result in the sensory cells falling deeper and deeper into the body cavity, giving rise to the chordotonal situation (Fig. 1). It is not difficult to envisage the selective advantages bestowed by this scheme, since although the trichoid sensillum is structurally able to monitor touch, stress and vibration stimulus modalities, the information content is greatly enhanced by specialising three types of receptors and supplying the information to the C.N.S. through three separate channels. Peak sensitivity is only approached by shielding the receptors from rough, random stimuli, that is in the chordotonal sensilla which are buried within the body cavity away from superficial touches and stresses. Under these conditions, a singular sensitivity is attained, with the chordotonal receptors responding to vibrations of amplitudes less than ten picometres in the subgenual organ of the cockroach (Autrum and Schneider, 1948). The same order of sensitivity to threshold stimuli is said to be present in the tibial organ receptors of crickets (Huber, 1974) and the tympanal organ receptors of noctuid moths (Roeder, 1974). Johnston's organ in the antenna of the mosquito is a structure containing more than thirty thousand chordotonal receptors and it is a most efficient auditory receptor with a threshold efficiency approaching that of the human ear. The vast numbers of receptor neurones involved suggests that sensitivity in these organs is brought to a peak by central averaging processes.

An increase in stimulus intensity applied to an insect mechanoreceptor generally results in an increase in its rate of discharge of action potentials. Certain sensilla are directionally sensitive, having a lower threshold to stimuli applied in one particular direction, such as the campaniform sensilla of the Dipteran haltares (Pringle, 1957) and the cervical hair cushions of bees (Thurm, 1963). Most Type I neurones are of phasico-tonic type, supplying information on the rate of change of a stimulus as well as on its intensity and duration, some being more phasic in their responses than others. In contrast, Type II neurones are more specialised to supply tonic information, in general having a much slower adaptation rate than the Type I neurones which innervate trichoid, campaniform and chordotonal sensilla. An exception to this is found in the trichoid sensilla of hair plates, which are able to supply tonic information for proprioreceptive purposes (Pringle, 1938c). When more than one cell innervates a sensillum, the neurones have different thresholds and adaptation characteristics, the best examples of which are the A1 and A2 cells of the noctuid tympanal chordotonals (Roeder, 1965). Innervation of any insect organ by a full range of Type I neurones endows the organ with sensitivity to touch, strain and vibration over a range of different sensitivities and phasico-tonic properties. In this way, the information content of mechanical changes in the environment is maximised and transmitted through separate channels to the insect's C.N.S. In the behavioural context, the input from any one receptor neurone is simply part of a composite pattern of inputs from a large group of diverse neurones. It is very unlikely that changes in the rate of firing of a single cell will effect any change in the active behaviour of an insect in its natural situation. Probably what is "seen" as meaningful information by the C.N.S. is changing patterns of inputs from groups of related receptors, relationship in this context being determined by the geometry of synaptic connections in the ganglionic neuropile. Such a situation would be no more than has been found to be true in vertebrates, where stimulation of single cutaneous afferents only gives rise to paraesthesiae - behaviourally meaningless sensations. An attempt to analyse the sensory contribution to behaviour in terms of single units has surely as little chance of success as an attempt to appreciate Beethoven's Ninth Symphony by listening to a single violin part. The factor of context should be given much more emphasis in the study of insect mechanoreceptors; failure to appreciate that the C.N.S. generally "listens" to a multiplicity of inputs "heard" in concert can lead to the misinterpretation of results from ablation experiments, to give but one example.

If there is a peripheral fusion of axons originating from the multiplicity of Type I receptor neurones in insect appendages, then the information that reaches the C.N.S. is much reduced. Such peripheral fusion was suggested by early observations using mainly light microscopy and if fusion exists, it tends to negate some of the argument in favour of the behavioural significance of centrally perceived multi-channel input patterns, as outlined above. However, now that electron microscopical techniques are available for resolving the membranes of the smallest axons, it is becoming apparent that very many axons can be crammed into a small space and that peripheral axonal fusion is unlikely to occur with any frequency (Sturckow, 1967; Nunnemacher and Davis, 1968). In addition, Chapman and Nicols (1969), using very elegant electrophysiological methods, found no evidence for axonal fusion in the leg nerves of cockroaches. Until some firm evidence is adduced in support of the fusion of peripheral sensory axons in insects, it can be taken that such fusion is improbable and that each sensory neurone has its own individual axonal input to the C.N.S., a conclusion that is of some importance when attempting to understand the afferent processes supporting insect behavioural mechanisms. In the appendages of many insects, a hundred or more mechanoreceptor neurones may be involved, each sending an axon into the neuropile of its appropriate ganglion. If the insect is simply stationary, or pinned down in the experimenters' apparatus, few of these receptors will be stimulated; in contrast, most of the receptors are constantly stimulated during the normal behavioural acts of locomotion, mating, feeding, grooming and so on. The manner in which the C.N.S. handles this multiplicity of input is a complete unknown in our understanding of insect mechanoreceptor mechanisms. At present we do not even know whether the insect C.N.S. possesses an "attention" system that is able to give selective

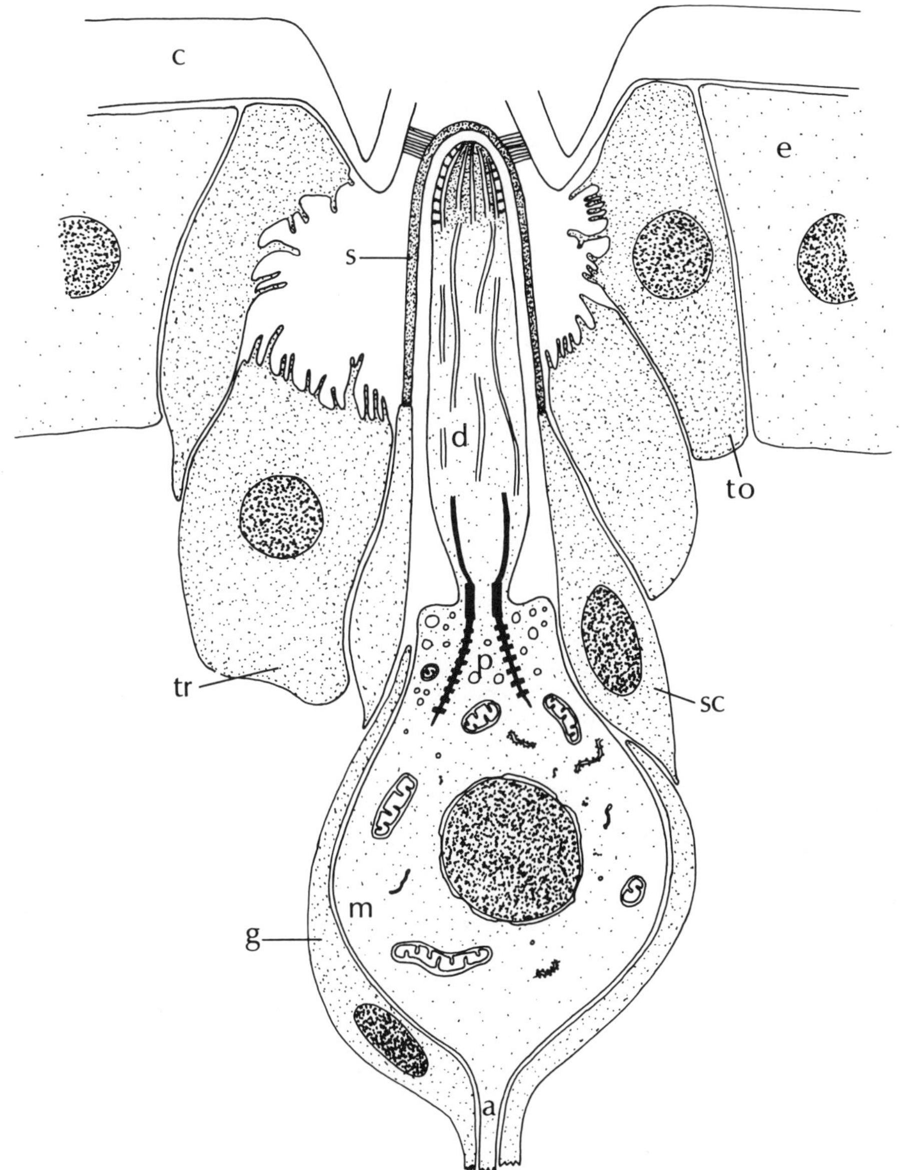


Fig 2 Ultrastructural details of Type I neurone anatomy. a. axon; c. cuticle; d. distal segment; e. epidermis; g. glial cell; m. sensory cell body; p. proximal segment; to. tormogen cell; tr. trichogen cell; s. scolopale; sc. scolopale secreting cell.

emphasis to one or other of the active channels, depending on circumstances. It could be that the various inputs are synaptically preconnected in a rigid, hierarchical manner but we simply do not know. The answer to this key question is surely the prelude to any real insight into the contribution of sensory physiology to behaviour.

Despite the wide range of morphological forms found in the cuticular components of Type I mechanoreceptors, their basic fine structural details are remarkably similar (Figure 2). There are three fundamental components:

(a) the sensory cell itself with some attendant glial cells;

(b) the scolopale-secreting cell, producing a dense sheath around the tip of the sensory cell;

(c) the trichogen and tormogen cells, secreting the cuticular components of the sensillum and investing an extra cellular fluid-filled space which invariably surrounds the receptor terminal of a Type I neurone.

The receptor terminal has a ciliary structure within its constricted basal region. This constriction divides the terminal into inner and outer segments, the inner segment being continuous with the cell body and containing abundant mitochondria, vesicles and ribosomes - evidence of much metabolic activity. In contrast, the outer segment has no mitochondria; its most conspicuous cytoplasmic components are microtubules and microfilaments running up to the tip, where there is a well-marked structure composed of dense-staining material and a variety of tubules and sometimes filaments. In well-fixed material, this dense-staining structure can be seen as linked to the terminal receptor membrane by fine bridges, like septate desmosomes (Rice *et al.*, 1973). The receptor terminal itself is not joined to the cuticular part of the receptor directly; instead, it is the scolopale sheath that is attached. Although these basic features are common to Type I neurones innervating trichoid, campaniform and chordotonal receptors, there is in practice a great deal of structural variation. The most striking variant is the elongation of the distal segment in chordotonal receptors, the elongated region having a peculiar swelling along its length (Howse, 1968). These details of Type I ultrastructure can be related to the physiology of the neurone, as will be described in the section on mechanotransduction below.

The question of the developmental origin of Type I nerve cells was solved by Schon (1911) for the chordotonals and by Wigglesworth (1953) for the trichoids and campaniforms. Both authorities found that the primary sense cells originated from the epidermis, with which they maintain contact through their receptive terminals, the axons elongating from the other pole of the cell and growing into the nearest nerve trunk and thence to the appropriate ganglion of the C.N.S., where they establish connections in the neuropile. Little is known of the mechanisms which guide the axons to their destination, though this information would certainly be of considerable interest. Presumably some trophic influence, released from nerves, guides the axons into the nearest nerve trunk. They are then directed to the C.N.S. but the factors within the neuropile that enable these elongated epidermal cell processes to establish the appropriate synaptic contacts are completely unknown. Progress has been made by Edwards and Palka (1971), who ablated the anal cerci of crickets during the first six stages of development and then permitted the cerci to regenerate during the final three stages. Using electrophysiological techniques, they demonstrated that new Type I neurones were formed, innervated the newly regenerated sensory bristles on the cerci and then sent axons inwards to establish normal synaptic connections with the giant interneurones of the terminal abdominal ganglion. The ability of such insect organs to regenerate sensory neurones which then recapitulate embryonic synaptogenesis is clearly of considerable interest to those concerned with the cellular basis of the development of behavioural patterns. Interesting developments in this field can be anticipated in the coming years.

A very different situation is presented by sensory neurones of Type II. These are very numerous in the softer regions of the insect body and are never associated with special cuticular structures as is invariably the case with Type I neurones. Type II neurones are found associated with the sub-epidermal nerve plexus and with the visceral nervous system on foregut, midgut and hindgut (Zarwarzin, 1916; Orlov, 1924; Kuwana, 1935; Rice, 1970 a, c; 1972), with joints in the limbs (Rogosina, 1928; Coillot and Boistel, 1969) and with stretch receptor strands (Slifer and Finlayson, 1956; Lowenstein and Finlayson, 1960; Weevers, 1966). Type II sensory cells are always associated with structures that either bend or stretch and are involved in monitoring these movements. The sensory processes of Type II neurones often ramify over a wide field, but despite such large receptive areas, the neurones are still capable of accurate localisation of stimuli by the use of overlapping receptor fields, as has been shown electrophysiologically in the cibarial pump receptors of the tsetse fly and the blowfly. Here, three neurones are involved, each with sensory processes branching over several thousand square microns of epithelium. The intensity of mechanical stimulation is reflected in the rate of action potential discharge by the three neurones. The position of the stimulus is registered by the ratio between the rates of firing of the three neurones (Rice, 1970a). All Type II neurones investigated to date respond in a phasicotonic manner but there is an important distinction between two main groups.

Type IIa innervate strand stretch receptors and nerve trunks; they are stimulated to increase their rate of firing by stretching during the relaxation of parallel muscles. These receptors show a progressive advance in the timing of their peak rate of firing as the rate of stimulus application is increased (Lowenstein and Finlayson, 1960). Type IIb are those innervating the body wall and cibarial pump; they are stimulated to increase their rate of firing by bending of the innervated surface during the contraction of parallel muscles. These receptors do not generally monitor the rate of stimulus application; rather they respond to an increased velocity of relaxation by an increase in negative rebound (Rice and Finlayson, 1972). In their relationship to muscle contraction, the two kinds of Type II neurones are similar to vertebrate muscle receptors - muscle spindles resembling Type IIa in being stimulated during muscle stretch and Golgi tendon organs resembling Type IIb in being stimulated during muscle contraction. However, Type IIb are not specialised to monitor muscle tension and in this important respect are quite different to vertebrate Golgi tendon organs. In soft-bodied insect larvae and in the abdomen of adult insects, many segments have both strand stretch receptors and numerous neurones on the body wall. Such an arrangement does not represent a duplication of functions, merely a means of accurately monitoring the dimensions and forces acting on each segment, since the two types of neurones will operate electrophysiologically in a push-pull fashion (Figure 3). This arrangement ensures that the C.N.S. is fed with positive information and does not have to rely on the absence of input as a signal in itself. This factor may explain why many ablation experiments produce less than the expected changes in behaviour. As in the case of overlapping receptor fields in the cibarial pump receptors described above, it is the combination of mechanoreceptor inputs that is important. This partly explains the insects' requirement for large numbers of mechanosensitive neurones having different receptive properties and response characteristics. The significance of one single input channel is low in the context of natural behavioural situations; it is the relationship between many inputs and their proportional rates of firing that provides a high information content. It must be emphasised that when attempting to account for simple behavioural acts in terms of reflex action, it is the overall sensory situation that must be considered. To take a single sensory input, isolate it and then trace its activity into and through the C.N.S. and to believe that this explains behaviour is an illusion. The C.N.S. "sees" even a highly specific mechanoreceptor input in very different ways, depending on the total sensory context. A simple example of this is provided by the behaviour that results from stimulating insect tarsal mechanoreceptors. If the animal is stationary and resting on a surface, then probing of the tarsus will elicit leg withdrawal and other evasive reactions. If the insect is stationary and suspended in the air without tarsal contact, probing a tarsus elicits grasping behaviour by that leg and the response often expands to involve other

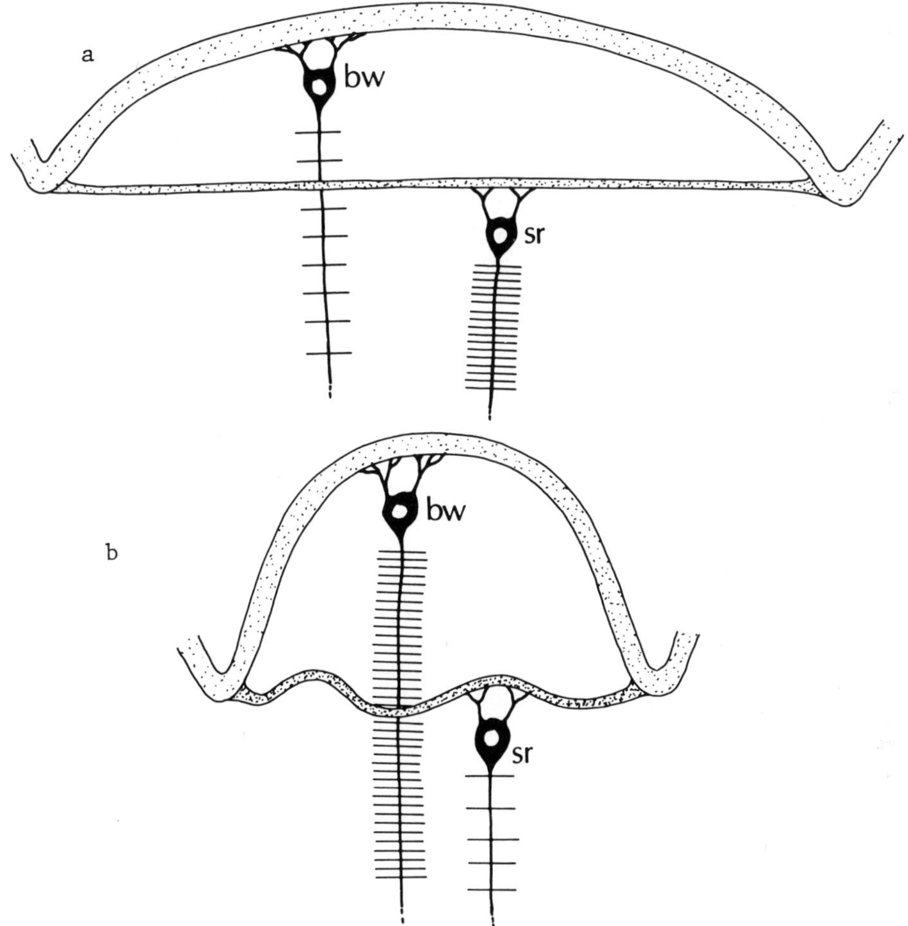


Fig 3 Push-pull operation of body wall mechanoreceptors.
a. Segment stretched and stimulating stretch receptor neurone;
b. Segment contracted and stimulating body wall neurone.

parts of the insect. If the insect is moving, either running or flying, probing of a tarsus often fails to elicit any detectable change in behaviour. Thus identical mechanoreceptor inputs can evoke contrary behavioural responses, depending entirely on the contextual situation, that is, whole sensory context governs the aspect given to particular sensory inputs. In summary, it can be stated that multiplicity of mechanoreceptors and their diversity form the basis for the provision of a continuous sensory context, a context in which variations in the proportional rates of firing of different neurones is the most significant informational and behavioural evoking factor. Indeed, it is the factor of context that makes any meaningful analysis of behaviour at the neuronal level so complex and difficult to handle. The classical techniques evolved by experimental physiologists, in which all variables are held constant except for the one under analysis, immediately negate contextual mechanisms and impose severe limitations on our understanding of the cellular bases of the insects' natural behaviour.

The origin of Type II sensory neurones has been widely assumed to be the same as that of Type I, i.e. differentiation *de novo* within the epidermis. There seems to be no experimental evidence to either support or contradict this notion. However, it is worthy of note that many mesodermal tissues such as midgut, ventral diaphragm, connective tissue and various muscles are innervated by Type II neurones, situations where Type I cells are never found. This could have arisen as a result of the migration of hypodermal Type II cells on to the mesodermal tissues; even so, the relationship between the ciliated Type I neurones and the non-ciliated Type II neurones would still be problematic. Alternatively, Type II neurones may have originated within the C.N.S. and then migrated outwards to innervate mesodermal and epidermal tissues, so that the development of the two different systems in insects would consist of the outward growth of Type II cells and the inward growth of Type I cells. What adds a certain amount of fascination to this subject is that the two types of insect sensory cell are so very different from one another in appearance and structure. Details of Type I structure have been given above. These contrast with the lack of ciliary structures, absence of specialised accessory cells, the presence of numerous branching sensory terminals containing mitochondria and neurotubules and the frequent occurrence of axon collaterals that so clearly characterise Type II neurone anatomy (Figure 4). From the physiological point of view, it is significant that the naked terminals of a Type II cell are bathed in haemolymph, while the naked terminal of a Type I cell is isolated; it is sealed off from the haemocoele by highly specialised accessory cells, which probably exert a marked influence on the composition and constancy of the ionic environment surrounding the terminal. The axons of both types of cell are covered by glial cells, which no doubt regulate their immediate ionic environment (Treherne, 1966), but in Type II cells, the primary receptor regions

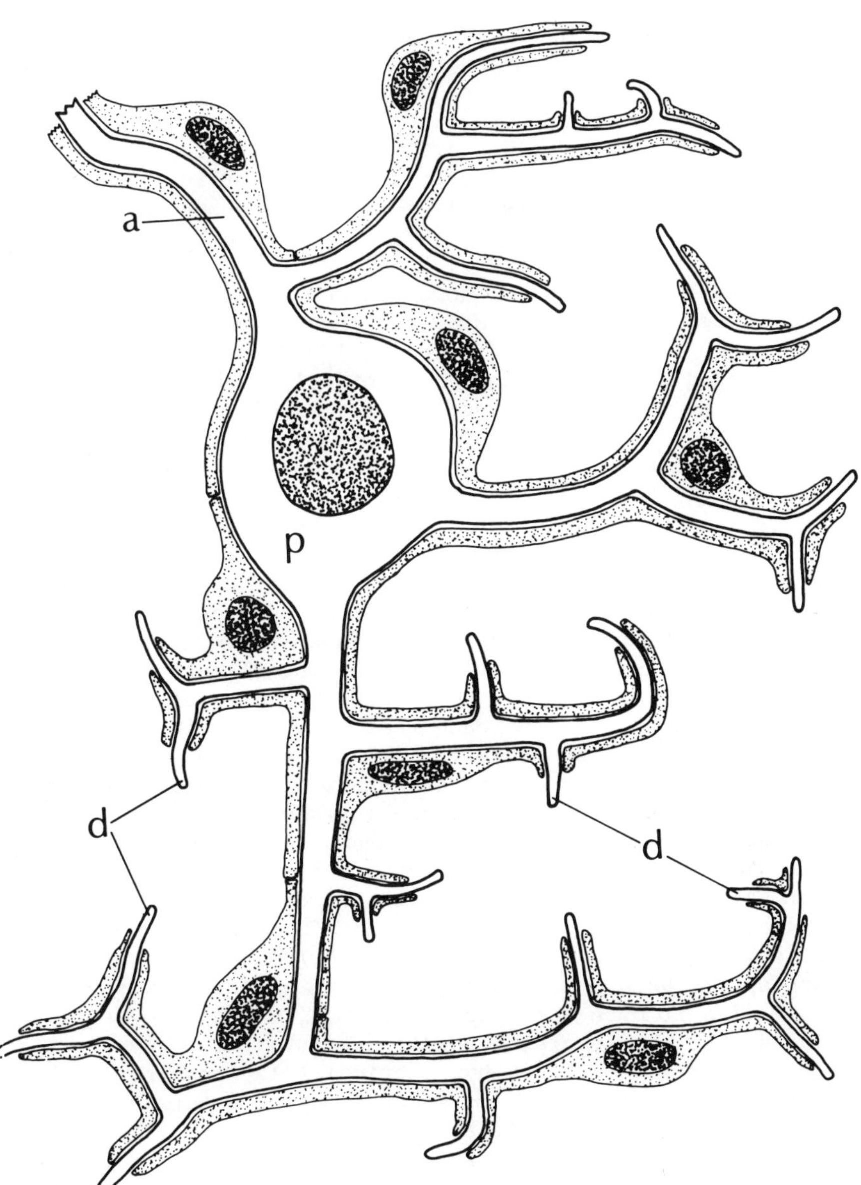


Fig 4 Ultrastructural details of Type II neurone anatomy. a. axon; p. perikaryon; d. naked dendrites.

are exposed to the haemolymph, while in Type I cells they are strictly segregated from the haemolymph and are bathed in a separate fluid.

Thus the origin of Type II cells remains an open question at the present time. It clearly ought not to be assumed that Type II have the same origin as Type I as there are significant structural and physiolgocal differences between the two types. A clue to this question may have been provided by the discovery of peripheral neurosecretory cells in the stick insect and blowfly (Finlayson and Osborne, 1968) and in the tsetse fly (Rice, 1969). Neurosecretory cells are generally found situated within the C.N.S. with only their processes extending into the peripheral nerves (Maddrell, 1967). It now appears that the somata of some neurosecretory cells may be situated anywhere between the C.N.S. and the periphery. The migratory ability of some insect neurosecretory cells could be based on the advantage bestowed by positioning the synthetic machinery of the cell body as close to the release regions as possible. Total separation from the C.N.S. by the neurosecretory cells of the corpus cardiacum would seem to represent the extreme of such a migratory process. The structure of peripheral neurosecretory cells is such that they are not readily distinguishable from any ordinary Type II mechanosensory neurone. The same multiplicity of branching processes, with naked terminals exposed to the haemolymph and lack of any specialised accessory cells, make them very similar in appearance. However, under the electron microscope, the cell processes are found to contain not only mitochondria and neurotubules, like Type II mechanoreceptors (Rice, 1970) but also numerous neurosecretory droplets together with cytological features that indicate that they are being secreted. In addition, peripheral neurosecretory cells possess only a rudimentary ability to respond to mechanical stimulation (Finlayson and Osborne, 1968). Apart from their marked secretory activity and lack of specific and consistent responsiveness to mechanical stimulation, there is little to distinguish peripheral neurosecretory cells from Type II mechanoreceptors. Whilst the resemblances between the two types of cells may be coincidental, it is tempting to speculate that they may indicate a more fundamental relationship. It could be that Type II mechanoreceptors became modified to take up a secretory function. However, I find it much more plausible that, if the two cell types are related, the neurosecretory cells antedate the mechanoreceptors. Figure 5 illustrates one such hypothetical relationship, in which central neurosecretory cell somata move gradually outwards, becoming more and more peripherally situated in nerves. Presumably, the primary situation is one where secretions are released from the cell in response to excitation transmitted outwards from the C.N.S. There is some evidence that certain peripheral neurosecretory cells may transmit action potential back into the C.N.S. (Rice, 1969; Finlayson and Osborne, 1970). If these early results should be confirmed by more detailed studies, they are of considerable interest in indicating that an efferent neurone may be able to change into an afferent

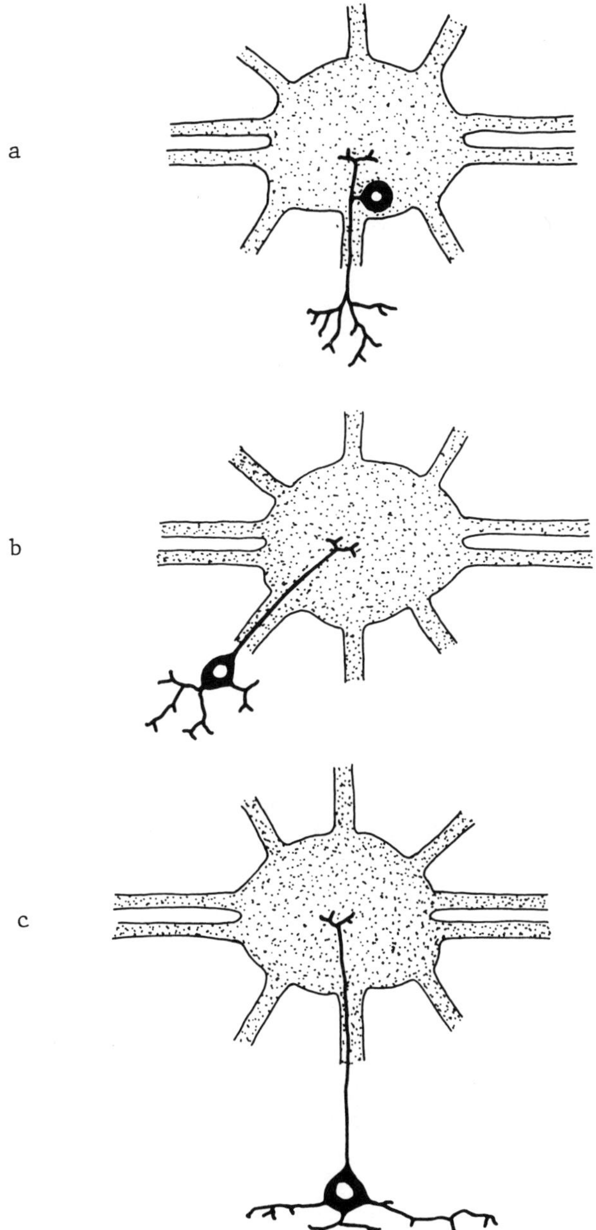


Fig 5 Hypothetical scheme of Type II neurone origin. a. typical central neurosecretory cell; b. typical peripheral neurosecretory cell; c. typical peripheral Type II mechanoreceptor.

neurone during the course of evolution. Peripheral neurosecretory cells may release material from their terminals into the haemolymph under the influence of some local mechanical or other stimulus and simultaneously signal this release to the C.N.S. by transmitting back trains of action potentials. It would not be difficult to imagine the evolutionary transformation of such a cell into a Type II mechanoreceptor, no longer secreting but continuing to signal back sensory information to the C.N.S. The synaptic connections of a vertebrate type of C.N.S. prohibits any such possibility, but the organisation of the insect neuropile would not preclude this possibility of efferent/afferent role swopping. If, in fact, Type II neurones do originate within the C.N.S. and migrate peripherally, it is interesting to speculate that during development they might initially provide a trophic influence to guide the axons of Type I neurones into the peripheral nerve trunks and towards the C.N.S. Such hypotheses are almost entirely speculative but should indicate that these gaps in our knowledge of insect mechanoreceptor relationships are wide open and ready for investigation.

## MECHANOTRANSDUCTION IN INSECT NEURONES

In both Type I and Type II mechanoreceptor neurones, the receptor terminals are "naked", that is, their plasma membranes stand alone, unprotected by any accessory cell membranes. In the Type I condition, the distal segment is situated in a fluid-filled space between the tormogen and trichogen cells, whilst in Type II cells the terminals are surrounded by haemolymph (see above). This "desheathing" of the sensitive part of a mechanoreceptor is quite characteristic and is also found in many vertebrate receptors (Pease and Quilliam, 1957; Merrillees, 1960; Cauna and Ross, 1960; Katz, 1961; Adal, 1969). In vertebrate mechanoreceptors, these desheathed regions have been shown to be areas where the threshold to mechanical stimulation is especially low (Katz, 1950a, b; Gray and Sato, 1955; Loewenstein and Rathkamp, 1958; Loewenstein, 1960). In vertebrates and in crustacea too, the picture that has emerged is of a decrease in ionic conductance in the naked receptor membrane when it is subjected to mechanical stimulation. The resultant ion movements generate receptor potentials that propagate decrementally across the soma on to the axon, where there is a spike-initiating zone. The magnitude of the generator potential at the spike-initiating zone regulates the frequency of action potential discharge along the axon (Katz, 1950b; Eyzaguirre and Kuffler, 1955a, b; Florey, 1955; Edwards and Ottoson, 1958; Diamond *et al.*, 1958). Recent work on insects by Guillet and Bernard (1972) has confirmed that the primary event in sensory transduction is also a decrease in ionic resistance of the terminal membrane. The basic problem remaining is to determine how mechanical stimulation causes a decrease in resistance of the terminal membrane and hence a receptor potential.

Currently, the most well-known theory of mechanotransduction in insect receptors is that of Thurm (1963; 1964; 1965; 1968). This theory has been applied to a variety of trichoid and campaniform sensilla but could not operate in chordotonal sensilla (Howse, 1968) and cannot be applied to any Type II receptors, which do not possess the structural requirements for the application of the mechanism proposed by Thurm (Rice, 1970). The proposed mechanism is similar to a piezo-electric effect, involving compression of a dense tubular body that is situated in the extremity of the distal segment of the receptive terminal. Compression is thought to cause a "protein-chemical process" that is somehow communicated to the proximal segment where there is an accumulation of mitochondria. At the proximal segment it was proposed that membrane permeability is altered, leading to "amplification and spatial extension of the signal" (Thurm, 1968). The irregular neurotubules that link the inner and outer segments of the receptor terminal were considered to provide the necessary link. However, it has been pointed out that these structures are also found in chemoreceptor neurones (Slifer and Sekhon, 1963) where there is no possibility of involvement of a compression mechanism. The function of these tubules is probably to transport metabolites between the two segments, as the outer segment has no mitochondria (Rice *et al.*, 1973). The compression theory of mechanotransduction has three main prerequisites:

i. the distal segment must enclose a dense tubular body that is compressed during mechanical stimulation of the sensillum;

ii. the energy released by compression of the tubular body must be communicated to the proximal segment;

iii. the energy is utilised at the proximal segment to generate a receptor potential.

Due mainly to the small size of the receptors concerned, it has proved difficult to find any firm experimental evidence to support any of these preconditions. All that can be stated is that certain Type I receptors do have a dense tubular body in the extremity of their distal segments.

It would be unfortunate if in studies on the ultrastructure of trichoid and campaniform sensilla the presence of a tubular body were to be automatically explained within the framework of the compression model, without further evidence. Although, from the physiological point of view, there is no reason why this should not be in order for rapidly-adapting receptors, for slowly-adapting receptors it is much more difficult to envisage how maintained compression of a tubular body could continue to supply excitation. Another difficulty is encountered by the discovery that the Type I neurones innervating certain trichoid sensilla do <u>not</u> possess a dense tubular body, but only a ring of neurotubules that are linked to the terminal membrane by small bridges. As more is discovered about insect mechanoreceptor neurones, there are less and less receptor types to which the compression hypothesis can be applied without tortuous reasoning. This situation led to the recent proposal of an alternative mechanism, which has been called the bend-stretch hypothesis (Rice *et al.*, 1973). This concept suggests that receptor potentials in all insect mechanoreceptors are caused by increases in ionic conductance of the plasma membrane of the naked terminal regions of the receptor neurones. It is envisaged that neurotubules make an important contribution in providing a cytoskeleton over which the receptor membrane is stretched during mechanical stimulation. There is considerable variation in the numbers and arrangements of neurotubules in the terminal cytoskeletons of various insect mechanoreceptors and this has been mathematically correlated with threshold sensitivities to bending of the receptor neurone terminals. It transpires that very little distortion of the endings is required to provide sufficient membrane stretch to account for the generation of receptor potentials at the distal segment of Type I neurones. Receptors with cytoskeletons that are elongated, loosely linked and weakly connected to the terminal receptor membrane are found to be those which have a higher threshold to mechanical stimulation - for example, Type II neurones, which have many receptor terminals that are normally subjected to fairly gross stimulation, and also Type I neurones innervating those trichoid sensilla which are normally subjected to large movements during the course of natural stimulation. On the other hand, those receptors which are normally subjected to very small movements, such as campaniform sensilla and those trichoid sensilla involved in only small deflections, are found to possess short, densely organised cytoskeletons that fill the receptor terminals. These highly sensitive receptors appear to be organised in such a way that the slightest deflection of the receptor terminal will cause differential movements of the receptor membrane and the cytoskeleton. The membrane, being weaker, takes most of the strain and is stretched. The exact amount of stretching exacted by unit movement will depend on the physical and spatial characteristics of membrane and cytoskeleton. Compliance of the neurotubular cytoskeleton is a key factor in this model, regulating not only the sensitivity of the receptor terminal but also the adaptation characteristics of the receptor.

The bend-stretch theory is attractive in that it suggests how the normal behavioural situations with which the various receptors are concerned, involving large or small movements, are reflected in the ultrastructure of the sensory terminals of their mechanoreceptive neurones (Figure 6). The model also provides a unified approach to the process of mechanotransduction in insect neurones and bases the process firmly on membrane properties, neurotubules operating in a supporting role. This is in contrast to the compression theory, where neurotubular compression is considered to be the primary event.

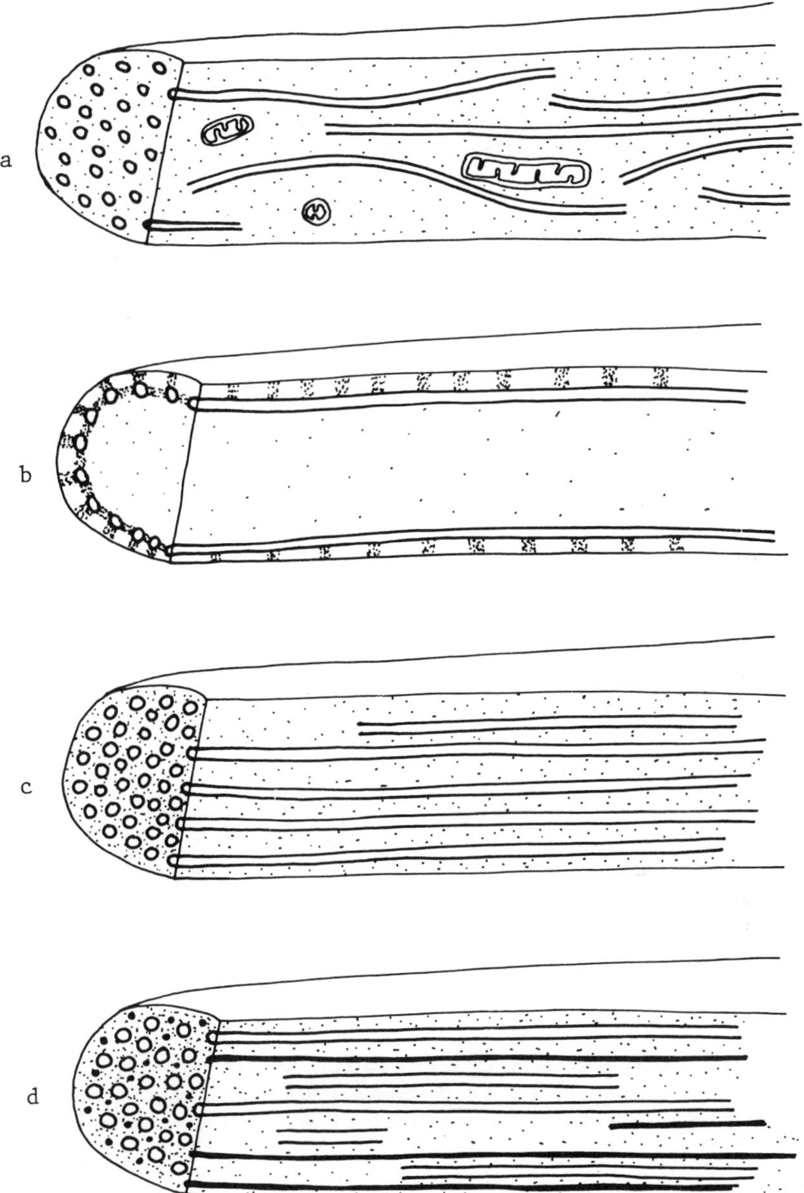


Fig 6 Range of neurotubular cytoskeletons in the receptor terminals of insect mechanoreceptor neurones.
a. from a Type II neurone; b. from a trichoid sensillum; c. from a leg campaniform sensillum; d. from a haltares campaniform sensillum.

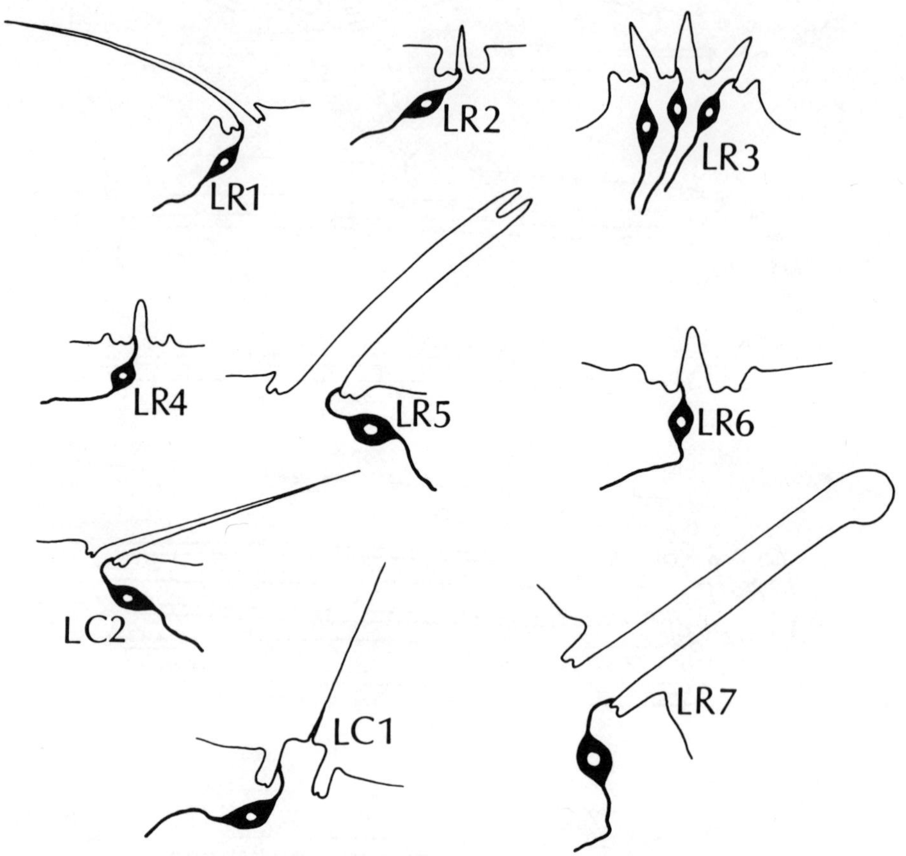


Fig. 7 Sensilla of the mouthparts of the tsetse.
LR1 from the labial bulb; LR2 from the labial shaft;
LR3 from the labial membrane; LR4 from the lateral labella;
LR5 from the lateral labella; LR6 from the terminal labella;
LR7 from the internal labella; LC1 from the labral canal;
LC2 from the cibarial pump.

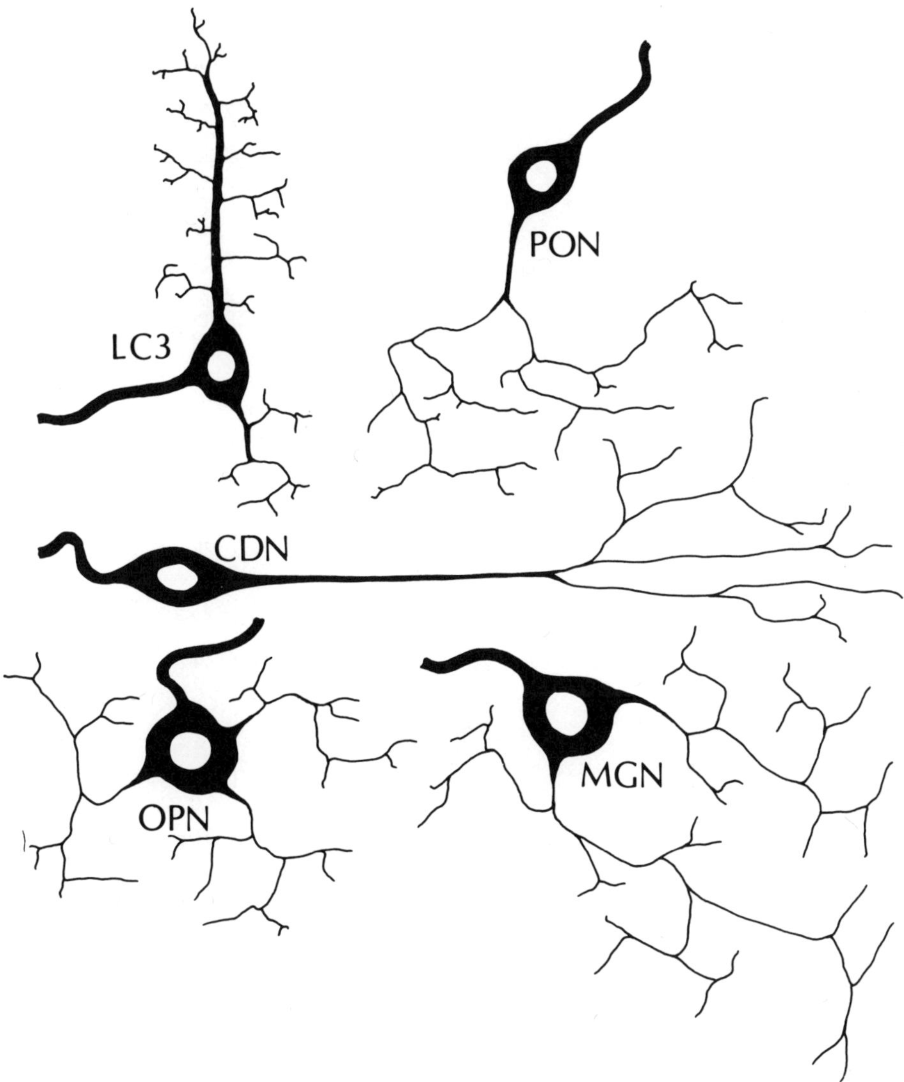


Fig 8 Type II neurones of the tsetse gut.
LC3 from Cibarial Pump; PON from Pre-cerebral Oesophagus;
CDN from Crop Duct; OPN from Oesophageal Pump;
MGN from Midgut.

TABLE I

MECHANORECEPTORS INVOLVED WITH TSETSE FLY FEEDING BEHAVIOUR

| Position | Designation | Number | Innervation |
|---|---|---|---|
| Labial bulb | LR1 | 2 | 1 Type I |
| Labial shaft | LR2 | 60 | 1 Type I |
| Labial membrane | LR3 | 2 | 3 Type I |
| Lateral labella | LR4 | 6 | 1 Type I |
| Lateral labella | LR5 | 8 | 1 Type I |
| Terminal labella | LR6 | 8 | 1 Type I |
| Internal labella | LR7 | 8 | 1 Type I |
| Labral canal | LC1 | 50 | 1 Type I |
| Cibarial lumen | LC2 | 10 | 1 Type I |
| Cibarial wall | LC3 | 6 | 1 Type II |
| Pre-cerebral oesophagus | PON | 6 | 1 Type II |
| Oesophageal pump | OPN | 6 | 1 Type II |
| Anterior midgut | MGN | 3 | 1 Type II |
| Crop duct | CDN | 2 | 1 Type II |

Physiologically, an increase in membrane conductance in response to membrane stretch is acceptable as a basis for both rapid and slow-adapting responses, while neurotubular compression is difficult to relate to slow-adapting responsiveness.

## MECHANORECEPTION IN TSETSE FLY FEEDING BEHAVIOUR

There are fourteen different kinds of mechanoreceptive sensilla on the mouthparts and anterior gut of the tsetse fly (Rice, 1969, 1970a, b, c; 1972; 1974; Rice *et al.*, 1973a, b). They range from long, robust trichoid sensilla to tiny, filament-like trichoid sensilla, to large Type II neurones with a multitude of sensory processes (Figures 7 and 8). These kinds of sensilla and the areas of the gut that they innervate are listed in Table I. Each type of receptor has its own structural and physiological peculiarities, related to their functions in co-ordinating the different stages of tsetse fly feeding behaviour. We can only review briefly here some of these sense organs and present a short outline of the part they play in patterning the various stages of penetrating the host and sucking blood. The general intention is to show something of the concerted operation of a group of varied mechanoreceptors during a complex behavioural act.

Tsetse flies are attracted to their hosts by olfactory and visual stimuli. Having settled on the host animal, they are stimulated to probe - that is to lower their probosces and penetrate the integument in search of blood - by mainly thermal and humidity stimuli. Penetration is achieved by the prestomal teeth and rasps on the labella, which are pulled across the skin by a repetitious everting movement caused by the muscles in the basal bulb of the proboscis (Jobling, 1933). Blood is detected by the ATP released from blood platelets which aggregate in the region due to the damage done to blood capillaries (Galun and Rice, 1972). The blood is then sucked up by the cibarial pump and passed, via the oesophagus, to the midgut and mainly into the crop. The crop of the tsetse fly accommodates a huge blood meal, often twice the weight of the fly itself. The time needed to take in such a gargantuan meal can be less than one minute. Rapid feeding has survival value for tsetse flies since, whilst they are stationary in the feeding posture, they are exposed to predation. This rapid feeding process depends on highly efficient penetrating and pumping mechanisms, involving excellent neuro-muscular co-ordination, which itself necessitates a complex and complete mechanoreceptive feedback system.

When the proboscis of the fly is lowered, contact with the host is registered by input from the LR6 sensilla, each of which is innervated by a single Type I neurone that sends its axon through the labial nerve to the sub-oesophageal ganglion. The consequences of this input are that efferent impulses are sent from the sub-oesophageal ganglion to operate the muscles that cause labellar eversion, so bringing into play the rasping mechanism. Feedback on the progress and orientation of rasping is provided by three kinds of receptors. The large, peg-like LR7 sensilla are grossly stimualted each time the labellar lobes are everted against the host's tissues. The LR4 and LR5 sensilla are stimulated by the progress of the labella through the penetrated tissues. The LR3 sensilla are stimulated by their being buried in the folds of the labellar membranes on each side, every time the labella are everted. Each LR3 sensillium is composed of three small trichoid processes radiating out of a single papilla, each of the three hairs being innervated by a single Type I neurone. These represent the smallest hair plates known, but they have none the less, a proprioreceptive function identical to that of the larger hair plates from the limb joints and cervical regions of other insects (Pringle, 1940; Mittelstaedt, 1950; 1957). Each labellum is independently controlled by its own muscles, and feedback from the labellar sensilla functions in enabling this control to be appropriately co-ordinated within the sub-oesophageal ganglion. This ensures that the correct amount of force is applied to each labellum so that the proboscis cuts into the host at an appropriate angle. Resistance in the hosts animal's skin is by no means uniform and feedback on the extent of labella eversion achieved by each muscle contraction is needed. This is supplied by the two LR3 hair plates, one situated on each side. They provide feedback on the actual amount of eversion achieved on each side during each rasping cycle, so enabling adjustment of the efferent outflow to the everter muscles. In the context of rasping behaviour, the sub-oseophageal ganglion uses three types of information:

i. the pattern of motor output to the everter muscles;

ii. the effectiveness of this in achieving labellar eversion;

iii. the effectiveness of the amount of labellar eversion achieved in rasping the host's skin (Figure 9).

It should be noted that mechanoreceptors are utilised in two distinct and separate ways; firstly, to monitor the extent to which the intended movement is achieved and secondly, to monitor the effect of the movement on the environment.

Other mechanosensitive sensilla are distributed in two lines along each side of the labial shaft. These LR2 setae are almost entirely submerged in deep cup-like depressions, but their tips project sufficiently to be stimulated by the tissues of the host as the proboscis is thrust progressively deeper into the skin. Each of these LR2 setae is innervated by its own Type I mechanoreceptive neurone, the axons of which run back into the sub-oesophageal ganglion. Once the proboscis is completely inserted, the basal bulb is pushed up against the skin and this is registered by the two LR1 sensilla. These are large trichoid sensilla situated on each side of the basal bulb of the proboscis. Thus, in total, there is an afferent input to the sub-oesophageal ganglion from seven distinct types of mechanoreceptors, involving nearly one hundred Type I neurones on

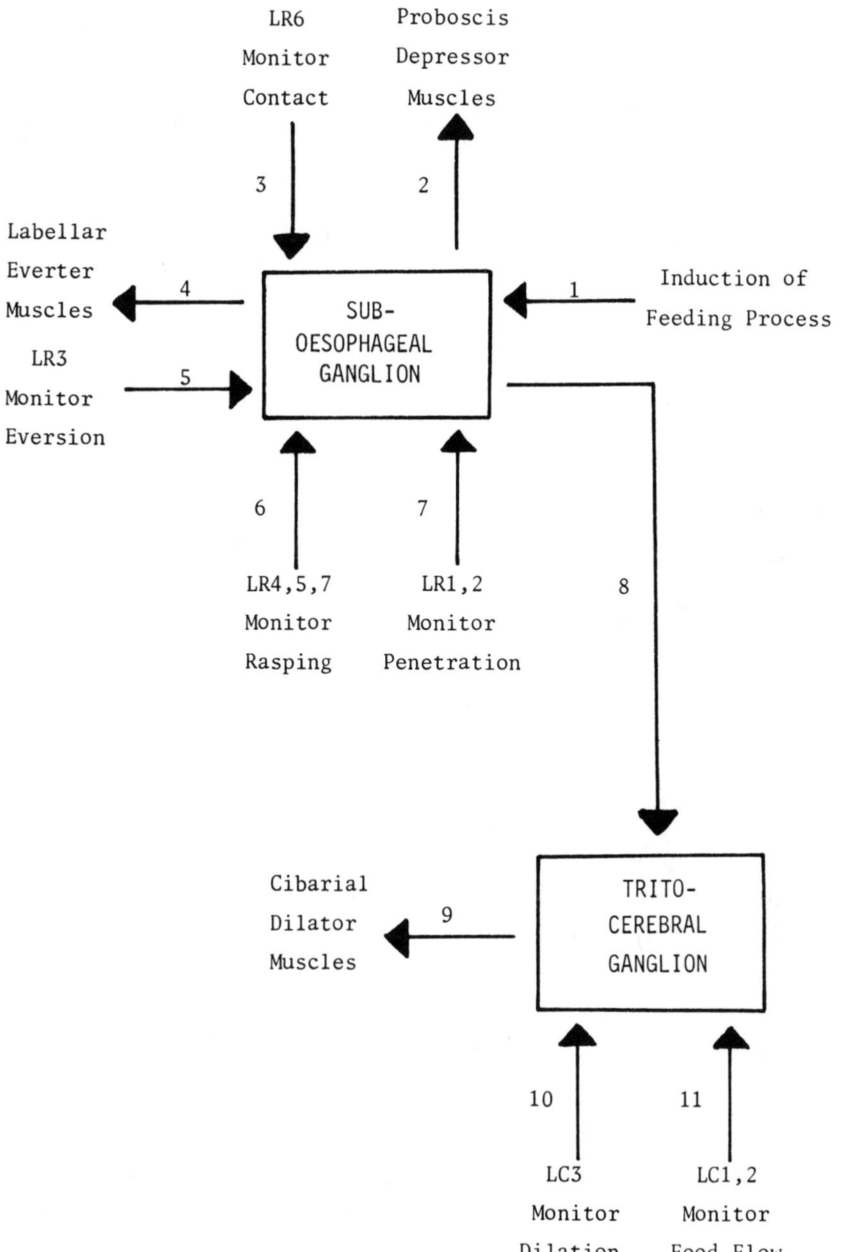


Fig 9 Sequential analysis of tsetse feeding behaviour. Control of probing and sucking is shown in terms of the eleven best-characterised neural events.

the proboscis. These provide the mechanosensory information needed to guide and co-ordinate rasping behaviour. The manner in which the separate inputs from the axons of these many receptors are co-ordinated within the neuropile of the ganglion is totally unknown. In the face of this multiplicity and quantity of sensory input, simple reflex models involving single inputs have only a restricted neuristic value. In order to comprehend the contribution of mechanoreceptors to probing behaviour it is essential to use models in which the changing inputs from a variety of receptors are incorporated. Work in this direction has only just begun.

As soon as a supply of blood has been broached, this is detected by chemoreceptor neurones in the LR5 and LR7 setae. Their input operates another centre in the sub-oesophageal ganglion which, via the circum-oesophageal connectives, activates the cibarial pumping centre in the tritocerebral part of the supra-oesophageal ganglion. Cibarial pumping aspirates blood through the proboscis, into the pump and on into the oesophagus (Rice, 1971). Three different kinds of mechanoreceptors are utilised to provide feedback on cibarial pumping, all their axons running, via the labro-cibarial nerve, to the tritocerebrum. In the food canal of the labrum there are many LC1 trichoid sensilla, each innervated by a single Type I mechanoreceptor. The very fine, filament-like setae of the LC1 sensilla are strongly stimulated when blood flows up the food canal. There are also other stouter and longer hairs, projecting into the lumen of the cibarial pump. These LC2 sensilla are grouped to monitor fluid movement in either direction through the pump and they too are innervated by Type I neurones. Both the LC1 and LC2 receptors provide information on the actual fluid flow achieved, that is, the effectiveness of cibarial pumping in removing blood from the host. In contrast, the LC3 receptors which are Type II neurones situated on the cibarial wall, monitor the movement of the pump. The LC3 receptors provide feedback on the effectiveness of the motor output to the cibarial dilator muscles. So here again it can be discerned that two, ethologically distinct, kinds of mechanoreceptors are being utilised. The first kind (LC3) check that the motor instructions issued do in fact cause the appropriate behavioural action; they can be termed self-assessor mechanoreceptors. The second kind (LC1 and LC2) monitor the effects of the behavioural action on the environment; these can be termed environmental-assessor mechanoreceptors. It seems that such an ethological classification of insect mechanoreceptors could have wide applications since, whenever motor instructions are issued by the C.N.S., these two distinct forms of feedback information are necessary for rapid co-ordination. If the sensory input during a behaviourally-induced movement is unusual, then the first piece of information that is needed is "was the movement itself unusual?" Only once this question has been answered can the unusualness of the sensory input be interpreted as being truly due to some unusual factor in the environment. On logical grounds it is impossible to use only one type of mechanoreceptor to ascertain both the nature of a piece of behaviour as well as its effects on the environment. It is a basic requirement to have independent methods of assessing the two kinds of effect, if an accurate estimate of the situation is to be made. Should the environmental-assessor (exteroreceptor) mechanoreceptor input become continuously unusual or inappropriate, despite the indication of the self-assessor (proprioreceptor) mechanoreceptor input that the intended behavioural act has been perfectly executed each time, this will lead to the adjustment of the motor output controlling the behaviour until a normal and appropriate environmental feedback is obtained. In short, possession of the two kinds of mechanoreceptive information is a prerequisite for adaptive behaviour and learning.

Behaviour as a whole can be described as consisting of an internal system of specific behavioural patterns composed of the activities of motor units and specific sensory mechanisms (Lashley, 1938; Tinbergen, 1951; Lorenz, 1960). A cybernetic approach to such systems was begun by von Holst and Mittlestaedt (1950), who suggested that, during postural adjustments, the C.N.S. must contain a pattern of the anticipated sensory feedback, whenever a motor output is produced. The authors called this idea the reafference principle, though probably the term "preafference" would be more descriptive of the mechanism envisaged. The behavioural significance of the mechanism is that by comparison, within the C.N.S., of the patterns of proprioreceptive feedback with the anticipated input patterns during a particular behavioural action, adjustments can be made in the motor outflow until the precise action intended is achieved. Once the actual sensory feedback patterns exactly equal the anticipated patterns, then the system is in equilibrium and no further movement results. The two types of information anticipated input pattern and actual input pattern, may be called alpha information and beta information respectively. Such ideas can be extended beyond the subject of posture and applied to complete behavioural processes such as mating and feeding, as long as a third variable - gamma information - is included. Gamma information can be specified as input from exteroreceptors (environmental-assessors) in contrast to beta information, which is derived from proprioreceptors (self-assessors). During any particular piece of behaviour, the three types of information will be present simultaneously in the ganglionic neuropile. The correlation between alpha and beta information will describe the effectiveness of a given motor output, and once that is known, the discrepancy between alpha and gamma will describe the state of the environment. This special use of priprioreceptive information, for non-postural purposes, ensures that a great deal of trial and error behaviour is avoided and throws a new light on the presence of such a multiplicity and variety of mechanoreceptors involved in proprioreception. The simplest example of this behavioural distinction between mechanoreceptors is to be seen in the limb receptors of insects. Here, hair plate sensilla supply beta information on the movement of the joints of the limb in response to a particular motor output, while gamma information is supplied by campaniform sensilla which monitor the resulting strains and tarsal receptors, which monitor changes in contact parameters. The chordotonal sensilla and Type II receptors in the limb will supply either beta or gamma information, depending on their position and response characteristics. In this way, it can be seen that the variety of mechanoreceptors in a limb are simply a reflection of the informational requirements of the C.N.S. computer.

These general principles can be used to interpret the variety of mechanoreceptors involved in tsetse fly probing and sucking behaviour. In the case of the LR3 receptors on the labella, these supply beta information on the effectiveness of labellar everter muscle contractions on each side. In contrast, the LR4, 5 and 7 receptors will supply gamma information on the environmental changes (penetration of the host) resulting from the pattern of labellar eversion that is achieved. Similarly, in the cibarial pump, the LC3 receptors supply beta information on the effectiveness of cibarial dilator muscle contractions, while the LC1 and LC2 receptors supply gamma information on the direction and amount of food flow achieved by the pumping action.

It is satisfying to be able to classify insect mechanoreceptors on ethological grounds as either proprioreceptors supplying beta information or exteroreceptors supplying gamma information. Not all insect mechanoreceptors will fit comfortably into this classification and some, such as certain limb mechanoreceptors, may have a dual role, supplying beta information in some situations and gamma information in others. However, the idea may be of some use, especially if subsequent studies demonstrate distinct specialisations in the central connections of the two kinds of receptors, as can be expected due to their distinct roles in behavioural regulation. Perhaps the main usefulness of the scheme is a conceptual one. It suggests the basic mechanism whereby the anticipated input from proprioreceptors and exteroreceptors (alpha) is compared with the actual input from proprioreceptors (beta) and exteroreceptors (gamma). The product of these comparisons is the central nervous system's notion of the environmental status. The insect's apparent "awareness" of its surroundings and "purposefulness" in action is thus interpreted as the product of a continuous process of balancing of the two types of sensory inputs against a parallel set of anticipated inputs. The patterns of sensory input that a given insect anticipates to result from a given behavioural act are determined by the synaptic interconnections between afferent and efferent centres in the neuropile of the ganglia and these in turn are mainly determined by natural selection. Those individuals that possess neuronal interconnections which anticipate most successfully, most of the time, what the effects of their actions will be on the environment, will have a higher survival chance and this is presumably the primary basis for the evolution of adaptive behaviour.

REFERENCES

1. ADAL, M.N. *J. Ultrastruct. Res.* *26*:332, 1969.
2. AUTRUM, H. & SCHNEIDER, W. *Z. vergleich. Physiol.* *31*:77, 1948.
3. BULLOCK, T.H. & HORRIDGE, G.A. Structure and Function in the Nervous System of Invertebrates. Freeman, San Francisco (1965).
4. CAUNA, N. & ROSS, L. *J. Biophys. Biochem. Cytol.* *7*:725, 1960.
5. CHAPMAN, K.M. & NICOLS, T.R. *J. Insect Physiol.* *15*:2103, 1969.
6. COILLOT, J.P. & BOISTEL, J. *J. Insect Physiol.* *15*:1449, 1969.
7. DIAMOND, J., GRAY, J.A.B. & INMAN, D.R. *J. Physiol.* *142*:382, 1958.
8. EDWARDS, C. & OTTOSON, D. *J. Physiol.* *143*:138, 1958.
9. EDWARDS, J.S. & PALKA, J.P. *Science, N.Y.* *172*:591, 1971.
10. EYZAGUIRRE, C. & KUFFLER, S.W. *J. Gen. Physiol.* *38*:87, 1955a.
11. EYZAGUIRRE, C. & KUFFLER, S.W. *J. Gen. Physiol.* *39*:121, 1955b.
12. FINLAYSON, L.H. *Symp. Zool. Soc. London.* *23*:217, 1968.
13. FINLAYSON, L.H. & OSBORNE, M.P. *J. Insect Physiol.* *14*:1793, 1968.
14. FINLAYSON, L.H. & OSBORNE, M.P. *J. Insect Physiol.* *16*:791, 1970.
15. FLOREY, E. *Z. Naturforsch B10*:591, 1955.
16. GALUN, R. & RICE, M.J. *Nature* *233*:110, 1972.
17. GRAY, E.G. *Phil. Trans. Roy. Soc. Lond.* *B243*:75, 1960.
18. GRAY, J.A.B. & SATO, M. *J. Physiol.* *129*:594, 1955.
19. GUILLET, J.G. & BERNARD, J. *J. Insect Physiol.* *18*:2155, 1972.
20. HOWSE, P.E. *Symp. Zool. Soc. London.* *23*:167, 1968.
21. HUBER, F. Personal communication. 1974.
22. JOBLING, B. *Parasitology* *24*:449, 1933.
23. KATZ, B. *J. Physiol.* *111*:248, 1950a.
24. KATZ, B. *J. Physiol.* *111*:261, 1950b.
25. KATZ, B. *Phil. Trans. Roy. Soc. London* *B243*:221, 1961.
26. KUWANA, Z. *Annot. Zool. Japan* *15*:247, 1935.
27. LAWRENCE, P.A. *J. Cell Sci.* *1*:475, 1966.
28. LASHLEY, K.S. *Psychol. Rev.* *45*:445, 1938.
29. LOEWENSTEIN, W.R. *Sci. Americ.* *203*:98, 1960.
30. LOEWENSTEIN, W.R. & RATHKAMP, R. *J. Gen. Physiol.* *41*:1245, 1958.
31. LORENZ, K. Methods of Approach to the Problems of Behaviour. The Harvey Lectures. Academic Press, N.Y. (1960).
32. LOWENSTEIN, O.E. & FINLAYSON, L.H. *Comp. Biochem. Physiol.* *1*:56, 1960.
33. MADDRELL, S. Neurosecretion in Insects. In: Insects and Physiology. Oliver and Boyd, London (1967).
34. MERRILLEES, N. *J. Biophys. Biochem. Cytol.* *3*:725, 1960.
35. MITTELSTAEDT, H. *Z. vergleich. Physiol.* *32*:422, 1950.
36. MITTELSTAEDT, H. Recent Adv. Invert. Physiol., Oregon Univ. Press, Eugene (1957).
37. NUNNEMACHER, R.F. & DAVIS, P.P. *J. Morph.* *125*:61, 1968.
38. ORLOV, J. *Z. wiss. Zool.* *122*:425, 1924.

39. PEASE, D.C. & QUILLIAM, T.A. *J. Biophys. Biochem. Cytol.* *3:* 331, 1957.
40. PRINGLE, J.W.S. *J. exp. Biol.* *15:*101, 1938a.
41. PRINGLE, J.W.S. *J. exp. Biol.* *15:*114, 1938b.
42. PRINGLE, J.W.S. *J. exp. Biol.* *15:*467, 1938c.
43. PRINGLE, J.W.S. *J. exp. Biol.* *17:*8, 1940.
44. PRINGLE, J.W.S. Insect Flight. Cambridge University Press. (1957).
45. PRINGLE, J.W.S. Proprioreception in Arthropods. In: The Cell and the Organism. J.A. Ramsay and V.B. Wigglesworth, Editors. C.U.P. (1961).
46. RETZIUS, M.G. *Biol. Untersuch.* *N.F.I.* 1890.
47. RICE, M.J. M.Sc. Qualifying Thesis, University of Birmingham. (1969).
48. RICE, M.J. *J. Insect Physiol.* *16:*277, 1970a.
49. RICE, M.J. *Trans. Roy. Soc. Trop. Med. Hyg.* *64:*189, 1970b.
50. RICE, M.J. Ph.D. Thesis, University of Birmingham. (1970c).
51. RICE, M.J. *Nature* *228:*1337, 1971.
52. RICE, M.J. *Trans. Roy. Soc. Trop. Med. Hyg.* *66:*317, 1972.
53. RICE, M.J. Recent Advances in the Physiology of the Tsetse Fly. Chapter 5 in: Parasitoses of Man and Animals in Africa E.A.M.R.C., Nairobi. (1974).
54. RICE, M.J. & FINLAYSON, L.H. *J. Insect Physiol.* *18:*841, 1972.
55. RICE, M.J., GALUN, R. & FINLAYSON, L.H. *Nature* *241:*286, 1973.
56. RICE, M.J., GALUN, R. & MARGALIT, J. *Ann. trop. Med. Parasit.* *67:*101, 1973a.
57. RICE, M.J., GALUN, R. & MARGALIT, J. *Ann. trop. Med. Parasit.* *67:*109, 1973b.
58. ROEDER, K.D. Nerve Cells and Insect Behaviour. Harvard Univ. Press. (1965).
59. ROEDER, K.D. Personal communication (1974).
60. ROGOZINA, M. *Z. Zellforsch.* *6:*732, 1928.
61. SCHON, A. *Zool. Jahrb. Anat.* *31:*439, 1911.
62. SCHWARTZKOPFF, J. Chapter 12 in: The Physiology of the Insecta I. Morris Rockstein, editor. Academic Press, N.Y. (1964).
63. SLIFER, E.H. & FINLAYSON, L.H. *Q. Jl. microscop. Sci.* *97:*617, 1956.
64. SLIFER, E.H. & SEKHON, S.S. *J. Morphol.* *112:*165, 1963.
65. SNODGRASS, R.E. *Smith. misc. Coll.* *77:*1, 1926.
66. STEINBRECHT, R.A. *J. Cell Sci.* *4:*39, 1969.
67. STURCKOW, B. *Z. vergleich, Physiol.* *54:*268, 1967.
68. TINBERGEN, N. The Study of Instinct. Oxford (1951).
69. THURM, U. *Z. vergleich, Physiol.* *46:*351, 1963.
70. THURM, U. *Science, N.Y.* *145:*1063, 1964.
71. THURM, U. *Cold Spring Harbour Sympos. Quantit. Biol.* *30:*75, 1965.
72. THURM, U. *Symp. Zool. Soc. Lond.* *23:*199.
73. TREHERNE, J. Neurochemistry of the Arthropods. C.U.P. (1966).

74. VON HOLST, E. & MITTELSTAEDT, H. *Naturwissenschaften* *37*:464, 1950.
75. WEEVERS, R. de G. *J. exp. Biol.* *44*:177, 1966.
76. WIGGLESWORTH, V.B. *Quart. J. microscop. Sci.* *94*:93, 1953.
77. WIGGLESWORTH, V.B. The History of Insect Physiology. In: The History of Entomology. R.F. Smith, T.E. Mittler & C.N. Smith, editors. Ann. Rev., Palo Alto (1973).
78. ZARWARZIN, A.A. *Z. wiss. Zool.* *100*:245, 1912.
79. ZARWARZIN, A.A. *Rev. Zool. Russe.* *1*:161, 1916.

# ARE CONNECTIONS STABLE IN THE ADULT MAMMALIAN BRAIN?

Patrick D. Wall
Cerebral Functions Research Group
Department of Anatomy
University College, London, England
and
Department of Zoology
Hebrew University, Jerusalem, Israel

One of the most striking aspects of sensory systems, which has been a repeated theme of this Conference, is the detail of maps contained within them. The visual system is a particularly impressive example but the auditory, somatosensory and other projection pathways also show an orderly spatial arrangement of cells and the axons which connect one group of cells to another. These maps have two features: 1) They retain some of the spatial relationships of the stimulus within the brain, so that the visual field is repeated in a neuronal form in retina, lateral geniculate and cortex. The maps may therefore transmit the information about the location of the stimulus. 2) A second possible function is that neighbouring cells tend to be handling very similar information and they are in an excellent anatomical position to interact with each other. The undoubted existence of such maps raises a number of challenging questions of some considerable importance. How are they formed during embryonic development? What is their function? Are they as rigid and exact as they appear?

Are they formed perfectly *ab initio* by preprogrammed instructions or do they crystallize out of more general organisations? Are they formed entirely by reference to internal properties within the developing brain or do they extract order from structures outside the brain or from the environment? Are the maps formed by the projection of connections from one group of cells to another or are they formed by the ongoing physiological interaction between cells? Like so many biological questions of this kind, the answer is probably that both factors in each of these questions plays a role.

Each question restates on a microscopic level the question of the relative role of nature and nurture.

I wish to present here a brief summary of a series of experiments that seem to show, within at least one mapped system, the somatosensory system, that the effective working mapped system may overlay a diffuse system which is normally inoperative. The first experiments (Wall & Egger, 1971) were on the linkage between the dorsal column nuclei and the lateral posterior ventral nucleus in the thalamus of the rat. Both of these structures contain an elaborate detailed map of the body surface. Heavily innervated structures occupy larger areas of the map than more sparsely supplied regions. Therefore, fingers and toes take up more than half the map, leaving more proximal parts of the limbs and the neck, thorax and abdomen to be represented in the minor part of the map. The nucleus which transmitted information from the hind legs to the thalamus, the nucleus gracilis, was surgically removed on one side. There were two immediate effects of the operation, one expected, the other unexpected. The expected result was that in the main leg area of the map, cells no longer responded to peripheral stimuli, while in the hand area of the map, cells responded in their normal fashion. The unexpected result seen immediately after removal was that in one small area of the nucleus, cells took on quite new properties. For example, many cells were observed which responded to stimuli on both sides of the body surface whereas in the intact nucleus such cells are very rarely observed. Evidently, the normal intact input to the nucleus suppresses some responses and connections exist which are normally inhibited. However these cells were a specialised exception and the majority acted as expected, that is to say the loss of their normal input resulted in the loss of their response to peripheral stimulation. We decided to allow animals to survive for long periods to see if time would reveal any connections which might not appear immediately after surgery. To our great surprise, what happened was that after three days the hand-arm area of the map gradually began to extend into the previous leg area. This process began three days after the operation and by ten to fourteen days, the expansion was complete. The hand now filled about half of the blank area previously occupied by leg cells. By various tests, it was possible to show that cells which had previously responded to afferents from the leg now responded to input from the hand and arm. Furthermore, the "new" receptive fields were beautifully organised with small areas, low thresholds, and no signs of any interposed cells adding to the complexity of the transmission system.

There are two possible classes of explanation for these new connections. One is that the intact axons from the arm nucleus sensed the presence of nearby denervated tissue and sent out sprouts to occupy the vacated territory. The other possibility is that the connections already existed in some inactive ineffective form and then matured and became effective as the dominant fibres degenerated. Sprouting to occupy denervated structures has been known for a long time to occur in muscle and in sympathetic ganglia. Clear evidence for such a process in the central nervous system is however very equivocal except in one well studied example. Cells in septal nuclei of the hypothalamus receive inputs from two sources. If either of the inputs is removed, the terminals of the other sprout and occupy the vacant sites. However there is no evidence that these sprouts move from one cell to another; they only spread over the surface of the cell they already contact. Furthermore, the earliest morphological signs of even this limited shift is not seen for some weeks. In our case, we observed that reactions to the new input began within days of the loss of their normal input. This biassed our thinking toward considering the possibility that the new connections might have existed before in a suppressed form.

We have now checked the existence of the phenomenon at two other locations in the somatosensory system, in the dorsal column nuclei (Basbaum, Millar & Wall, 1974) and in the spinal cord (Basbaum & Wall, 1972). We performed these experiments in the cat rather than in the rat because the rat brain gives some signs of retaining embryonic properties in the adult. The preparation here was to cut all of the dorsal roots, bringing afferent fibres from one hind leg with the exception of one relatively small root. We allowed the animals to survive for some months and then examined the nature of the map in the partially deafferented dorsal column nuclei. We found again that no empty areas of the nucleus existed. The map was now distorted by a huge representation of the area normally subserved by the remaining root and by a great expansion of the abdominal area of the map. The denervated cells had evidently become occupied by the nearest remaining intact afferents, either the one root from the leg or the supply from abdomen and thorax. In these nuclei, unlike in the thalamus, the new connections are capable of occupying the entire evacuated territory.

The situation in the spinal cord is even more dramatic. Dorsal roots innervate most intensively the area immediately around their entry zone. Therefore, it is not surprising that if one examines a spinal cord with a large number of roots cut, leaving one root intact, one observes three zones within the spinal cord. 1) In the region of entry of the intact root, cells respond to peripheral stimuli in a fairly normal fashion. 2) At some distance from the intact root, cells in the grey matter either fail completely to respond to peripheral stimuli, or they respond in a very delayed and sluggish manner to inputs which reach the denervated segment by polysynaptic pathways within the spinal cord and brain stem. 3) In an intermediate area between the normal and denervated zones, cells respond to peripheral stimuli in an abnormal way, showing that they have been released from an inhibition normally evoked by the intact roots. This demonstrates that (as in the example of the results of partial denervation of the thalamus) the physiological interaction of excitation and inhibition is one of the factors which forms the shape and nature of the receptive fields of sensory cells. These are the acute immediate changes which follow deafferentation. However by one month, some quite different changes appear in the completely deafferented zone. It looks as though a "bonanza" has taken place, in which there has been a race to occupy the empty territory. On the medial side of the dorsal grey matter, cells now respond to caudal segments; and in the lateral grey, cells respond to fibres originating from rostral segments. In the transition zone between medial and lateral, there is a mixture of cells, showing a gross disturbance of the normally orderly map, so that one cell responds to abdomen and its neighbour to toe. A few extreme examples have been seen in which single cells have double or occasionally triple receptive fields in widely separated parts of the body surface. Such cells are never seen in the normal animal. We must now accept that new physiological connections can be formed in the adult mammal when partial deafferentation occurs.

The nature of the receptive fields is important. They are discrete, tending to have smaller areas than those of cells in the normal animal. Their pressure thresholds are low. On electrical stimulation of the receptive field by intradermal needles, the cells in spinal cord and dorsal column nuclei respond with a short latency period which is consistent with their being monosynaptically connected to the afferents. In spite of their low threshold and apparent monosynaptic connections, repeated stimulation frequently results in habituation.

We are left with the possibility that these "new" connections are either the result of sprouts from existing intact afferent axons, or they result from changes in the effectiveness of previously ineffective synapses. There is evidence for relatively ineffective synapses (Merrill & Wall, 1972). Cells exist in lamina IV of cat, rat and monkey dorsal horn which have discrete small peripheral receptive fields with an abrupt edge. They respond to hair movement and light touch and do not increase their response if the intensity of stimulus is increased. Electrical stimulation of the skin in the receptive field, or of the nerve supplying it, shows that the cells respond to large myelinated fibres only - not to small myelinated or unmyelinated afferents. There is evidence that this type of relatively specialised cell has no natural sub-liminal fringe. If the excitability of the cell is varied, the size of the receptive field does not change. In other words, there are no signs that large afferent fibres impinge on the cell and produce excitatory post synaptic potentials which fail to reach threshold. The following methods have been used to change the cells' excitability 1) anaesthesia 2) abolition of descending inhibition 3) temperature variation 4) strychnine. None of these shift the edge of the receptive field. All of the afferents which excite the cell following natural stimulation run in a fraction of one root, "a microbundle". This was shown both by surgical sectioning of roots and by reversible electrical block. In this preparation in which the cell has been deafferented and therefore no longer responds to natural stimulation, it turns out that electrical stimulation of neighbouring roots produces a monosynaptic response in the cell. Evidently there are afferents which, if driven into synchronous activity by electrical stimulation, are capable of stimulating the cell; these are large myelinated afferents, judging from their threshold and conduction velocity. All large myelinated afferents are low threshold mechanoreceptors. Therefore these fibres must be activated by natural stimuli, yet they neither fire the cells nor increase their tendency to fire spontaneously. We have no idea as yet how these fibres remain ineffective - obviously, there could be either a pre- or post-synaptic explanation. We only know of their existence from the evidence just presented and by the fact that antidromic microelectrode stimulation shows that a nerve such as the sural nerve has terminals in regions of grey matter where no cells can be shown to respond monosynaptically to the sural nerve.

We now have an interesting situation.

1) If nerve cells are destroyed in the adult mammalian brain, there is no evidence that these cells are ever replaced by regeneration.
2) If axons are cut across in the mammalian central nervous system there is little or no evidence that the cut axons send out sprouts and successfully reconnect to their former target cells.
3) If axons are cut and degenerate, there is good evidence that intact neighbours sprout and occupy the synaptic sites left vacant. There is some doubt about the range and success of this sprouting.
4) There is some evidence that certain axons amongst cells make a type of very ineffective or totally ineffective synapse.
5) When degeneration occurs, there are presynaptic changes as shown by Merrill and Wall, 1972 and there are post-synaptic changes in which the morphology of the dendrites of the partially deafferented cell is altered.
6) Changes of the post-synaptic morphology or of the physiology of its membrane, "denervation sensitivity", might make the cell either i) attractive to sprouting axons or
   ii) responsive to previously ineffective terminals.

It is quite clear that the connectivity within the mammalian adult nervous system is more plastic than was once thought and it is also clear that this modifiability may occur even in those structures with detailed maps where one might expect rigidity and permanence of connection.

## REFERENCES

1. BASBAUM, A., MILLAR, J. & WALL, P.D. In press, 1974.
2. BASBAUM, A. & WALL, P.D. In press, 1974.
3. MERRILL, E.G. & WALL, P.D. *J. Physiol.* *222*:825, 1972.
4. WALL, P.D. & EGGER, M.D. *Nature, Lond.* *232*:542, 1971.

PHEROMONE COMMUNICATION IN MOTHS AND BUTTERFLIES

Dietrich Schneider

Max-Planck-Institut für Verhaltensphysiologie

Seewiesen, Germany

## INTRODUCTION

Insects as well as many animals of other classes, use chemical signals - so called pheromones (Karlson and Lüscher, 1959; Karlson, 1960; Karlson and Butenandt, 1960) - for intraspecific communication. Our interest is to gain an understanding of communication in the form of exchange of biologically meaningful signals between conspecifics (Schneider, 1965; Wilson, 1970), in moths and butterflies. Originally it was assumed that pheromones are species-specific, that is, each species produced, for example, its own sexual attractant. While this appears to be true in many cases, recent investigations have shown that very often the situation is much more complex. Closely related species may have the same pheromone and therefore need additional means, for example differences in their diel rhythm, behavioral differences and/or different amounts of the attractant (Kaae *et al.*, 1973), to secure their reproductive isolation. Furthermore, it has been found that many species use more than one compound to attract the sexual partner. In field experiments, the addition of other compounds to the main pheromone can increase the catching rate of one species and block the attraction of another. In some cases, two closely related species were found to utilize the same two isomers of an acetate in different ratios (Minks *et al.*, 1973; Klun *et al.*, 1973). To what extent interspecific attraction (but not necessarily mating attempt) occurs under normal field conditions is not known, but cross-attraction was observed in field experiments (Ganyard and Brady, 1972).

The state of the art with regard to pheromone biology in insects was recently reviewed in a number of articles and books: Butler, 1967,

1970; Blum, 1969, 1970; Eiter, 1970; Shorey, 1970, 1973; Jacobson, 1972; Priesner, 1973; Karlson and Schneider, 1973; MacConnell and Silverstein, 1973; Barth and Lester, 1973. The function of insect olfactory receptors has been considered by Kaissling, 1971 and Schneider, 1974.

## PHEROMONE COMMUNICATION AND OLFACTORY RECEPTION IN MOTHS

The pheromone communication system in the moth as shown schematically in Fig. 1 illustrates the extent of our present understanding of the different functions involved. No attempt will be made here to present a complete picture, but rather to emphasize some functions and to present some examples.

Some time after emergence from the pupa, the virgin female moth expands her sexual attractant glands. The performance of this "calling" behavior (Fig. 2) depends upon a number of factors, some of which are known. As a rule, calling is only observed before copulation. In the female of the domesticated silkmoth *Bombyx*, calling is more or less continuous, while in most other moths studied to date, calling depends upon a diel rhythm which appears to be correlated with the activity rhythm of the male of this species (Bartell, 1968; Traynier, 1970; Shorey, 1973; Fatzinger, 1973). In the well studied cabbage looper moth (*Trichoplusia ni)*, it was found that the duration of calling and the amount of attractant emitted depended upon the wind speed (Kaae and Shorey, 1972). This phenomenon can be understood in relation to the distribution of the luring odor (see below).

In some cases (for reference see Shorey, 1973), the female moths fly to the larval food plant before they start calling. A particularly striking food-plant odor dependency was reported for the North American Saturniid *Antheraea polyphemus* (Riddiford, 1967; Riddiford and Williams, 1967). The female of this moth only called in the presence of the odor of the preferred food plant: oak. The critical compound is t-2-hexenal, which is found in most green leaves. Pure hexenal brings abut the same effect as oak leaves, while other leaves - in spite of the fact that they contain hexenal - do not induce calling. The odor signal is perceived with antennal receptors. With regard to the failure of leaves such as birch to elicit calling, one is led to assume that leaves of plants other than oak contain, in addition to the omnipresent hexenal, some other compounds which prevent calling. The experiments of Riddiford and Williams(1971) have enabled us to advance a tentative functional scheme on the basis of experiments with this and other species. (Fig. 3): The hexenal receptor cells activate neurosecretory brain cells, the axons of which run to the corpora cardiaca, where their neurosecretion subsequently activates local hormone cells. The latter produce a "calling hormone" which circulates in the hemolymph and is the prerequisite for expansion of

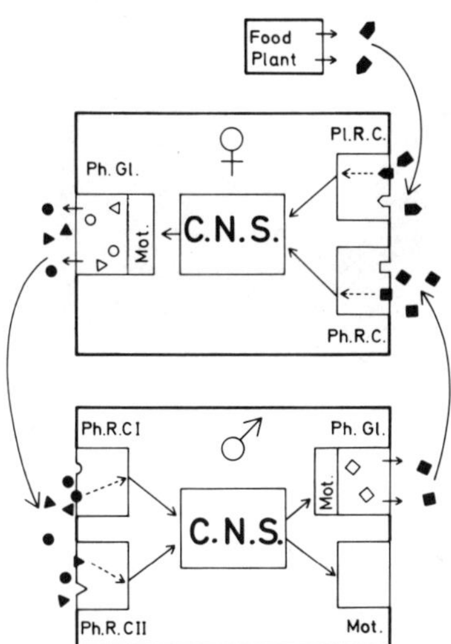


Fig. 1 Functional scheme of the pheromone communication system between a female and a male moth (Including the foodplant odor signal for the female's calling behavior). Arrows indicate the direction of the information flux. Small symbols (circles, triangles, squares, pentagons) symbolize odor molecules (filled) or their respective precursors (open). Open niches in the receptor cells represent the acceptors (receptor sites). - CNS = central nervous system; Mot (♀) = expansion mechanism for the lure gland; Mot (♂) = motor system (wings and legs) for approach to the female; Mot Ph. Gl. = motor system to expand the male hairpencil gland; Ph. Gl. = pheromone gland (♂ and♀); Ph.R.C. I and II (♂) receptor cells for two female sex attractants; Ph.R.C. (♀) = receptor cell for the male aphrodisiac; Pl.R.C. (♀) = plant odor receptor cell.

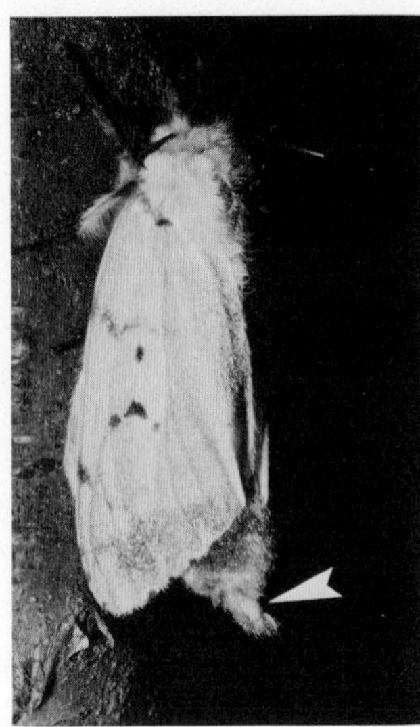

Fig. 2 Female gypsy moth (*Lymantria dispar*) in calling position with expanded lure gland. Length of the forewing - 30 mm.

the lure gland. This gland is shifted outward by hemolymph pressure as the result of muscular contractions in the abdomen, and can be retracted by a retractor muscle. Since hormonal effects are slow and lasting, quick expansion and retraction of the glands are presumably controlled through neural pathways.

The glands which produce the female attractant pheromones are composed of specialized intersegmental epidermis cells with deeply fluted distal cell membranes, underlying a cuticle with some pores (Steinbrecht, 1964a; for further references see Percy and Wheatherstone, 1971; Jefferson and Rubin, 1973). Little is known of pheromone biosynthesis. In the gypsy moth (*Lymantria dispar*) for instance, the attractant is an epoxide (disparlure) which apparently is synthesized from its olefinic precursor (Bierl *et al.*, 1972; Cardé *et al.*, 1973; Kasang *et al.*, 1974). In this species, as well as in *Bombyx*, where the precursor of the alcoholic pheromone might be a fatty acid, the weight ratio of precursor: pheromone is of the order of 10:1. Transformation of the precursor to the final product might take place in the cell or even in the cuticle. The pheromone quantity per gland (the so called female equivalent) is of the order of 1 μg (approximately $10^{15}$ molecules) in some species (Steinbrecht, 1964b; Shorey and Gaston, 1965), but less in the majority of cases. The number of pheromone molecules emanating from the gland surface was estimated in *Bombyx* to be of the order of $10^{11}$ molecules/sec, corresponding to a pheromone molecule density of $10^8/cm^3$ in a moderate

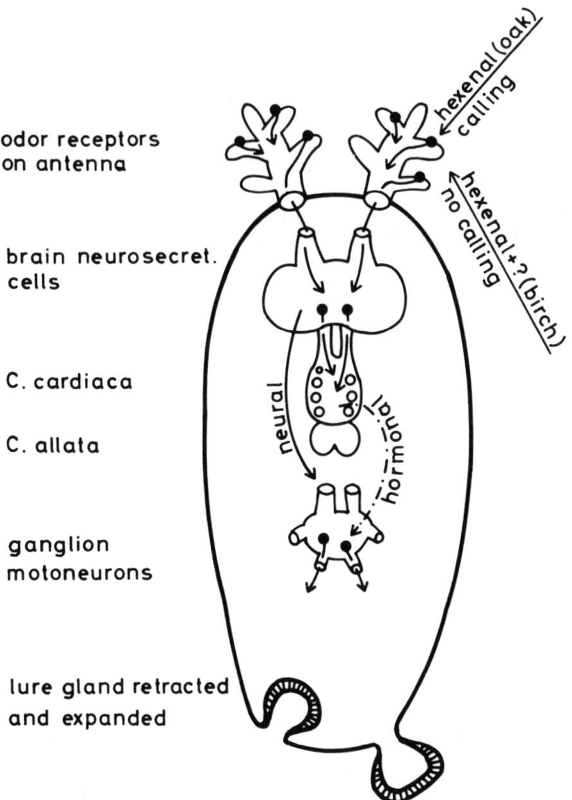


Fig. 3 Functional scheme of the olfactory, neurohormonal, hormonal, and neural control of the calling behavior of the female giant silkmoth *Antheraea polyphemus* (after Riddiford and Williams, 1967/71; see text).

airstream passing over the female gland (calculated from Kaissling and Priesner, 1970; see also Priesner, 1973).

The transfer medium is air, which carries the pheromone to the receptors of the male moth antenna. Reports on effective attraction distances vary from several kilometers to a few tens of meters (for reference see Priesner, 1973), depending on the pheromone output rate, the physical transfer conditions, and eventually on the male moth's behavior threshold, which in *Bombyx* was found to be reached at $10^3$ bombykol molecules/$cm^3$ of air (Kaissling and Priesner, 1970).

On the receiving side, the signal molecules are first adsorbed on the cuticle of the receptor hair and then migrate by surface diffusion through pores and tubules to the membrane of the receptor cell dendrite, where they interact with postulated acceptors (receptors). While the surface diffusion and penetration of the cuticle by the pheromone is well documented (Kasang, 1971, 1973; Kasang and Kaissling, 1972; Steinbrecht and Kasang, 1972), pheromone molecules have for technical reasons not yet been seen *in flagranti* on the dendritic membrane or in the tubules leading to this membrane. The result of this so far postulated signal-acceptor interaction can be seen as a depolarization of the dendritic membrane (the receptor potential of a single cell, or, in an overall recording, the electroantennogram, EAG), leading to the elicitation of nerve impulses. The amplitude of the receptor potential and consequently the frequency of the impulses are an exponential function of the stimulus strength. In *Bombyx* (Kaissling and Priesner, 1970) and presumably in other moths also, single pheromone molecules elicit single impulses, but the behavior threshold of the male insect is not reached before several hundred cells are activated. The nerve fibers (axons) run without branching through the antennal nerve to the deutocerebrum (Steinbrecht, 1969) where they synaptically contact secondary olfactory cells. As in the vertebrates, the total number of secondary olfactory cells in insects is less than the number of receptor cells (Pareto, 1972; Boeckh, 1974). The neuroanatomy of the moth brain is not well known yet. Prediction as to possible nerve connections for the processing and distribution of the olfactory information would therefore be very difficult.

The number of olfactory receptor cells in each antenna of the *Bombyx* male is about 50,000 of which more than 30,000 are specialized for the female pheromone (Schneider and Kaissling, 1957; Schneider and Steinbrecht, 1965; Kaissling and Priesner, 1970; Steinbrecht, 1970, 1973); in some wild silkmoths, these figures are more than twofold higher (Boeckh *et al.*, 1960). While our understanding of the specificity of the pheromone receptor cells in the males of *Bombyx* and *Lymantria* is quite advanced, we know very little of the specificity of the other odor receptor cells. These cells which do not respond to the pheromone have been found in an earlier study to be present in rather large numbers of physiological cell types with different, but overlapping, response spectra for general odors (Schneider *et al.*, 1964). Here it remains to be seen whether these cells respond to as yet unknown odorants which are biologically significant.

Odor molecules must for a number of reasons interact directly with the proposed acceptors. The cell's (or cell type's) specificity is defined by the whole set of compounds to which the cell responds, and necessarily also by the respective stimulus response characteristics (Kaissling, 1973). Since some odor receptor cells seem to have more than one type of acceptor in their membrane, the respective specificity of one acceptor is only part of the cell's specificity (Kafka *et al.*, 1973). Interaction probably is by weak physical (polar and dispersion) forces (Kafka, 1970).

The specificity of the odor receptors generally is rather high because the effectiveness of the "wrong" geometrical isomer is in some cases only 1/100 - 1/1000 of that of the pheromone, and even chirally different molecules elicit different cell responses in the receptor cell and can be distinguished behaviorally (Kafka *et al.*, 1973; see also Riley *et al.*, 1974).

So far, nothing is known of the fate of the odor molecule after it has delivered its message. Metabolic processes which change the odor molecule in antennal tissue are probably not fast enough to be either directly related to the transduction or to immediate inactivation of the odor molecule (Kasang, 1971, 1973; Ferkovich *et al.*, 1973).

The eventual outcome of all these processes in the pheromone receptor cells, which send their messages to the brain via their axons in the nerves of both antennae, is a motor reaction of the male insect. The domesticated and flightless male silkmoth *Bombyx*, when stimulated with the female sexual attractant, first lifts its antennae and then starts marching upwind, while vibrating its antennae and fluttering its wings (Schwinck, 1954, 1955). Wild moths only react if they are stimulated at certain hours of the day; they then lift their antennae like *Bombyx* and sooner or later fly upwind in the aerial pheromone trail or odor plume. If they lose it, they may start undirected circling, searching flights, as do other insects (Steiner, 1953). Systematic studies of all factors involved in the final approach of the male to the female in the field have not been conducted. Since odor alone does not give the animal a directional clue, it presumably uses its optomotor system to steer upwind (Kennedy and Marsh, 1974). But wingless moths are able to follow a terrestrial pheromone trail like ants and termites (Shorey and Farkas, 1973).

Male *Bombyx* marching upwind toward a piece of paper which holds the attractant find it simply by not leaving the bombykol odor plume. While doing so, they are indifferent to the visible female calling in an airtight glass box next to the artificial bait (Fig. 4). This experiment is a repetition of the classical J.H. Fabre experiment (1879) with the wild silkmoth *Saturnia pyri*.

*Bombyx* males are extremely excited when they reach the bombykol impregnated filter-paper and try to copulate with it. If several males arrive together, they may try to couple with each other.

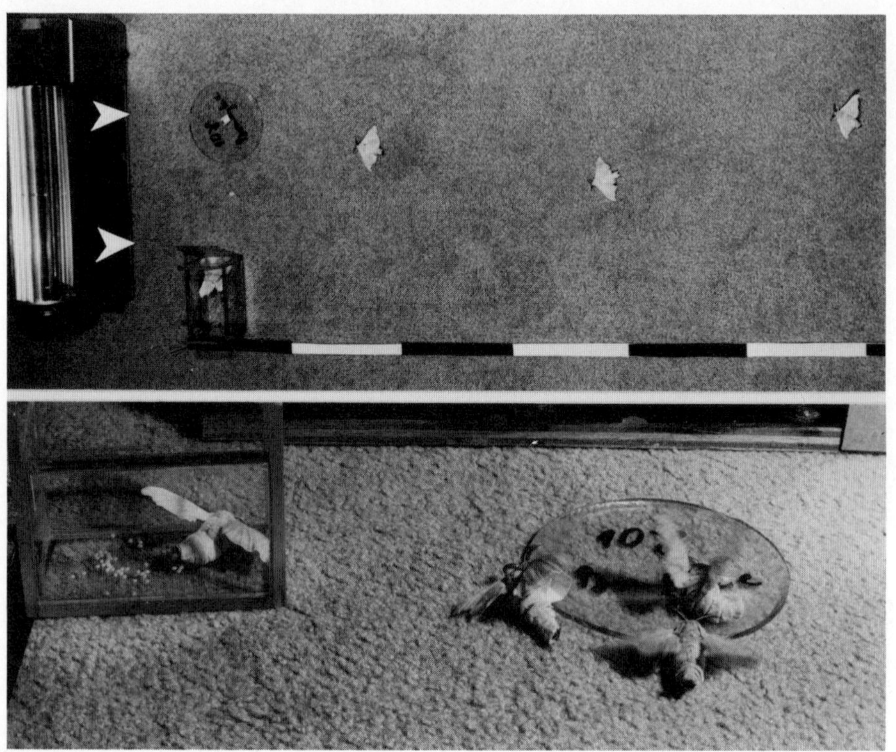

Fig. 4 *Bombyx mori* sex attractant orientation. Top: a fan produces an air current from left to right (arrows). In front of the fan, a filter paper which contains 10 µg of the synthetic sexual attractant (bombykol) is mounted on a glass plate. Three of the flightless males march - while fluttering their wings - toward the bombykol source, ignoring a virgin, "patiently" calling female in an airtight glass box. Length of black and white scale segments: 10 cm each. Bottom: Close-up view of the three males near the bombykol source. The left male has seized the filter paper; the upper male bends his abdomen in an empty copulatory attempt. - The female has her lure glands expanded after laying some (unfertilized) eggs.

Our understanding of the orientating mechanism is not well developed. While osmo-tropotaxis (Lindauer and Martin, 1963; Martin, 1964) is involved, more complex mechanisms (currently under study in our laboratory) play an additional role.

Theoretical considerations of the composition of such an odor plume lead to unexpected predictions, at least in an idealized case (Wright, 1958; Bossert and Wilson, 1963; Wilson and Bossert, 1963). The gradient of decreasing odor concentration is very steep near the odor source when there is a reasonable air flow speed (Fig. 5). Next to the source the air may contain up to $10^8$ pheromone molecules/$cm^3$, while at a few to 30 meters distance (as a result of air turbulence) the concentration range is $10^3$-$10^4$ molecules/$cm^3$. The odor plume then extends with little reduction of concentration (depending upon the rate of air flow and dilution, see also Sower *et al.*, 1973) to more than 100 meters. Effective luring at longer distances is only possible if either the source is more effective than is known at present, or the pheromone catching rate of the male antenna is better than in *Bombyx*. The sensitivity of the attractant receptor cell reaches its theoretical physical limits and the neural noise-spontaneous firing of the odor receptor cells - (Kaissling and Priesner, 1970), 0.1 impulses/sec., is rather low for such a sensitive system. However, theoretically, a reduction of this spontaneous activity by a factor of ten would allow the receptor system to respond to a greater dilution range of the phermone and allow the male to approach from up to 3 times the distance.

In the light of this theoretical background, it is interesting to note that *Trichoplusia ni* females relate their pheromone-releasing behavior to the wind velocity (Kaae and Shorey, 1972). At low wind speed, when the odor is persistent and dilution is low, the females call for longer periods. In addition, most females vibrate their wings (fanning!) when calling at low wind speeds and do not at high wind speeds.

This completes the story with respect to chemical information transfer from the female to the male which eventually mates with her. The message is biologically highly meaningful; the male moth understands the "language" of his mate.

While this functional cycle seems in some moths to be completed with the male's approach and instant mating after he reaches the female, some groups of moths do have male pheromones, which are apparently designed for short distance effects. In fact, male scent scales and scent brushes or hair pencils (androconia and coremata) have been described in many lepidoptera. Many male Noctuids, Sphingids and Arctiids have large hairpencils which they can expand for the dissemination of an odor. These scents are usually physiologically detectable by humans, while most of the female moth pheromones have no odor for us.

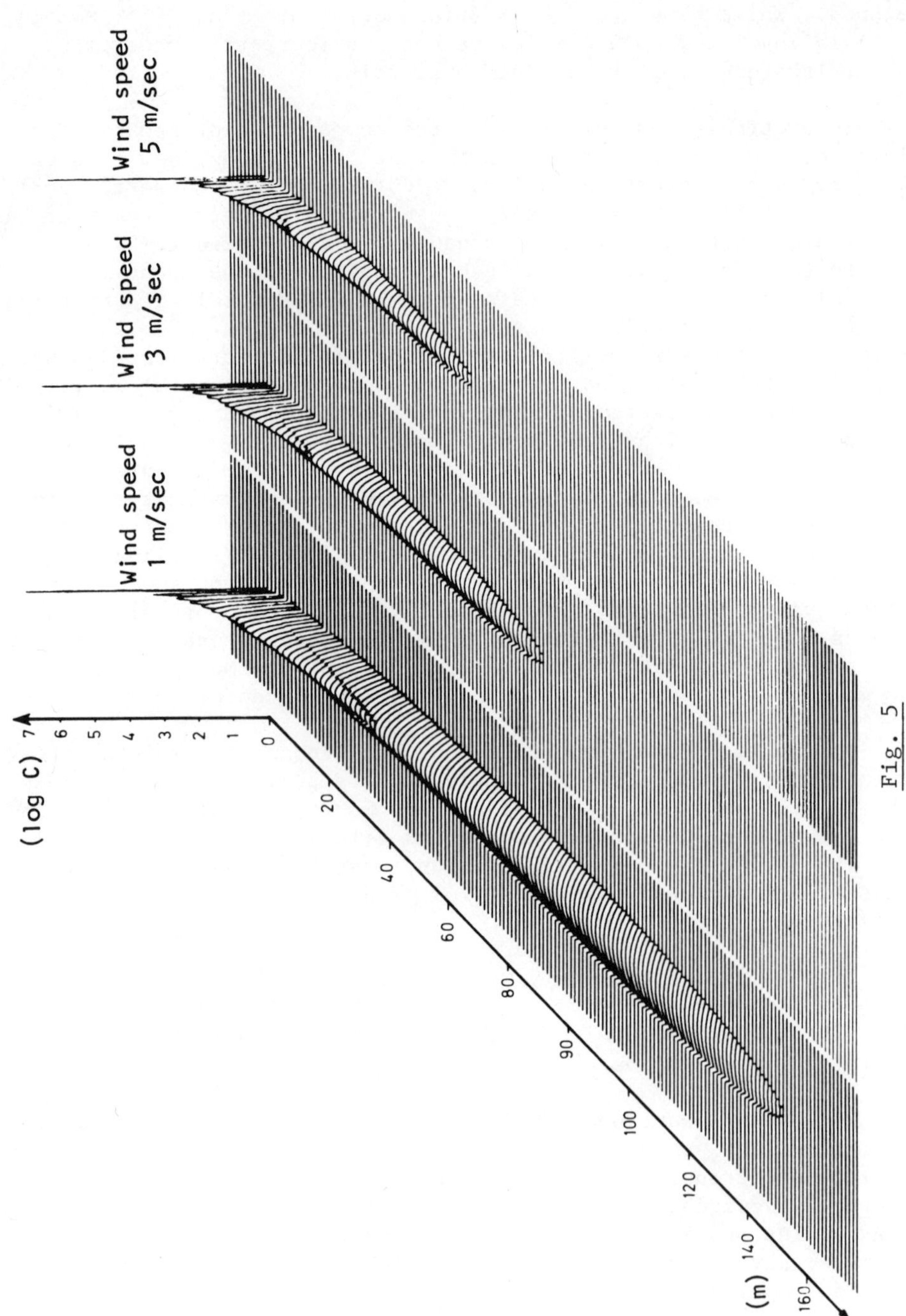
Wind speed
5 m/sec
Wind speed
3 m/sec
Wind speed
1 m/sec
(log C)
7
6
5
4
3
2
1
0
20
40
60
80
90
100
120
140
160
(m)

Fig. 5

Fig. 5

Odor plumes. Computer plots of aerial odor trails (odor plumes) at wind speeds of 1, 3, and 5 m/sec (courtesy of E. Kramer, Seewiesen). The plots are based on the quotient Q/K which determines the length of the trail (Bossert and Wilson, 1963). Q = odor emission at the source (molecules/sec); K = threshold concentration to elicit the male's pheromone response (molecules/$cm^3$ of air). In this diagram Q/K is $2.4 \times 10^8$ ($Q = 2.4 \times 10^{11}$; $K = 1 \times 10^3$).

Note: The z-axis (vertical axis) is *not* an expression of the vertical expansion of the aerial trail but indicates the odor concentration on each point of the horizontal plane which intersects the odor source at point 0. In the plots, the odor plume has a concentration of $>10^3$ molecules/$cm^3$ in a plume which reaches approximately 145, 85, and 75 meters, and $>10^4$ molec/$cm^3$ for plumes extending to approximately 33, 10, and 5 m, respectively (see text).

With some of the Noctuids, it was reported that the male during his final approach to the female briefly expands his hairpencils and that his arrestant or aphrodisiac pheromones (for instance 80% benzaldehyde plus 20% isobutyric acid in three *Leucania* species; or 95% pinocarvone in *Apamea monoglypha*, Birch, 1970; Aplin and Birch, 1968, 1970) prevent the female flight reaction otherwise observed and induce her to accept the male.

This generalization that among the moths, only the females produce attractant pheromones and the males produce aphrodisiacs - either from wing glands, hair-tufts or hairpencils - does not apply to the two species of wax-moths *Achroea grisella* and *Galleria mellonella*. Here, male wing-gland pheromones (aldehydes) at low concentrations attract the female moths and exhibit a seductive effect at high concentrations (Röller *et al.*, 1968; Dahm *et al.*, 1971; Leyrer and Monroe, 1973).

## PHEROMONE COMMUNICATION IN BUTTERFLIES

Among the butterflies, which in general are more visually orientated than most moths, female pheromones are probably present at least in some species but have never been isolated. It is for instance well known to collectors that the males of the Florida Zebra (*Heliconius charitonius*) are attracted to the female chrysalid just before the latter emerges (Mitchell and Zim, 1964) and the females of a European fritillary butterfly (*Argynnis paphia*) expose abdominal glands which might produce a pheromone, to their males before copulation (Treusch, 1967).

Male butterfly pheromones, which fall into the category of arrestant scents or aphrodisiacs, have been described in a number of cases and are presumably present in many species. So far, the best known group in this respect are the milkweed butterflies, tigers, or monarchs (Danaidae). Here, the males have paired abdominal hairpencils (Fig. 6) which produce a number of compounds of which at least one (a ketone: pyrrolizinone, Meinwald *et al.*, 1966, 1969) was proved to be an effective aphrodisiac (Brower *et al.*, 1965; Pliske and Eisner, 1969; Myers and Brower, 1969; Myers, 1972). The role of some other compounds of the hairpencils is still unknown except for a viscous terpenoid diol, which serves as a "fixative" for the ketone in *Danaus gilippus* (Pliske and Eisner, 1969). While the ketone or its derivatives - which are widely distributed in this family - and also the diol have no detectable odor to humans, freshly everted hairpencils of most Danaid species have a distinct scent which to the human observer is more or less species-specific. So far, these scents have not been analyzed chemically.

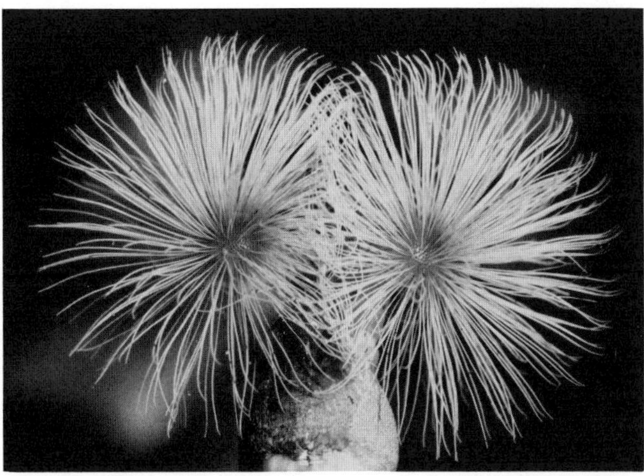

Fig. 6 Danaid hairpencils. Two fully expanded abdominal hairpencils of a male *Danaus formosa mercedonia* from Uganda. Diameter of each sphere of hairs: 10 mm.

The ketone elicits a marked electrophysiological response in antennal odor receptors of both sexes in all the Danaids which have so far been studied (Schneider and Seibt, 1969; Schneider, 1971; Seibt *et al.*, 1972; see also Myers and Brower, 1969). The electrophysiological effect of the other odorous compounds is weak but may nonetheless be important for species recognition. The state of our knowledge of the distribution of pyrrolizines and an aromatic compound is shown for 22 Danaid species in Fig. 7.

Heterocyclic nitrogen-containing compounds are rare among insects and have only been found, in addition to in the Danaids, as trail substances in two ants and in the male hairpencils of two Arctiid moths.

The striking fact that the hairpencils of indoor-raised Danaids of several species do not contain the ketone (which led in *D. gilippus* to a drastic reduction in the mating success of the males: Pliske and Eisner, 1969; Schneider and Seibt, 1969; Seibt *et al.*, 1972; Meinwald *et al.*, 1971), drew attention to earlier field observations that male Danaids were attracted to special plant species of some families. Interestingly, the plants (some Boraginaceae, Compositae, Leguminosae) have one property in common - they produce esters of a pyrrolizine base which in vertebrates are

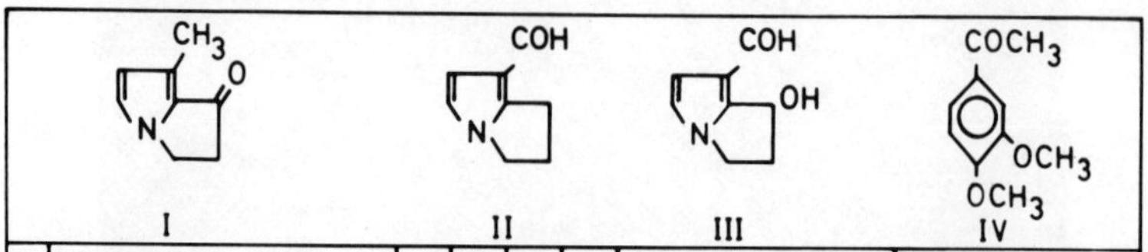

| $CH_3$, O, N | COH, N | COH, OH, N | $COCH_3$, $OCH_3$, $OCH_3$ |
|---|---|---|---|
| I | II | III | IV |

| | species | I | II | III | IV | range | sub-fam. |
|---|---|---|---|---|---|---|---|
| 1 | L. ceres | + | - | - | - | Am | Lycoreinae |
| 2 | D. plexippus | - | - | - | - | Am Pac Atl | |
| 3 | D. gilippus | + | - | - | - | Am | |
| 4 | D. chrysippus | + | - | - | - | Af As Au | |
| 5 | D. affinis | + | + | - | - | Au Pac Indo | |
| 6 | D. limniace pet. | + | | | - | Af | |
| 7 | D. formosa | - | | | - | Af | |
| 8 | D. hamata | + | - | + | | Au Ind Pac | Danainae |
| 9 | D. pumila | - | - | + | | Pac | |
| 10 | A. niavius | + | - | - | + | Af | |
| 11 | A. tartarea | - | | | + | Af | |
| 12 | A. ochlea | + | | | - | Af | |
| 13 | A. echeria | + | | | - | Af | |
| 14 | A. oscarus | - | | | - | Af | |
| 15 | A. albimaculata | + | | | - | Af | |
| 16 | E. sylvester | (+) | - | + | | Au | |
| 17 | E. core | - | - | - | | Au | |
| 18 | E. nemertes | - | - | + | | Pac | |
| 19 | E. treitschkei | - | - | + | | Pac | Euploeinae |
| 20 | E. boisduvali | - | - | - | | Pac | |
| 21 | E. tulliolus | - | - | + | | Au Pac | |
| 22 | E. levinii | - | - | + | | Pac | |

Fig. 7 Danaid hairpencil substances. Only substances of which the pheromone function was proven (No. 3), or is probable, are listed. Symbols: "+" or "-" represent substances present or absent. Danaid genera: 1 = *Lycorea*; 2 - 9 = *Danaus*; 10 - 15 = *Amauris*; 16 - 22 = *Euploea*.

Af = Africa; Am = America; As = Asia; Atl = Atlantic; Au = Australia; Ind = India; Indo = Indonesia; Pac = Pacific. References for species: No. 1: Meinwald *et al.*, 1966; No. 2: Meinwald *et al.*, 1968; No. 3: Meinwald *et al.*, 1969; No. 4: Meinwald *et al.*, 1971; No. 5, 8, 9, 16 - 22: Edgar *et al.*, 1971, 1973; No. 6, 7, 10 - 15: Meinwald *et al.*, 1974.

known for their hepatotoxic properties.

The final proof for the uptake of a plant product as a precursor of the ketone came from an experiment by Edgar *et al.* in 1973 in Australia. Three male laboratory-raised *D. chrysippus* were allowed to lick from dry *Heliotropium* branches; a few days later the hairpencils were found to contain the ketone, which was absent in control animals.

Early in 1973, we observed male *D. chrysippus* in Kenya, assembling in numbers on dry parts of a *Heliotropium* (Fig. 8). In extensive experiments (Schneider *et al.*, 1974) we obtained electrophysiological and chemical evidence that the ketone is indeed only synthesized in the hairpencils of this species if the indoor-raised animals either have access to this plant, or are fed a methanol extract of the plant, or are fed a pyrrolizine alkaloid ester (see Fig. 9) isolated from this *Heliotropium* species from Kenya (J. Meinwald and W.R. Thompson, unpublished).

Consequently, one may state that this latter compound is the precursor of the ketone and an essential substance for the production of a pheromone. This substance is actively searched for by odor receptors on the butterfly antenna. These conclusions are supported by the important observation that the hairpencils of several wild Australian Danaids (including *D. chrysippus*) contained these esters which very probably were ingested from plants (Edgar and Culvenor, 1974; Bull *et al.*, 1968).

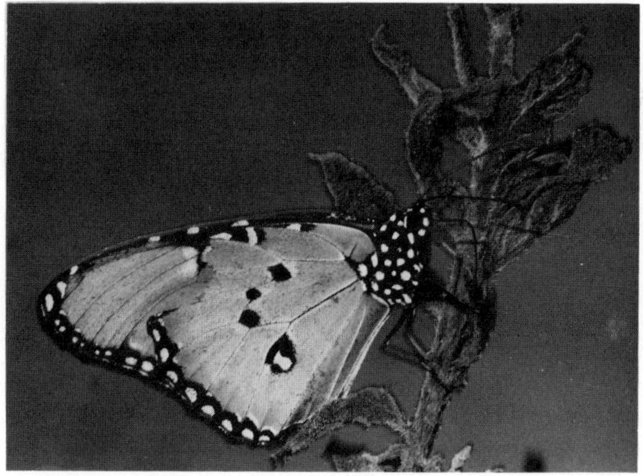

Fig. 8 *Danaus chrysippus dorippus*. Male butterfly sucking on dry parts of *Heliotropium* spec. (Boraginaceae) in the East African Rift Valley, south of Nairobi, Kenya. The males were observed to approach these plants in an upwind flight.

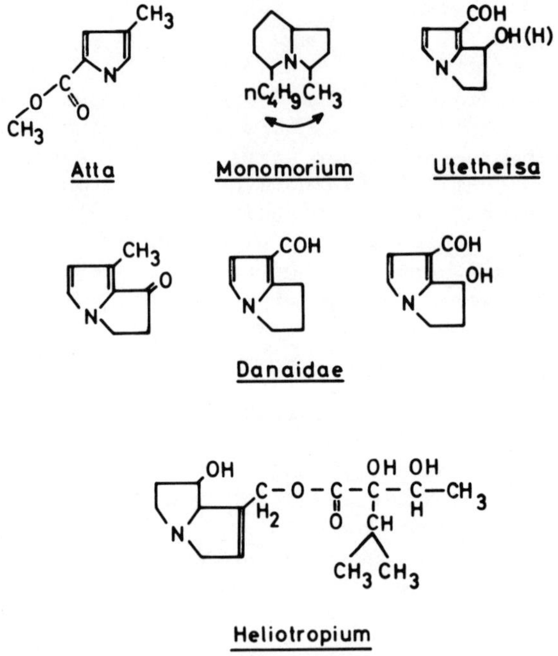

Fig. 9 Nitrogen-containing pheromones and a pheromone precursor.

Top row: Trail substances in the leaf-cutting ant *Atta texana* (Tumilson *et al.*, 1971, 1972), the pharao ant *Monomorium pharaonis* (Ritter *et al.*, 1973), and the supposed hairpencil pheromone of the tiger-moth *Utetheisa* (Culvenor and Edgar, 1972).

Middle row: Hairpencil compounds of Danaid butterflies (cf. Fig. 7).

Bottom row: Pyrrolizine alkaloid ester from *Heliotropium* spec., cf. Fig. 8 (Meinwald and Thompson, 1973). This compound was found to be the precursor of the ketone (left, middle row).

The behavioral attractivity of the *Heliotropium* has its correlate in the response of the antennal odor receptors: air blown over the slightly moistened *Heliotropium*, or over the pure pyrrolizine ester as an odor source, elicits a significant electrophysiological response as shown in the electroantennogram.

The Danaid butterfly family is not only biologically dependent upon these hepatotoxic plant products for the synthesis of the male pheromone but biologically also closely connected to plants which produce heart toxins. The milkweeds (Asclepiadaceae), which are the larval foodplants for at least two of the three Danaid subfamilies, contain toxic cardiac glycosides (cardenolides) which make the larva and the butterfly unpalatable to predators (cf. Reichstein *et al.*, 1968; Brower, 1969; Rothschild, 1972). These butterflies then serve as models for a number of palatable butterflies which mimic the Danaid wing pattern and in some cases also their peculiar slow flight habits. The interrelationships of the Danaids with the plant families is summarized in Fig. 10.

| | sub-families | plants | toxins |
|---|---|---|---|
| larval food plants | Lycoreinae | Asclepiadaceae | cardiac-glycosides |
| | Euploeinae | Apocynaceae | alkaloids, glucosides |
| | Danainae | Asclepiadaceae | cardiac-glycosides |
| ♂ (♀) imago attractant | Danaus chrysippus<br>D. gilippus?<br>D. limniace?<br>Amauris ochlea?<br>A. niavius? | Heliotropium<br>(Boraginaceae)<br>Senecio?<br>(Compositae)<br>Crotalaria?<br>(Leguminosae) | pyrrolizin alkaloids |

Fig. 10 Interrelationship of Danaid butterflies with flowering plants. Toxins of the larval foodplants render the larvae and butterfly unpalatable to bird predators. Pyrrolizine alkaloid esters attract the males (and to some extent also the females, cf. Edgar *et al.*, 1973). The males of *D. chrysippus* suck these alkaloids from *Heliotropium* to biosynthesize hairpencil ketone (I, Fig. 9). Four other species of Danaids were unable to produce the ketone when raised in captivity without access to *Heliotropium*. Supposed further sources for the pyrrolizine pheromone precursors are for instance *Senecio* and *Crotalaria* (cf. Edgar and Culvenor, 1974).

## REFERENCES

1. ALPIN, R.T. & BIRCH, M.C. *Nature 217:*1167, 1968.
2. ALPIN, R.T. & BIRCH, M.C. *Experientia 26:*1193, 1970.
3. BARTELL, R.J. *Proc. Ecol. Soc. Austr. 3:*155, 1968.
4. BARTH, R.H. & LESTER, L.J. *Ann. Rev. Entomol. 18:*445, 1973.
5. BIERL, B.A., BEROZA, M. & COLLIER, C.W. *J. Econom. Entomol. 65:*259, 1972.
6. BIRCH, M.C. *Anim. Behav. 18:*310, 1970.
7. BLUM, M.S. *Ann. Rev. Entomol. 14:*57, 1969.
8. BLUM, M.S. In: Chemicals controlling insect behavior (Ed. M. Beroza), Academic Press, New York-London, p. 61, 1970.
9. BOECKH, J. *J. Comp. Physiol. 90:*183, 1974.
10. BOECKH, J., KAISSLING, K.-E. & SCHNEIDER, D. *Zool. J. Anat. 78:*559, 1960.
11. BOSSERT, W.H. & WILSON, E.O. *J. Theor. Biol. 5:*443, 1963.
12. BROWER, L.P. *Scient. Am. Feb. 1969:*22, 1969.
13. BROWER, L.P., BROWER, J. VAN ZANDT & CRANSTON, F.P. *Zoologica (New York) 50:*1, 1965.
14. BULL, L.B., CULVENOR, C.C.J. & DICK, A.T. The pyrrolizidine alkaloids. North-Holland Publ. Co., Amsterdam, 1968.
15. BUTLER, C.G. *Biol. Rev. 42:*42, 1967.
16. BUTLER, C.G. In: Advances in Chemoreception I. (Ed. J.W. Johnston *et al.*), Appleton-Century Crofts, New York, p. 35, 1970.
17. CARDÉ, R.T., ROELOFS, W.L. & DOANE, C.C. *Nature 241:*474, 1973.
18. CULVENOR, C.C.J. & EDGAR, J.A. *Experientia 28:*627, 1972.
19. DAHM, K.H., MEYER, D., FINN, W.F., REINOLD, V. & RÖLLER, H. *Naturwiss. 58:*265, 1971.
20. EDGAR, J.A. & CULVENOR, C.C.J. *Nature 248:*614, 1974.
21. EDGAR, J.A., CULVENOR, C.C.J. & ROBINSON, G.S. *J. Austr. Entomol. Soc. 12:*144, 1973.
22. EDGAR, J.A., CULVENOR, C.C.J. & SMITH, L.W. *Experientia 27:* 761, 1971.
23. EITER, K. In: Chemie der Pflanzenschutz- und Schädlingsbekämpfungsmittel I (Ed. R. Wegler), Springer Verlag, Berlin-Heidelberg-New York, p. 497, 1970.
24. FABRE, J.H. Souvenirs Entomologiques. Ch. Delagrave, Paris, 1879.
25. FATZINGER, C.W. *Ann. Ent. Soc. Am. 66:*1147, 1973.
26. FERKOVICH, S.M., MAYER, M.S. & RUTTNER, R.R. *J. Insect Physiol. 19:*2231, 1973.
27. GANYARD, M.C. & BRADY, U.E. *Ann. Ent. Soc. Am. 65:*1279, 1972.
28. JACOBSON, M. Insect sex pheromones. Academic Press, New York-London, 1972.
29. JEFFERSON, R.N. & RUBIN, R.E. *Ann. Ent. Soc. Am. 66:*277, 1973.
30. KAAE, R.S. & SHOREY, H.H. *Ann. Ent. Soc. Am. 65:*436, 1972.
31. KAAE, R.S., SHOREY, H.H. & GASTON, L.K. *Science 179:*487, 1973.
32. KAFKA, W.A. *Z. vergl. Physiol. 70:*105, 1970.

33. KAFKA, W.A., OHLOFF, G., SCHNEIDER, D. & VARESCHI, E. *J. Comp. Physiol.* *87:*277, 1973.
34. KAISSLING, K.-E. In: Handb. Sensory Physiol. Vol. IV, Part 1, (Ed., L. Beidler) Springer Verlag, Berlin-Heidelberg-New York, p. 351, 1971.
35. KAISSLING, K.-E. & PRIESNER, E. *Naturwiss.* *57:*23, 1970.
36. KARLSON, P. *Ergebn. Biol.* *22:*213, 1960.
37. KARLSON, P. & BUTENANDT, A. *Ann. Rev. Entomol.* *4:*39, 1959.
38. KARLSON, P. & LÜSCHER, M. *Naturwiss.* *46:*63, 1959.
39. KARLSON, P. & SCHNEIDER, D. *Naturwiss.* *60:*113, 1973.
40. KASANG, G. In: Gustation and Olfaction (Ed., G. Ohloff & A.F. Thomas), Academic Press, London-New York, p. 245, 1971.
41. KASANG, G. *Naturwiss.* *60:*95, 1973.
42. KASANG, G. & KAISSLING, K.-E. In: Olfaction and Taste IV (Ed., D. Schneider), Wissensch. Verl. Ges., Stuttgart., p. 200, 1972.
43. KASANG, G., SCHNEIDER, D. & BEROZA, M. *Naturwiss.* *61:*130, 1974.
44. KENNEDY, J.S. & MARSH, D. *Science* *184:*999, 1974.
45. KLUN, J.A., CHAPMAN, O.L., MATTES, K.C., WOJTKOWSKI, P.W., BEROZA, M. & SONNET, P.E. *Science* *181:*661, 1973.
46. LEYRER, R.L. & MONROE, R.E. *J. Insect Physiol.* *19:*2267, 1973.
47. LINDAUER, M. & MARTIN, H. *Naturwiss.* *50:*509, 1963.
48. MAC CONNELL, J.G. & SILVERSTEIN, R.M. *Angew. Chem.* *85:*647, 1973.
49. MARTIN, H. *Z. vergl. Physiol.* *48:*481, 1964.
50. MEINWALD, J., BORIACK, C.J., SCHNEIDER, D., BOPPRÉ, M., WOOD, W.F. & EISNER, T. *Experientia,* 1974. In press.
51. MEINWALD, H., CHALMERS, M., PLISKE, T.E. & EISNER, T. *Tetrahedron Lett.* 47:4893, 1968.
52. MEINWALD, J., MEINWALD, Y.C. & MAZZOCCHI, P.H. *Science* *164:*1174, 1969.
53. MEINWALD, J., MEINWALD, Y.C., WHEELER, J.W., EISNER, T. & BROWER, L.P. *Science* *151:*583, 1966.
54. MEINWALD, J. & THOMPSON, W.R. 1973. Unpublished.
55. MEINWALD, J., THOMPSON, W.R., EISNER, T. & OWEN, D.F. *Tetrahedron Lett.* *38:*3485, 1971.
56. MINKS, A.K., ROELOFS, W.L., RITTER, F.J. & PERSOONS, C.J. *Science* *180:*1073, 1973.
57. MITCHELL, R.T. & ZIM, H.S. Butterflies and Moths. Golden Press, New York, 1964.
58. MYERS, J. *Am. Zool.* *12:*545, 1972.
59. MYERS, J.H. & BROWER, L.P. *J. Insect Physiol.* *15:*2117, 1969.
60. PARETO, A. *Z. Zellforsch.* *131:*109, 1972.
61. PERCY, J.E. & WHEATHERSTONE, J. *Can. Ent.* *103:*1733, 1971.
62. PLISKE, T. & EISNER, T. *Science* *164:*1170, 1969.
63. PRIESNER, E. *Fortschr. Zool.* *22:*49, 1973.
64. REICHSTEIN, T. VON EUW, J., PARSON, J.A. & ROTHSCHILD, M. *Science* *161:*861, 1968.

65. RIDDIFORD, L.M. *Science 158:*139, 1967.
66. RIDDIFORD, L.M. & WILLIAMS, C.M. *Science 155:*589, 1967.
67. RIDDIFORD, L.M. & WILLIAMS, C.M. *Biol. Bull. 140:*1, 1971.
68. RILEY, R.G., SILVERSTEIN, R.M. & MOSER, J.C. *Science 183:* 760, 1974.
69. RITTER, F.J., ROTGANS, I.E.M., TALMAN, E., VERWEIL, P.E.J. & STEIN, F. *Experientia 29:*530, 1973.
70. RÖLLER, H., BIEMANN, K., BJERKE, J.S., NORGARD, D.W. & MC SHAN, W.H. *Acta Ent. Bohemoslov. 65:*208, 1968.
71. ROTHSCHILD, M. *New Scientist May, 1972:*318, 1972.
72. SCHNEIDER, D. *Sympos. Soc. Exp. Biol. 20:*273, 1965.
73. SCHNEIDER, D. In: Gustation and Olfaction (Ed., G. Ohloff & A.F. Thomas), Academic Press, New York-London, p. 45, 1971.
74. SCHNEIDER, D. *Scientific American 231(No. 1):*28, 1974.
75. SCHNEIDER, D., BOPPRÉ, M., MEINWALD, J., BORIACK, C. & THOMPSON, W.R. Unpublished results, 1974.
76. SCHNEIDER, D. & KAISSLING, K.-E. *Zool. J. Anat. 76:*223, 1957.
77. SCHNEIDER, D., LACHER, V. & KAISSLING, K.-E. *Z. vergl. Physiol. 48:*632, 1964.
78. SCHNEIDER, D. & SEIBT, U. *Science 164:*1173, 1969.
79. SCHNEIDER, D. & STEINBRECHT, R.A. *Symp. Zool. Soc. (London) 23:*279, 1965.
80. SCHWINCK, I. *Z. vergl. Physiol. 37:*19, 1954.
81. SCHWINCK, I. *Z. vergl. Physiol. 37:*439, 1955.
82. SEIBT, U., SCHNEIDER, D. & EISNER, T. *Z. Tierpsychol. 31:* 513, 1973.
83. SHOREY, H.H. In: Control of Insect Behavior by Natural Products (Ed., D.L. Wood *et al.*), Academic Press, New York-London, p. 249, 1970.
84. SHOREY, H.H. *Ann. Rev. Entomol. 18:*349, 1973.
85. SHOREY, H.H. & FARKAS, S.R. *Ann. Ent. Soc. Am. 66:*1213, 1973.
86. SHOREY, H.H. & GASTON, L.K. *Ann. Ent. Soc. Am. 58:*604, 1965.
87. SOWER, L.L., KAAE, R.S. & SHOREY, H.H. *Ann. Ent. Soc. Am. 66:*1121, 1973.
88. STEINBRECHT, R.A. *Z. Zellforsch 64:*227, 1964a.
89. STEINBRECHT, R.A. *Z. vergl. Physiol. 48:*341, 1964b.
90. STEINBRECHT, R.A. *J. Cell Sci. 4:*39, 1969.
91. STEINBRECHT, R.A. *Z. Morph. Tiere 68:*93, 1970.
92. STEINBRECHT, R.A. *Z. Zellforsch 139:*533, 1973.
93. STEINBRECHT, R.A. & KASANG, G. In: "Olfaction & Taste IV" (Ed., D. Schneider), Wissenschaftl, Verlagsges., Stuttgart, p. 193, 1972.
94. STEINER, G. *Naturwiss. 40:*514, 1953.
95. TRAYNIER, R.M.M. *Can. Entomol. 102:*534, 1970.
96. TREUSCH, H.W. *Naturwiss. 54:*592, 1967.
97. TUMLINSON, J.H., SILVERSTEIN, R.M., MOSER, J.C., BROWNLEE, R.G. & RUTH, J.M. *Nature 234:*348, 1971.
98. TUMLINSON, J.H., MOSER, J.C., SILVERSTEIN, R.M., BROWNLEE, R.G. & RUTH, J.M. *J. Insect Physiol. 18:*809, 1972.

99. WILSON, E.O. In: Chemical Ecology (Ed., E. Sontheimer & J.E. Simenone), Academic Press, New York-London, p. 133, 1970.
100. WILSON, E.O. & BOSSERT, W.H. *Recent Progr. Hormone Res.* *19:* 673, 1963.
101. WRIGHT, R.H. *Can. Entomol.* *90:*81, 1958.

# CHEMORECEPTION AND SELECTION OF OVIPOSITION SITES BY PHYTOPHAGOUS INSECTS

S. Gothilf

Israel Institute for Biological Research

Ness Ziona, Israel

In most phytophagous insects, the host range of the species is determined by the adults, which select the host as the appropriate site for egg laying. In some insects the eggs are laid quite far from the host, for example, in the case of locusts, even in the ground, in which case the larvae have to make the host selection. Even when eggs are laid on the host, larvae often select a certain organ or tissue of the host plant for feeding.

The physiology of the chemo-sensory organs of larvae and the feeding behavior have been studied extensively in quite a number of insects. However, the primary and most important stage of host selection, namely, locating the host for egg laying by the females, has been scarcely investigated.

In analysing the oviposition behavior of the hornworm, *Manduca sexta* (L), Yamamoto and his colleagues (1969) constructed a scheme to show the major components of oviposition behavior of the hornworm which is reproduced in Fig. 1. Comparison of Yamamoto's data with observations on oviposition behavior of other insects suggests that the sequence of behavior delineated in Fig. 1 is true for other lepidoptera as well as for other insects.

Dispersal flight is common to alate insects; after such flight, and probably influenced by host odors, the insect starts searching. The pattern of the searching flight of *M. sexta* as observed in a cage, is circular; the moth may approach objects and plants. The fact that approach is affected by visual cues is known for a few insects. The females of *Pieris brassicae* tend to approach green plants even when the plant is covered with glass (David & Gardiner

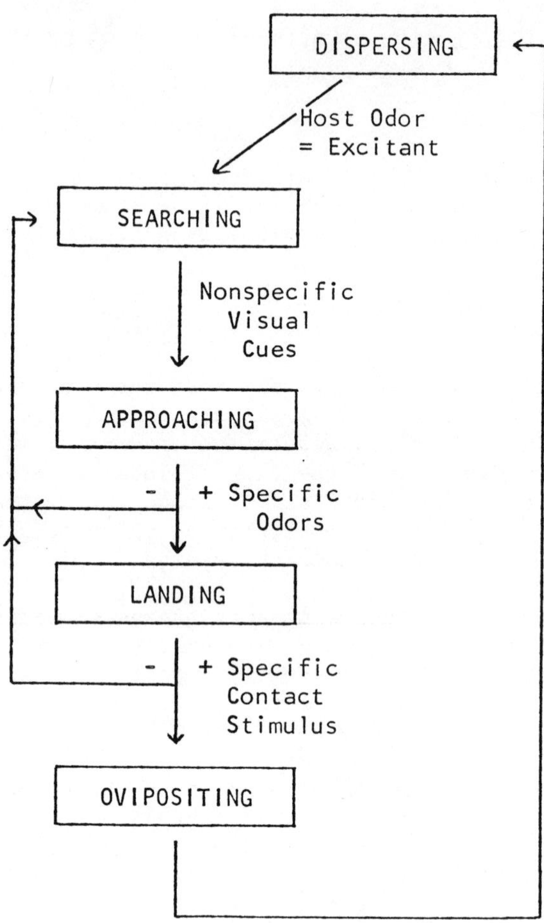


<u>Fig. 1</u> Scheme showing major behavioral components of oviposition behavior of *M. sexta* adult. (From Yamamoto *et al.*, 1969)

1962). For *Trichoplusia ni*, yellow paper is more attractive than paper of other colors (Shorey 1964).

Females of the hornworm veer away from a non-host plant at a distance of 4 - 15 cm, but will land on the appropriate host. There is no doubt as to the stimulatory effect of plant odors at this stage. The question is, from what distance does the insect detect the host? Thorsteinson (1960) remarked that insects are probably unable to recognize the host at a distance of more than a few cm. However, *Scolytus*, and apparently other bark beetles as well, can orient towards weakened or freshly cut trees by following the gradients of volatile attractants from distances of 1000 ft or more (Meyer and Norris 1967; Baker and Norris 1968). Shorey (1964) showed in *Trichoplusia ni* that humidity is also important in stimulating the females to land on the plant. Likewise, a combination of odor and moisture was more attractive to *Manduca sexta* than odor alone (Sparks 1973). So far there is no data available on the structure and reaction of the female's olfactory receptor cells which are responsible for host recognition. It should be noted that the discriminatory ability of insects is highly developed - females can recognize and land on their specific host even when the plant is in the midst of others belonging to different botanical groups.

Once the female has landed on the host, both chemical and mechanical contact stimuli are needed to induce oviposition. David and Gardiner (1962) observed that females of the large white butterfly drum with their forelegs on the upper side of the leaf before laying eggs, as if to taste the leaf. This was confirmed by Ma and Schoonhoven (1973), who described a type of trichoid sensillum which appears in greater number in females, especially on the fifth tarsomere of the forelegs. Each hair contains five receptor cells - 4 chemoreceptors and 1 mechanoreceptor. By recording the electrical response from these sensillae, they found that one cell responded to components of mustard oil which are specific to plants of the family Cruciferae. This botanical group serves as host for the white butterfly. Mustard oil was the first plant substance considered to be a specific chemical stimulus which enables cruciferous feeders to recognize their host (Verschaeffelt 1910). Plant chemicals which have been identified as oviposition stimulants are listed in Table 1. The term "stimulant" is used here in a broad sense, since the methods applied in these studies do not permit accurate designation (according to Dethier *et al.* 1960) of the chemicals, whether attractants which draw the insects from a distance or oviposition stimulants for females which have already encountered the odor source, or both. At least for the bark beetle, it is strongly indicated that the volatile components of the oleoresin attract the pioneer female to the breeding site from a distance (Rudinsky 1966). Degradation products of dying wood, such as vanillin and syringaldehyde, are believed to be oviposition attractants for other species of this group (Meyer and Norris 1967). It should be pointed out, however, that the female beetles bore galleries and feed before laying eggs, therefore, whether the attractive chemicals are oviposition or food attractants is not established.

In addition to known, naturally-occurring, oviposition stimulants, there are a number of chemical oviposition stimulants whose relation to the host plant is doubtful. Such chemicals, and the corresponding reacting insects are:

Glyceryl-triacetate - Corn earworm (Jones *et al.* 1970)
t-6-Nonen-1-ol acetate - Melon fly (Keiser *et al.* 1973) and
2-Chloro-ethanol - Queensland fruit fly (Fletcher and Watson 1974).

The insects listed in Table 1 are oligophagous in the sense that each oviposits and feeds only on closely related plants. This is the common definition of oligophagy. Polyphagous insects, on the other hand, feed on a large variety of plants belonging to different families. Obviously, such definitions are arbitrary; therefore, phytophagous insects are usually classified according to plant chemicals which stimulate feeding and oviposition. Thus, Dethier (1947) suggested that the term "monophagy" be restricted to insects which are stimulated by one chemical or by a few closely related chemicals perceived as one by the insect; oligophagous insects are those which are stimulated by different chemicals distinguished by the insect, and polyphagous insects will accept any food provided it does not contain inhibitory or repellent compounds. Thorsteinson (1960) also proposed a classification of host preference, based on the presence of chemical stimulants in plants. Such classification seems to be valid provided it is supported by enough data on the insect's sensory reaction to chemicals of plants accepted or not accepted by it. However, there is not sufficient information available on this subject, especially with regard to host finding by gravid females.

The carob moth, whose oviposition behavior we are currently investigating, feeds on fruits of a variety of trees, such as almond, accacia, carob, citrus, quince, palm dates, etc. When laying eggs on the carob, the females prefer pods infested by the fungus *Phomopsis ceratoniae*. We have found that the ether extract of the volatile fraction of such carob pods contains various alcohols of which ethanol, n-propanol, iso-propanol, n-butanol and iso-butanol, are oviposition stimulants (Gothilf *et al.* 1974). These alcohols are less stimulating than the total extract which contains additional components still unidentified. It is obvious at this stage that selection of oviposition sites by this polyphagous insect is affected by a number of chemicals. Humidity was found not to influence the insect response. The difference between electroantennogram response to total extract of the fungus-infested carob pods (about 3 mv) and the response to each of the stimulating alcohols (about 1 mv) suggests that olfactory cells having a variable spectrum of sensitivity

TABLE I

NATURALLY OCCURRING CHEMICAL OVIPOSITION STIMULANTS

| Chemical stimulant | Responsive insect | Reference |
|---|---|---|
| Mustard oil (sinigrin, allyl isothiocyanate etc.) | Diamond-back moth | Gupta & Thorstein 1960 |
| | Cabbage root fly | Traynier 1965 |
| | The large white butterfly | David & Gardiner 1962 |
| | | Ma & Schoonhoven 1973 |
| α - Farnesene | Codling moth | Wearing & Hutchins 1973 |
| Terpenes (pinene, limonene, camphene, terpineol etc.) | Bark and timber beetles | Rudinsky 1966 |

are involved. Once the carob stimulants are identified, we will try to find out what are the stimulatory chemicals which induce egg laying on other hosts. Such a comparative study should contribute to a better understanding of the mode in which a polyphagous insect selects its host for egg laying.

ACKNOWLEDGEMENT

The experimental work reported here was done in the laboratory of Professor M.V.L. Bennet at the Albert Einstein College of Medicine, New York. I am indebted to him for agreement to use unpublished figures. I wish to thank Professor R. Werman for helpful discussions and for his critical reading of the manuscript.

## REFERENCES


1. BAKER, J.E. & NORRIS, D.M. *Ann. Entomol. Soc. Amer.* *61:*1248, 1968.
2. FLETCHER, B.S. & WATSON, C.A. *Ann. Entomol. Soc. Amer.* *67:*21, 1974.
3. GOTHILF, S., LEVI, E., COOPER, R. & LAVIE, D. Submitted for publication.
4. GUPTA, P.D. & THORSTEINSON, A.J. *Ent. exp. & appl.* *3:*305, 1960.
5. DAVID, W.A.L. & GARDINER, B.O.C. *Bull. Ent. Res.* *53:*91, 1962.
6. DETHIER, V.G. Chemical Insect Attractants and Repellents. The Blakkton Co., Philadelphia. (1947).
7. DETHIER, V.G., BROWN, L.B. & SMITH, C.N. *J. Econ. Entomol.* *53:*134 (1960).
8. HOVANITZ, W. & CHANG, V.C.S. *J. Res. Lepid.* *3:*159, 1964.
9. JONES, R.L., BURTON, R.L., BOWMAN, M.C. & BEROZA, M. *Science* *168:*856, 1970.
10. KEISER, I., KOBAYASHI, R.M., MIYASHITA, D.H., JACOBSON, M., HARRIS, E.J. & CHAMBERS, D.L. *J. Econ. Entomol.* *66:*1355, 1973.
11. MA, W.C. & SCHOONHOVEN, L.M. *Ent. exp. & appl.* *16:*343, 1973.
12. MEYER, H.S. & NORRIS, D.M. *Ann. Entomol. Soc. Amer.* *60:*642, 1967.
13. MEYER, H.S. & NORRIS, D.M. *Ann. Entomol. Soc. Amer.* *60:*858, 1967.
14. RUDINSKY, J. *Science* *152:*218, 1966.
15. SHOREY, H.H. *Ann. Entomol. Soc. Amer.* *57:*165, 1964.
16. SPARKS, M.R. *Ann. Entomol. Soc. Amer.* *66:*571, 1973.
17. THORSTEINSON, A.J. *Ann. Rev. Entomol.* *5:*193, 1960.
18. TRAYNIER, R.M.M. *Nature* *207:*218, 1965.
19. VERSCHAEFFELT, E. *Proc. Acad. Sci., Amsterdam* *14:*536, 1910.
20. WEARING, C.H. & HUTCHINS, R.F.N. *J. Insect Physiol.* *19:*1251, 1973.

# TASTE RECEPTORS

Lloyd Beidler

Florida State University

Tallahassee, Florida, U.S.A.

*When they came to Marah, they could not drink the water of Marah because it was bitter; therefore it was named Marah. And the people murmured against Moses, saying, "What shall we drink?" And he cried to the Lord; and the Lord showed him a tree, and he threw it into the water, and the water became sweet.*

Exodus 15:22

## TASTE CELL STIMULI

A typical feature of all cells is the difference in concentration of ions between the interior and exterior; this gives rise to a potential difference that can be measured by inserting a microelectrode inside the cell and an indifferent electrode on the outside. It is this potential difference of a sensory cell that changes when an adequate stimulus is applied. The cell membrane is primarily composed of protein and lipid, with which a wide variety of chemicals can interact, and the application of some chemical species to the environment of a cell will result in a change in the transmembrane potential. It is a peculiarity of the taste cell that it is in direct contact with the outside environment, namely the oral cavity; the chemical nature of this environment changes with food intake. A large variety of chemicals can, therefore, interact with the taste cell membrane as they do with many other membranes. However, the taste cell has the added feature that such interactions lead to a partial depolarization of the cell membrane which results in the initiation of nerve impulses in the nerve with which it synapses.

Thus, it appears that it is the transduction process rather than the typical initial adsorption which is peculiar to taste cells and allows them to respond to a very large variety of chemicals.

This extraordinary characteristic of mammalian taste receptors - their ability to react to a large number of chemicals - has been related in a book written by Cohn in 1914. This book, entitled "Die Organischen Geschmackesstoffe" describes thousands of chemicals known to elicit a taste sensation in man. Today thanks to the organic chemists, this list must run into tens of thousands, most consisting of chemicals not found in nature, but the result of chemical synthesis in the laboratory. Thus, many have no biological function.

The molecular weight of taste stimuli may range from unity of the hydrogen ion to the 44,000 daltons of the recently described glycoprotein of the Nigerian berry, Miracle Fruit. Both charged and uncharged atoms and molecules may stimulate the taste receptors.

Although the receptors respond to a wide variety of chemicals they also display high selectivity. The quality of taste sensation may vary with a slight change in molecular configuration (Shallenberger & Acree, 1971) as shown in the alpha and beta form of mannose,

| | |
|---|---|
| α - D - mannose | Sweet |
| β - D - mannose | Bitter |

or the d and l form of asparagine

| | |
|---|---|
| D - asparagine | Sweet |
| L - asparagine | Bitter |

The genetic basis of the ability of taste receptors to respond to a specific molecular structure is only well known for those molecules similar to phenylthiourea which possess a C-N =S component. Human thresholds for these molecules are distributed in a bimodal fashion, the percentage of people possessing a low threshold depending upon the racial background (Kalmus, 1971).

It was known by the early students of electricity, such as Galvani and Volta, that taste receptors can also be stimulated electrically. Anodal stimulation elicits a taste sensation at low current density. This fact is often used to determine which pole of a battery is positive: if the tongue is touched to the positive pole, a taste sensation results. Von Bekesy (1966) proposed that individual human fungiform papillae containing three to five taste buds with a population of 150 - 250 taste cells can be electrically stimulated to produce but one taste quality, the type of which depends upon the individual papilla. Since it is known that each taste cell can respond to molecular stimuli that represents more than one taste quality, and since each taste nerve innervates more than one taste receptor, these experiments suggest that much information processing may occur in the nerve network immediately below the taste bud, before the taste messages enter the central nervous system.

Does electric current stimulate directly the taste receptors or does it excite the nerve endings? A number of years ago Nejad (1961) and Warren (1965) both indicated that a dual function curve describes the relationship between electrophysiological latency of taste response and the current density applied to the surface of the tongue. As the current density increases, the latency decreases.

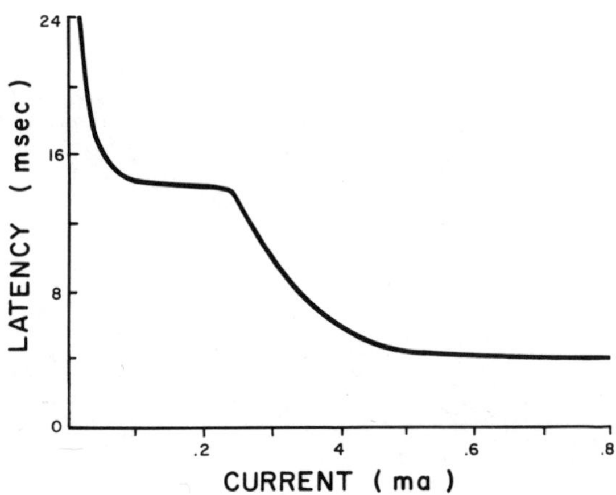


Fig. 1 Plot of latency of electrophysiological response of taste nerve as a function of anodal current applied to the surface of the tongue. The curve indicates a two step process. The 14 - 15 msec latency of the plateau of the first curve is similar to that recorded when the tongue is stimulated maximally with chemicals.

It was argued that low electrical current stimulates the taste cells, probably by ionophoresis, while a higher current density stimulates the nerve innervation of these cells. Thus a tongue treated to deactivate or remove the taste buds will not respond to applied low current density but the free nerve endings do respond at higher current densities.

## TASTE CELL ANATOMY

The foci of taste in mammals are specific papillae containing taste buds. These papillae may be seen on the front of the tongue as red dots. Each human papilla contains three to five taste buds, and each taste bud, 30 - 50 cells. These slender taste cells are about 50 microns in length and synapse with nerves that penetrate the taste buds from beneath. The apical end of each taste cell forms a number of fine microvilli that protrude to the surface of the tongue and interact with the taste stimuli.

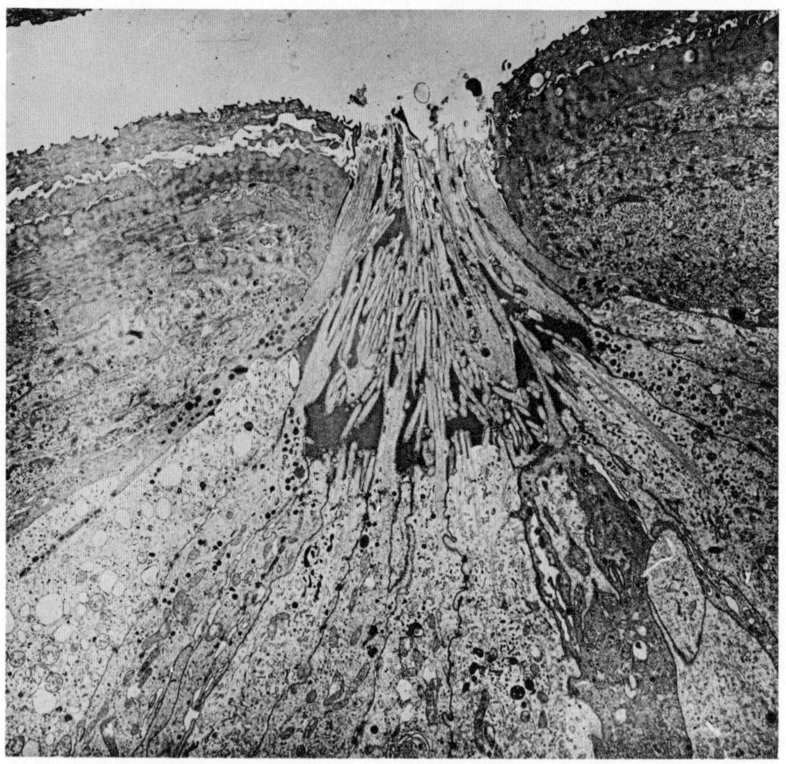

Fig. 2 Electron microscope photo of taste pore showing microvilli of taste cells communicating with tongue surface. Magnification - 8,750 x.

A single taste nerve may divide and its branches innervate several taste cells. The morphology of the synapse shows no synaptic ribbons and only a few vesicles. This lack of classical synapse morphology may be related to the short life of the taste cell.

The chromosomes of individual taste cells have been shown by a tritiated thymidine labelling technique to be formed by mitotic division of epithelial cells surrounding the taste bud, which then move into the buds and differentiate into taste cells. The half life of mammalian taste cells is about ten days. It has been suggested that taste microvilli might have a much more rapid turnover. From such studies we conclude that the taste system, including both the taste receptors and the nerve innervating them, is very dynamic and that new receptor membranes are made available for chemical interaction. The short duration of contact between innervating nerve and the taste cell may account for the fact that the typical synapse morphology as seen with the electron microscope is often missing in taste buds. It is known, for example, that auditory receptors do not show a classical synapse morphology at birth but it slowly appears thereafter.

One taste nerve may branch to innervate not only several cells within a single taste bud, but also more than one taste papilla. Thus one would expect interactions between papillae that would influence the neural response of a single taste nerve fiber. This was suggested by Rapuzzi (1965) who found experimental evidence for interaction between two neighboring taste papillae in the frog. That such interactions were due to taste receptors and not other sensory structures was not determined. A few years later Miller (1971) recorded potentials from a single nerve fiber that innervated more than one fungiform papilla of the rat tongue. He found both inhibitory and excitatory interactions between two papillae when stimulated simultaneously, using a precise microstimulator, by two different taste solutions. Thus, the information concerning a taste stimulus that is relayed by a single taste fiber to the central nervous system is obtained from not only several taste cells of a single taste bud but also from cells from several different taste buds of neighboring papillae. This not only complicates the system of neural coding of taste quality but also makes difficult the study of taste interactions with single cells.

## RESPONSE OF SINGLE TASTE CELLS

It is possible, but difficult, to penetrate single taste cells with microelectrodes and record transmembrane potentials. This was first performed by Kimura & Beidler (1961) who showed that a single taste cell can respond to a wide variety of stimuli representing more than one taste quality. For example, many of the cells may respond to salts, sugars, and acids, although no two taste cells respond in exactly the same manner to a series of stimuli. In performing such experiments it is important to know precisely the microelectrode location. This was not determined in these early experiments, but later Tateda & Beidler (1964) used micropipette iron stains to determine whether or not the electrode was within the taste bud. After more sophisticated methods of cell staining were developed by other investigators, Sato and Beidler (1973) recorded potentials from single cells of the frog fungiform papillae and used Procion yellow to demonstrate that the measured potentials arose from taste receptor cells. Measurement of the transmembrane resistance by Sato and Beidler (1973) and Ozeki (1971) added further evidence that cell membrane depolarization does occur when a chemical stimulus is applied and that this depolarization is related to an increase in membrane permeability. It is interesting to note, however, that the change in ion permeability does not occur at that part of the cell membrane where the stimulus is adsorbed. The magnitude of a response to sucrose, for example, is not influenced by concentration changes of sodium, potassium or calcium applied exterior to the cell membrane. Presumably the depolarization measured occurs at a site distant from the microvilli, probably near the synapse at the base of the receptor cell. Thus, the membrane differs in its properties from one part of the cell to another. This is not unusual, since many cells show such a localization of specific function, a notable example being the nerve where the membrane of the axon differs from the membrane of the synapse.

## MECHANISMS OF TASTE CELL TRANSDUCTION

What is the mechanism by which chemical stimuli interact with the taste cell? Direct evidence is difficult to obtain. However, much quantitative taste data indicate that the chemical stimulus merely adsorbs to the membrane of the microvilli of the taste cell. The epithelium of the tongue surface is rather impermeable to most chemicals, whereas the taste bud contains a pore into which microvilli can project and enter the medium of the saliva, which is in direct contact with chemicals of the oral cavity. Quantitative measurements show that the magnitude of adsorption binding is very small, only several kilocalories per mole for most stimuli.

The relationship between the stimulus concentration and magnitude of response can be expressed by the hyperbolic relationship

$$R = \frac{C\ K\ R_S}{1 + C\ K}$$

where C = concentration, K = association constant, R = response magnitude and $R_S$ = response magnitude at high concentration (Beidler, 1971). This equation adequately describes much of the taste data measured after a steady state response is obtained. The equation is similar in mathematical form to that of the Michaelis-Menton equation, but otherwise there is no relationship, since the taste equation is concerned with an equilibrium reaction whereas the Michaelis-Menton equation describes kinetic events using velocity measurements. Thus the two equations are analogs mathematically but are not related physicochemically. Recently Heck and Erickson (1973) suggested that the response might be related to the rate of stimulus adsorption. However, no quantitative measurements were made to verify this suggestion and there are many facts that cast doubt on its validity. For example, the application of some stimuli will produce a taste that is long-lasting even after the tongue is continuously washed with water. The rate of adsorption is greatly reduced even though the taste response is maintained. Thus it is more likely that the magnitude of taste response is related to the number of receptor sites occupied by a taste stimulus at any given moment rather than the rate of occupancy of the sites.

## STIMULUS BINDING AND TRANSDUCTION

If weak stimulus adsorption to the taste membrane is the initial event, then it should be possible to isolate the membrane molecules involved. During the past decade, there have been many experiments wherein proteins from the tongue were isolated and their interaction with taste stimuli measured. Specific tongue proteins have been found that interact well with sugars, for example (Dastoli, Lopiekes & Price, 1968). Unfortunately, there is as yet no direct evidence that such proteins indeed play a role in the taste mechanism. Since adsorption of chemicals to membranes is a common property of most cells, one must look elsewhere for specificities in the taste mechanism. What events occur between the time the receptor membrane interacts with the chemical and the time a nerve impulse appears in the innervating taste nerve? Little is known concerning this transduction. A number of methods have been utilized to try to study the transduction process. One of the most successful is the use of sulfhydryl inhibitors. Moderate concentrations of PCMBS (parachloromercuribenzenesulfonic acid) applied to the tongue surface for several minutes causes the response to sugars to decrease dramatically, with no decrease in response to salts. The penetration of such inhibitors has been extensively studied in red blood cells. Knowledge gained from these taste studies would indicate that inhibition of the taste receptor does not occur at the receptor site but rather at some later step in the transduction process. If high concentrations of the inhibitor are applied, then both the salt and sugar responses decline. If an inhibitor that penetrates rapidly, such as mercuric chloride, is applied then both responses decline rapidly.

Perhaps sulfhydryl groups are important in the change of protein conformation that is presumed to occur in the transduction process. Thus, there are two important parameters in taste stimulation. The first is the affinity of a stimulus for a particular receptor site of the taste cell membrane. Second is the intrinsic activity of the stimulus molecule that determines its effectiveness in producing a response after adsorption takes place. The affinity is related to the association constant of the taste equation and intrinsic activity is one of several parameters related to the maximum amplitude of response at high concentration of a given stimulus. It is contended here that it is not the affinity a stimulus has for a receptor site within the membrane that is of prime importance or peculiar to a taste cell in comparison to other cells, but rather the transductive events that follow.

The membrane of a given taste cell can respond to a wide variety of stimuli, as noted above. Since a number of different receptor sites exist on each taste cell membrane, it is possible to adapt a given taste cell with one stimulus and produce no effect on its response to another different stimulus. Thus the lack of cross-adaptation is no indication of whether both stimuli are stimulating the same taste cell. Competitive inhibition with the same receptor site of a taste cell can occur and has been shown to be useful in our understanding of the transduction process.

Although single taste cells respond to many chemical stimuli of diverse taste quality, it is possible to inhibit or modify the quality of human taste. A number of early writings mention modifications of taste by various botanical substances. The Old Testament states that Moses placed parts of a tree or shrub into bitter water to make it more palatable for his followers. The identity of this plant is unknown. An old Persian document states that the leaf of a tree grown along the Caspian Sea can temporarily destroy the sense of taste. This leaf has been studied and its active ingredient inhibits sweet taste in a manner similar to the well-studied ingredient of the leaf of the plant from India, *Gymnema sylvestre*. Indeed, many years ago the powdered leaf of this Indian plant was made and sold in tablet form by a major pharmaceutical company in Germany for the treatment of diabetes. Perhaps the most interesting plant is *Synsepalum dulcificum*. Natives of Nigeria chew its red berry to make food more palatable. It makes all sour foods taste sweet. The active ingredient is a glycoprotein of 44,000 daltons molecular weight. The effect of all the above taste inhibitors or modifiers may last up to two hours, depending upon the dosage. An American company, Miralin, currently sells a tablet containing an extraction of the miracle fruit from Nigeria. It is used by diabetics and those on diet to decrease their sugar intake without the need of artificial sweeteners.

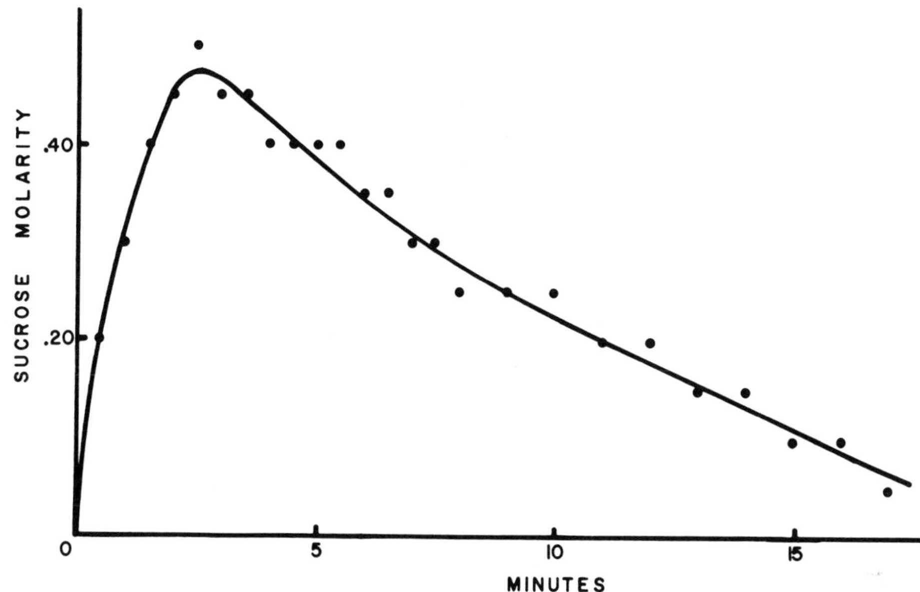


Fig. 3 Sweetness of 0.01 M citric acid at various times after miracle fruit application compared to a sucrose concentration of equal sweetness. The duration of taste modification is dependent upon the amount of applied miracle fruit.

Researchers who are chemically oriented would like to know more about the relationship between the chemical structure of the stimulus and its ability to stimulate taste receptors. A number of studies have been undertaken to determine these relationships. Perhaps the most productive study has been that of Shallenberger and Acree (1967) who first showed a relationship between sweet substances and their structure, using thresholds as an indicator. They concluded that the sweet stimulus molecule binds to the taste receptor site at two points separated by about three Å. Hydrogen bonds are involved and their magnitudes of binding are in agreement with those suggested by electrophysiological experiments (Shallenberger & Acree, 1971). Unfortunately, it is known that not all sweet receptor sites are identical. Some cells respond better to fructose than to sucrose and others do just the reverse. The lack of homogeneity in receptor sites of sweet substances makes structure-function relationships difficult to determine.

*"...its leaves cause the perception of taste be changed, it is so that food can not be differentiated".*

Tohefeh Hahim Moamen
by Mohammad Moamen Hoseini Tabib

## REFERENCES


1. BEIDLER, L.M. Taste receptor stimulation with salts and acids, In: Handbook of Sensory Physiology, Vol. IV, Chemical Senses, Part 2. p. 200. (Ed., L.M. Beidler), Springer-Verlag, Berlin, 1971.
2. VON BEKESY, G. *J. of Applied Physiol 21:*1, 1966.
3. COHN, GEORG. Die Organischen Geschmacksstoffe. Franz Siemenroth SW 11, Hafenplatz 9, 1914.
4. DASTOLI, F.R., LOPIEKES, D.V. & PRICE, STEVEN *Biochem. 7:* 1160, 1968.
5. HECK, G.L. & ERICKSON, R.P. *Behavioral Biology 8:*687, 1973.
6. KALMUS, H. Genetics of taste, In: Handbook of Sensory Physiology, Vol. IV Chemical Senses, Part 2. p. 165. (Ed., L.M. Beidler), Springer-Verlag, Berlin, 1971.
7. KIMURA, KATSUMI & BEIDLER, L.M. *J. Cell & Comp. Physiol. 58 (2):*131, 1961.
8. MILLER, I.J. *J. Gen. Physiology 57(1):*1, 1971.
9. NEJAD, M.S. Factors involved in the mechanism of stimulation of gustatory receptors and bare nerve endings of the tongue of the rat. Ph.D. Dissertation, Florida State University, 1961.
10. OZEKI, M. *J. Gen. Physiol. 58:*688, 1971.
11. RAPUZZI, G. & CASELLA, C. *J. Neurophysiol. 28:*154, 1965.
12. SATO, TOSHIHIDE & BEIDLER, L.M. *Brain Research 53:*455, 1973.
13. SHALLENBERGER, R.S. & ACREE, T.E. *Nature 216:*480, 1967.
14. SHALLENBERGER, R.S. & ACREE, T.E. Chemical structure of compounds and their sweet and bitter taste. In: Handbook of Sensory Physiology, Vol. IV Chemical Senses, Part 2. p. 221. (Ed., L.M. Beidler), Springer-Verlag, Berlin, 1971.
15. TATEDA, HIDEKI & BEIDLER, L.M. *J. Gen. Physiol. 47(3):*479, 1964.
16. WARREN, J.F. JR. A study of the responses of taste receptors of rat tongue to electrical stimulation. Master's Thesis. Florida State University, 1965.

BEHAVIORAL ASPECTS OF CHEMORECEPTION IN BLOOD-SUCKING INVERTEBRATES

Rachel Galun

Israel Institute for Biological Research

Ness Ziona, Israel

Feeding is accomplished through a series of behavior patterns, which, while related and perhaps interdependent, can be considered not only as parts of a single act, but also as separate phenomena, each controlled by a particular set of physical and chemical conditions (Lindstedt, 1971). The generalized feeding pattern in blood-sucking invertebrates is shown graphically in Fig. 1.

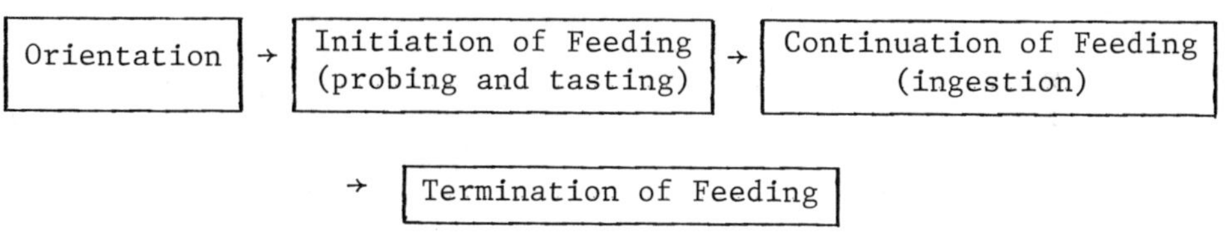


Fig. 1 Generalized feeding response.

The following abbreviations are used in this paper: AMP: adenosine 5'-monophosphate; CAMP: 3', 5' cyclic-adenosine monophosphate; ADP: adenosine diphosphate; ATP: adenosine triphosphate; IDP: inosine diphosphate; ITP: inosine triphosphate; GTP: guanosine triphosphate; CDP: cytidine diphosphate; CTP: cytidine triphosphate; DPNH: reduced diphosphopyridine nucleotide; GSH: reduced glutathione.

The stages in this response are as follows. The insect first must orient itself with respect to the food source; this is accomplished by active movement toward the warm-blooded host, stimulated by a complex of airborne signals emanating from the host. Though these stimuli may show some specific variations, they conform to a common general pattern in which the dominant elements are carbon dioxide, water vapor, fatty acids and their derivatives (especially lactic acid), ammonia, amines and thermal stimuli. Once the insect lands on the host, initiation of feeding is activated by a different combination of stimuli. Probing into the host tissue requires thermal, tactile and sometimes also chemical stimuli.

After probing, two distinct phases can be observed in many bloodsucking insects. The first is questing, sampling or tasting phase, in which the diet comes in contact with the chemoreceptor cells situated in the insect's food canal. If the proper chemical stimulus occurs there, the second phase - sucking by regular pumping - commences.

The two phases in feeding can be illustrated by recording changes in electrical resistance between an electrode touching the insect and a second one submerged in the diet or implanted in the host (Figs 2, 3).

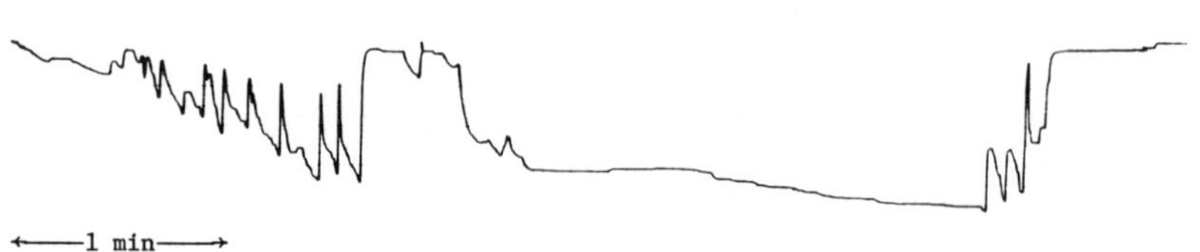


Fig. 2 Record of changes in electrical resistance between tsetse fly and its rabbit host during the feeding process. The initial frequent changes in resistance corresponds to sampling and tasting phase. The long homogenous decrease in resistance corresponds to the second feeding phase - pumping and sucking.

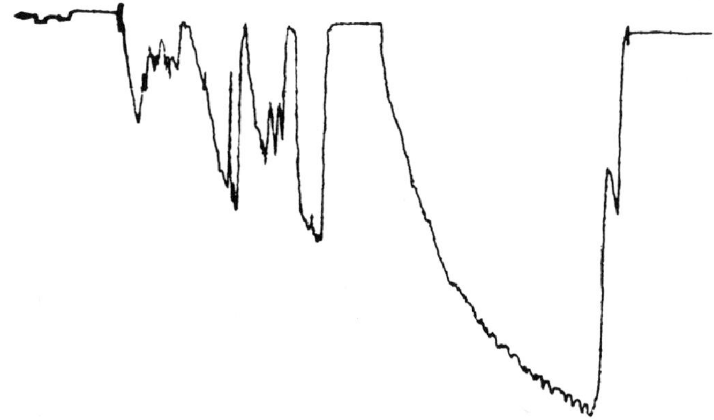

Fig. 3 Record of changes in electrical resistance between tsetse fly and its diet. The diet is whole beef blood presented to the fly through a membrane. The two phases are clearly seen also under these conditions - indicating that the factors required for the first phase are present in shed blood.

During the initial phase, a continuous high resistance is measured, interrupted by transient periods of low resistance which are correlated with sampling activity. This phase was described for *Rhodnius*, mosquitoes and tsetse flies (Smith & Friend, 1971; Owen, 1963; Margalit *et al.*, 1972). Its related physical and chemical factors are not well understood.

Mosquitoes and *Rhodnius* do not possess any chemoreceptors on the parts of the proboscis which come into contact with the diet or with the host tissues during the initial phase. The tsetse fly does have several mechano- and chemoreceptors on the labella. The function of the mechanoreceptors in this phase was described in the present symposium by Dr. Rice. Tasting takes place not only on host tissue or on whole blood, but plasma or saline isotonic with blood also initiate this phase, while water alone is not sampled at all by several parasites (Galun & Kindler, 1965). Thus, osmostimulation is probably important for the initiation of this phase, as well as thermostimulation.

As regards the second phase, the factors which initiate continuation of feeding-pumping and ingestion of the meal have been identified for many parasites. Some data are presented in Table 1.

TABLE I

CHEMICALS IDENTIFIED AS CHEMOSTIMULANTS OF HAEMATOPHAGOUS PARASITES

| Animal | Phagostimulants | References |
|---|---|---|
| Medical leech | arginine > histidine > cysteine > glutamate > aspartate > lysine; glucose = galactose = sorbose (only in the presence of $Na^+$) | Galun & Kindler 1965b, 1968b |
| Soft ticks | GSH > ATP > DPNH > ADP > ITP = GTP; leucine, phenyl alanine, alanine, isoleucine, proline (only in the presence of glucose) | Galun & Kindler 1965a, 1968a |
| *Rhodnius* bug | ATP > ADP = CTP = GTP = CDP = ITP > cAMP > IDP = GDP > AMP | Friend & Smith 1971 |
| Mosquitoes and tsetse flies | ATP > ADP > AMP = cAMP | Galun 1967, Galun & Margalit 1969 |
| Rat flea | ATP | Galun 1966 |

Several conclusions may be drawn from these data:

1. The range of phagostimulatory compounds tends to narrow with evolution, ending with ATP as the only phagostimulant, as observed in fleas (Galun 1966).

2. Like most carnivores and omnivores, haematophagous creatures respond positively to molecules of relatively small size which are widely distributed in animal tissues and blood. All the stimulatory compounds are found in concentrations of $10^{-4}$ to $3 \times 10^{-3}$ M in plasma or blood cells (Table 2).

This however cannot serve as an absolute guideline; for example ATP and GSH which are so abundant in the red blood cell are not available to the insects' chemoreceptors because they are tightly bound in the cell. It is the ATP of the platelets and probably the GSH of the tissues which come in contact with the chemoreceptors (Galun and Rice 1971).

TABLE II

COMPOSITION OF HUMAN BLOOD

| Compound | Blood cells mg/100 ml | Plasma mg/100 ml |
|---|---|---|
| glucose | 70 | 100 |
| amino acids | | |
| arginine | 0.3 | 2.3 |
| methionine | 0.5 | 0.5 |
| histidine | 1.1 | 1.4 |
| ATP | 70 | 0 |
| GSH | 80 | 0 |

Once gorging has started, it was found in *Rhodnius* to proceed to repletion also in the absence of further phagostimulation with ATP (Friend and Smith 1972). On the other hand, in the leech, if after commencement of feeding arginine solution is replaced by saline, the leech stops sucking. Thus this animal seems to require continuous sensory input from the oral chemoreceptors for feeding (Galun and Kindler 1968b). In any event, neither *Rhodnius* nor the leech, nor for that matter mosquitoes or tsetse flies, terminate feeding due to adaptation of chemoreceptors. The volume of meal activates various abdominal proprioreceptors which provide negative feedback to feeding behavior. Perforating the gut to prevent stretching prolongs feeding in tsetse or leeches; cutting the ventral nerve cord in mosquitoes results in massive hyperphagia (Rice 1972, Galun and Kindler 1968b, Gwadz 1969).

The two phases of feeding in the tsetse could be associated with the two distinct groups of sensory receptors found on the mouth parts of the fly. The first group - the labial receptors, whose axons run in the labial nerve to the subesophageal ganglion - is involved in the first phase of questing and tasting. The second group - the labrocibarial receptors, whose axons run via the labrocibarial and tritocerebral nerves to the tritocerebrum - controls the second phase of pumping and ingestion of the food (Rice *et al.* 1973a). Using scanning and transmission electron microscopy all the mouth-part sensilla of the tsetse fly have been cataloged.

The labium is equipped with seven different types of sensilla; four of these are at the distal tip of the labium, i.e., in the labella (Table 3).

Only two of the labellar sensilla contain chemoreceptive cells. One type contains three dentritic processes - one mechanoreceptor and two chemoreceptors. The second sensilla contains two dentrites - one mechano- and one chemoreceptor.

Thus altogether the labella carry only 24 chemosensory neurons, situated so that they can detect tissue or blood components and initiate tasting. This number is small in comparison to the 1,600 labellar chemoreceptors described in *Phormia* (Wilezek, 1967). It is reasonable to assume that the tsetse is likely to accept only a limited range of phagostimulants. As noted earlier, the stimulants responsible for the phagostimulation phase are not known yet. As soon as adequate stimulus is detected by the labial receptors, the fly begins tasting: the cibarial pump is operated in short bursts, so that if blood is present it will be sucked up into the cibarium. Inside the cibarium, the fly is equipped with a variety of mechanoreceptors and one group of chemoreceptors (Table 3, Rice *et al.*, 1973b). This group is the most proximal labrocibarial sensilla and they occur in all the Diptera. In the tsetse fly, they are composed of four basiconic pegs, each having a depression in the center filled with some amorphous material. Each peg is innervated by a uniterminal neuron, the dendrite of which passes up the central tube to the tip. These are the only chemoreceptors within the food canal and thus they have a unique role to play - that of deciding whether the fluid sucked up should be swallowed or not. These four chemoreceptive neurons are highly specific - they react only to isomolar solutions of adenine nucleotides, as can be observed from the gorging response of the tsetse fly (Table 4).

The amorphous material filling the depression in the peg may contain a platelet releasing factor which activates the blood platelets to release their nucleotides at the proper location - the receptor surface. The axons of these chemoreceptive neurons run into branches of the frontal connective and hence to the tritocerebrum. Axons from the tritocerebrum innervate the various muscles of the cibarial pump (Table 5).

Thus the recognition of the presence of blood by the larocibarial chemoreceptors initiates continuous cibarial pumping.

TABLE III

SENSE ORGANS ON THE TSETSE MOUTHPARTS*

| Position | Number | Neurons each | Input to |
|---|---|---|---|
| 1. Internal labella | 8 | 2 Chemoreceptors<br>1 Mechanoreceptor | Sub-oesphageal ganglion |
| 2. Distal ext. labella | 8 | 1 Mechanoreceptor | " |
| 3. Medial ext. labella | 8 | 1 Chemoreceptor<br>1 Mechanoreceptor | " |
| 4. Proximal ext. labella | 6 | 1 Mechanoreceptor | " |
| 5. Labial membrane | 2 | 3 Mechanoreceptors | " |
| 6. Labial shaft | 80 | 1 Mechanoreceptor | " |
| 7. Labial bulb | 2 | 1 Mechanoreceptor | " |
| 8. Labrum | 60 | 1 Mechanoreceptor | Tritocerebrum |
| 9. Anterior lat. cibarium | 5 | 1 Mechanoreceptor | " |
| 10. Anterior med. cibarium | 10 | 1 Mechanoreceptor | " |
| 11. Posterior cibarium | 4 | 1 Chemoreceptor | " |

* From Rice, 1972

TABLE IV

FEEDING RESPONSE OF THE TSETSE FLY *G. AUSTENI**

| | % Response | | | |
|---|---|---|---|---|
| Compound | $10^{-2}$M | $10^{-3}$M | $10^{-4}$M | $10^{-5}$M |
| ATP | - | 93(57/61) | 95(21/22) | 39(5/13) |
| ADP | | 55(12/22) | | |
| AMP | 92(11/12) | 39(5/13) | | 23(3/13) |
| cAMP | | 30(5/17) | | |
| TPN | | 54(6/11) | | |
| IMP | 0(0/12) | | | |
| GMP | 8(1/12) | | | |
| GTP | | 5(1/21) | | |
| CTP | | 0(0/11) | | |
| UTP | | 0(0/11) | | |
| GSH + glucose | | 10(2/23) | | |
| Saline | 10% (1/10) | | | |

*From Galun and Margalit, 1969

TABLE V

EFFECTOR MECHANISM OF THE TSETSE MOUTHPARTS*

| Axons to | From |
|---|---|
| 1. Proboscis depressor muscles | Sub-oesophageal ganglion |
| 2. Proboscis elevator muscles | " " |
| 3. Proboscis protractor muscles | " " |
| 4. Proboscis retractor muscles | " " |
| 5. Labella retractor muscles | " " |
| 6. Salivary pump muscles | " " |
| 7. Fulcrum depressor muscles | Tritocerebrum |
| 8. Cibarial dilator muscles | " |
| 9. Precerebral oesophagus muscles | " |

*From Rice, 1972

In summary, the feeding behavior of the tsetse fly can be delineated sequentially as follows:

Host tissue stimuli

↓

detected by labial sensilla

↓

intermittent cibarial pumping

↓

food flow

↓

food stimuli
(nucleotides from platelets)

↓

detected by labrocibarial sensilla

↓

continuous cibarial pumping

↓

ingestion of meal

↓

meal volume stimuli

↓

detected by stretch receptors

↓

termination of meal

Fig. 4 Feeding behavior of the tsetse fly

## REFERENCES

1. ALBRITTON, E.C. Standard Values in Blood. Sounders Co. Philadelphia, 1952.
2. FRIEND, W.G. & SMITH, J.J. *J. Insect. Physiol.* *17*:1315, 1971.
3. FRIEND, W.G. & SMITH, J.J. Feeding stimuli in hematophagous insects. In: Insect and Mite Nutrition (Ed. J.G. Rodriguez), 1972.
4. GALUN, RACHEL. *Life Sciences* *5*:1335, 1966.
5. GALUN, RACHEL. *Bull. Wld. Hlth. Org.* *36*:590, 1967.
6. GALUN, RACHEL & KINDLER, S.H. *Science* *147*:166, 1965a.
7. GALUN, RACHEL & KINDLER, S.H. *Comp. Biochem. Physiol.* *17*:69, 1965b.
8. GALUN, RACHEL & KINDLER, S.H. *J. Insect. Physiol.* *14*:1409, 1968a.
9. GALUN, RACHEL & KINDLER, S.H. *Experentia* *24*:1140, 1968b.
10. GALUN, RACHEL & MARGALIT, J. *Nature* *222*:583, 1969.
11. GALUN, RACHEL & RICE, M.J. *Nature* *233*:110, 1971.
12. GWADZ, R.W. *J. Insect. Physiol.* *15*:2039, 1969.
13. LINDSTEDT, K.J. *Comp. Biochem. Physiol.* *39A*:353, 1971.
14. MARGALIT, J., GALUN, RACHEL & RICE, M.J. *Ann. of Trop. Med. and Parasitol.* *66*:525, 1972.
15. OWEN, W.B. *J. Insect. Physiol.* *9*:73, 1963.
16. RICE, M.J. *Trans. R. Soc. Trop. Med. Hyg.* *66*:317, 1972.
17. RICE, M.J. *Proc. East African Med. Res. Coum. Conf.*, 1972.
18. RICE, M.J., GALUN, RACHEL & MARGALIT, J. *Ann. of Trop. Med. and Parasitol.* *67*:101, 1973a.
19. RICE, M.J., GALUN, RACHEL & MARGALIT, J. *Ann. of Trop. Med. and Parasitol.* *67*:109, 1973b.
20. SMITH, J.J. & FRIEND, W.B. *J. Insect Physiol.* *16*:1709, 1970.
21. WILEZEK, M. *J. Morphol.* *122*:175, 1967.

# ON THE EVOLUTION OF RECEPTORS ASSOCIATED WITH FEEDING

Howard M. Lenhoff
Department of Developmental and Cell Biology
University of California
Irvine, California, U.S.A.

I would like to present a hypothesis that some neurotransmitter and hormone receptors to amino acids, related metabolites and peptides may have evolved from receptors that originally functioned to stimulate feeding and drinking. This hypothesis is based upon a number of interrelated discoveries showing that feeding and digestion in many lower forms is controlled by specific small molecules.

In order to develop this thesis and to provide the supporting evidence, I shall summarize the information available under the following topic headings:

I. Chemical control of the feeding response of some cnidaria.

A. Gluthathione activation of feeding in hydra including a description of the phenomenon, data on conformation of the molecule, a report on *in vivo* studies on the mechanism of activation, the pH profile of the glutathione receptor, and the proposed mechanism.

B. Chemical control of feeding in other cnidaria and by more than one molecule.

II. Evolution of feeding receptors in cnidaria.

III. Evolution of cellular receptors to peptides, amino acids and their analogs.

## CHEMICAL CONTROL OF FEEDING

During the past two decades, a number of examples have been reported in which the feeding behavior of cnidaria is controlled by specific small molecules. The most thoroughly investigated case is the control of feeding in the freshwater hydra (Loomis, 1955; Lenhoff, 1968). This work has recently been reviewed in detail (Lenhoff & Lindstedt, 1974; Lenhoff, 1974); thus, only the most salient points are presented here.

### Feeding in Hydra

The freshwater hydra are among the simplest of the metazoa. Structurally, they are like a two-ply cylinder closed at the basal end, the other end containing a sphincter-like mouth surrounded by a ringlet of thin long tentacles. The inner "ply" is the endodermal cell layer which contains primarily the ameboid-like cells involved in digestion. Among the cells of the outer "ply", the ectoderm, are the *nematocytes*. These cells contain within their cytoplasm complex harpoon-like structures, the *nematocysts*. These are used to lasso, wound or paralyze potential prey animals. Most of the nematocysts are concentrated in the slender tentacles surrounding the mouth.

During normal feeding, four different behavioral stages can be observed in hydra. First, the hydra, usually affixed to a solid surface, periodically sweeps its tentacles in a concerted fashion toward the verticle axis of its body tube; this step is called a tentacle "concert" (Rushforth & Hofman, 1972). Secondly, when an unsuspecting prey accidently strikes a tentacle, nematocysts in the stricken area discharge and lasso, wound and/or paralyze the prey. Thirdly, contraction of the tentacles toward the mouth, and opening of the mouth is induced by only one of the numerous compounds emanating from the mouth of the prey. The fourth and last step is the actual swallowing of the captured prey.

The third step, the bending of the tentacles and the opening of the mouth, is called the *feeding response* (Ewer, 1947), and has been shown to be stimulated specifically by the reduced tripeptide glutathione (Loomis, 1955). We focused on this step for both practical and theoretic reasons: Practically, this behavioral response was quantifiable: i.e., merely by measuring the times at which the mouth opened and closed, we had an accurate measure of the response, and likewise, the response was controlled by one molecule, a molecule that we could experimentally modify. Theoretically, we believe that by focusing our efforts on understanding how a receptor is activated by a specific molecule, we may be investigating a fundamental cellular phenomenon, one that is basic to similar phenomena in the activation of taste, smell, hormone and neurotransmitter receptors.

## Conformation of the Glutathione Molecule

The unique specificity of the hydra receptor for the size and shape of the glutathione molecule was first indicated by Loomis' discovery that reduced asparthione (β-aspartylcysteinylglycine), which is structurally similar to reduced glutathione except that the glutamyl moiety lacks one methylene group, does not activate a feeding response. This rigid specificity was further documented by studies in which glutathione analogs and related amino acids were used (Cliffe and Waley, 1958; Lenhoff and Bovaird, 1961). Data from all these investigations, summarized in Table I, established the following. (a) The thiol group is not required for activation; ophthalmic acid (γ-glutamyl-α-amino-η-butyrylglycine), norophthalmic acid (γ-glutamylalanylglycine), and S-methylglutathione also activated feeding. (b) The hydra recognized the specific structure of the intact tripeptide backbone of glutathione; the analogs just mentioned activated feeding, and tripeptide analogs with large and charged substituents at the sulfhydryl grouping of glutathione competitively inhibited glutathione action. (c) The receptor has a high affinity for the glutamyl part of the tripeptide; glutamic acid and glutamine were the only amino acids to show competitive inhibition. (d) The α-amino of glutathione is probably required for the association of glutathione with the receptor; glutamic acid competitively inhibited, whereas α-ketoglutaric acid and β-glutamic acid did not.

## *In vivo* Studies on Mechanism of Action

The glutathione-elicited feeding response in *H. littoralis* has been used as a model for the investigation of the mechanism of activation of a specific chemical receptor site (Lenhoff, 1969). These studies required animals that could respond to glutathione in a dependable and quantitative fashion. Of the cnidaria investigated thus far, *H. littoralis* and *H. attenuata* have proved to be the only ones in which reliable quantification of the feeding response was possible. Details of the procedures and of the present assay methods are given elsewhere (Lenhoff, 1961b). The major parameter of measurement was the "duration of the feeding response", that is, the length of time the animal's mouth remained open in the presence of reduced glutathione. This assay, although a measure of behavioral response, is both accurate and objective. The assays were carried out at constant temperature and pH and in a solution of known ionic composition. The experimental hydra were placed directly into a solution of glutathione in order to activate all functioning glutathione receptor-effector systems and thus gain further control over the animals. These conditions differ, of course, from those in nature, where hydra are presented with an oriented gradient of glutathione and of other substances emitted from the prey, in a solution of unknown composition.

TABLE I

PEPTIDES AND AMINO ACIDS SERVING AS EITHER ACTIVATORS OR COMPETITIVE INHIBITORS OF THE GLUTATHIONE-ACTIVATED FEEDING RESPONSE[a]

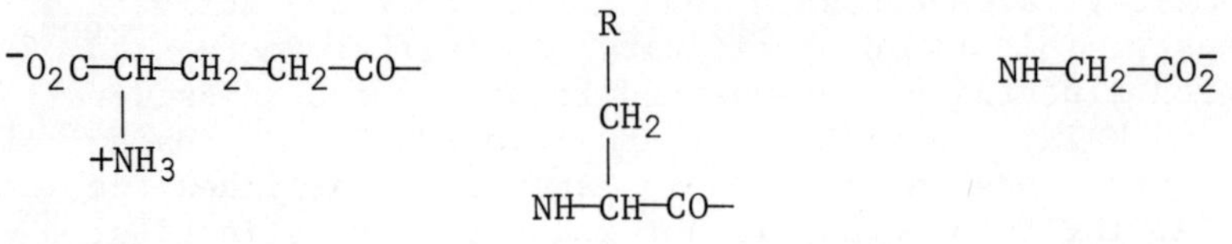

| A | B | C |
|---|---|---|
| $^{-}O_2C{-}CH(NH_3^+){-}CH_2{-}CH_2{-}CO{-}$ | $NH{-}CH(CH_2{-}R){-}CO{-}$ | $NH{-}CH_2{-}CO_2^-$ |
| γ-glutamyl— | alanyl | —glycine |

| Activators | Inhibitors: Tripeptide | Inhibitors: Others |
|---|---|---|
| R = —H | R = $—SO_2H$ | Glutamic acid |
| R = $—CH_3$ | R = $—SO_3H$ | Glutamine |
| R = —SH | R = $—S—COCH_3$ | Cysteinylglycine |
| R = $—S—CH_3$ | R = —S(*N*—ethylsuccinimido) | |
| | R = —S—SG | |
| | R = SH and A = $^{-}O_2C{-}CH(NH_3^+){-}CH_2CO{-}$ | |

[a]The formula represents the basic tripeptide backbone of glutathione and its analogs. For example, when the R of the alanyl component (component B) is —SH, the formula represents reduced glutathione and, hence, is an activator. On the other hand, if R = —S—SG, then the formula represents oxidized glutathione, an inhibitor of the feeding response. A, B, and C refer to the three component amino acids of the tripeptide backbone of γ-glutamylalanylglycine. In the last line of the middle column, A represents β-aspartyl rather than γ-glutamyl. From Lenhoff (1961a).

By controlling our experimental system in the manner described, we procured reproducible results with as few as five animals per measurement.

Using such an assay, we have found, for example, that both environmental calcium ions (Lenhoff & Bovaird, 1959) and sodium ions (Asbill, Danner & Lenhoff, unpublished) are absolute requirements for activation by glutathione to take place. Environmental potassium ions, on the other hand, are inhibitory. All of these effects can be easily reversed by either adding or removing the respective ions. Perhaps these ions act by affecting the cellular membrane potential of hydra.

An indication of the relative speed at which the equilibrium between glutathione and the receptor was attained was determined by means of a simple set of experiments. Hydra placed in a glutathione solution would open their mouths within a minute, and would close their mouths within a minute after the glutathione was removed (Lenhoff, 1961b). These same animals could repeat this opening and closing sequence many times during an hour (Lenhoff, 1961b). Hence we can conclude (a) that glutathione has to be present constantly in the solution, and thus at the receptor site, in order for a response to take place, and (b) that the equilibrium between glutathione and the receptor is rapidly attained.

Other *in vivo* experiments indicate that glutathione is not consumed during activation of the feeding response, that the response eventually stops for some intrinsic reason, and that following this cessation ther is a "recovery" period for the animal to respond fully to glutathione again.

## pH Profile of the Glutathione Receptor

From measurements of the duration of mouth opening, it is possible to determine the dissociation constant between glutathione and the receptor and also to use those equilibrium data to elucidate the nature of the receptor site in the same way that an enzymologist uses data on $K_M$ (the dissociation constant of the enzyme-substrate complex) to help determine the active site of an enzyme.

I have reported elsewhere (Lenhoff, 1965, 1968) the assumptions made in determining the dissociation constant, $K_A$, between the activator $A$ and the receptor $R$. The effect of the activation is signified by $\varepsilon$ and the maximum effect, by $\varepsilon_M$. The equation derived

$$\frac{(A)}{\varepsilon} = \frac{1}{\varepsilon}(A) + \frac{K_A}{\varepsilon_M}$$

is analogous to the second form of the Lineweaver-Burk (1934) plot, the equation developed by Beidler (1954) for mammalian taste chemoreception, and, of course, a form of the Langmuir adsorption isotherm.

Previous data (Lenhoff, 1969) show that this equation can be used to interpret the plot of $(A)/\varepsilon$ against $(A)$; we obtain straight lines at most glutathione concentrations. From such plots we can determine, for example, at pH 7, a dissociation constant of $10^{-6}$ *M*. Such a low $K_A$ is meaningful from at least four viewpoints. (a) The smallness of the constant indicates a high affinity of the receptor for glutathione; (b) concentrations around $10^{-6}$ *M* are well within the physiological range to be expected under natural conditions of feeding; (c) this constant provides a means of characterizing the receptor - that is, the glutathione receptor of *H. littoralis* may be said to have a dissociation constant of $10^{-6}$ *M* under the given conditions. The constant is a characteristic of the receptor and remains nearly the same no matter what the nutritional state of the hydra (Lenhoff, 1961a, b). Similarly, experiments in which the buffer anion is varied alter the maximum response, but not the dissociation constant (Lenhoff, 1969); (d) changes in the $K_A$ with pH can be used to determine the p*K*'s of the ionizable groups on glutathione or at the receptor site which are involved in the combination with glutathione.

The p*K* measurements were made by means analogous to those used by enzymologists in determining the p*K*'s of ionizable groups at the active site of enzymes. For our purposes, we needed an equilibrium equation, like Dixon's (1953) for enzymes, which would take into account the influence of pH on the dissociation constant. This modified equation (Lenhoff, 1965, 1968, 1969) involved the assumption that if the activator, receptor site, or activator-receptor complex ionizes, then, in the expression for equilibrium, each component ($A$, $R$, $AR$) equals its concentration multiplied by a term which is a function of pH. For example, if the activator ionized, then the total concentration of free activator, $A_t$, would be $A$ times the pH function of $A$, or $f_a$ (pH). The logarithimic form of the equation is

$$\mathrm{p}K_A = \mathrm{p}K^0{}_A + \log f_{ar}(\mathrm{pH}) - \log f_r(\mathrm{pH}) - \log f_a(\mathrm{pH})$$

Here $\mathrm{p}K_A$ refers to the negative logarithm of the dissociation constant of $AR$, while $\mathrm{p}K^0{}_A$ is the same constant if none of the components has ionic groups; if no component ionizes, then $\mathrm{p}K_A$ and $\mathrm{p}K^0{}_A$ are equal. (The derivation of this equation is explained elsewhere (Lenhoff, 1968).

The foregoing equation indicates that a plot of $\mathrm{p}K_A$ against pH will consist of a series of straight lines joined by short curved parts, and holds true for the glutathione-hydra system. The results followed almost exactly the predictions from the modified Dixon equations. The following interpretations were made (Lenhoff, 1969). (a) Ionizable groups at the receptor site participated in binding glutathione, because significant variations in $pK_A$ occurred with change in pH. (b) The concave downward inflections at pH's 4.6, 4.8, 6.5 and 7.6 represented p*K*'s of ionizable groups at the receptor site. These p*K*'s probably do not represent ionizable groups of glutathione, which have p*K*'s either below pH 4 (2.1 and 3.5) or above pH 8 (8.7 and 9.6) (Wieland, 1954). If the receptor site is protein, then the p*K*'s determined may represent two β-carboxyls of peptide aspartic acid (or γ-carboxyls of peptid glutamic acid), an imidazole group, and a terminal α-amino group, respectively. (c) The horizontal lines indicate pH values which do not affect the combination of glutathione with the receptor site. (d) The quenching of the charges (Dixon and Webb, 1958) at around pH 4 and 8 indicated that receptor-site groups having p*K*'s of 4.6 and 7.6 may be associated with complementary charged groups of glutathione.

## Proposed Mechanism

A proposed mechanism (Lenhoff, 1969) for binding glutathione to the receptor site suggests that the charged groups at the receptor site bind complementary charged groups on glutathione. This mechanism takes into account previous data which show that the receptor recognizes the tripeptide backbone of glutathione and that the free α-amino of the glutamyl moiety of glutathione is implicated in binding to the receptor. Thus, the positively charged α-amino of glutathione might neutralize a negatively charged carboxyl of the receptor, while the terminal carboxyl of the glycyl moiety of glutathione might bind to a positively charged group of the receptor's terminal α-amino. Similarly, the groups represented by p*K*'s at pH 4.8 and 6.5 may be involved in the binding or may be sufficiently close to the receptor site to be displaced somewhat during the binding process. These displacements were represented by concave upward bends at pH 5.2 and 7.0 (Lenhoff, 1974, Fig. 3).

The proposed binding mechanism indicates the rigid specificity of the receptor for glutathione but does not tell us what happens after the combination occurs. Since, during activation, there was no detectable chemical alteration of glutathione, and glutathione had to be constantly present at the receptor site, it would appear that glutathione operates by causing a reversible modification (possibly allosteric) of the tertiary structure of the receptor, which renders the receptor active (see Lenhoff, 1961a, 1969).

# CHEMICAL CONTROL OF FEEDING IN OTHER CNIDARIA AND BY MORE THAN ONE MOLECULE

It has been shown that the feeding responses of at least 20 cnidaria are controlled by specific chemicals. In addition to reduced glutathione, five specific amino acids have been shown to activate various phases of cnidarian feeding behaviors: proline, valine, leucine, glutamine, asparagine and tyrosine (see Lenhoff, 1974).

The two compounds most commonly observed to specifically activate feeding are reduced *glutathione* and *proline*. Reduced glutathione is the activator in all hydra tested, in two marine siphonophores— the Portuguese man-of-war *Physalia physalis* (Lenhoff & Schneiderman, 1959) and *Nanomia cara* (Mackie & Boag, 1963) — in the hydroid *Campanularia flexuosa* (Lenhoff & Schneiderman, 1959) and in the zoanthis *Zoanthus* sp. (Reimer, 1971a). Proline activates a feeding response in two gymnoblastic hydroids — *Cordylophora lacustris* (Fulton, 1963) and *Pennaria tiarella* (Pardy & Lenhoff, 1968).

Perhaps the most interesting recent cases are those involving two chemical activators. There are at present four well-documented cases, each one very different from the others:

Either proline or glutathione. The coral Cyphastrea responded to low concentrations ($10^{-7}$to $10^{-3}$M) of proline or of a proline analog. Yet the coral would also respond to reduced glutathione or its analog at much higher concentrations ($10^{-4}$M) (Mariscal & Lenhoff, 1968).

Synergistic effects of proline and glutathione. A further variation of the involvement of both proline and glutathione was described by Reimer (1971b). She showed that the Hawaiian zoanthid, *Palythoa psammophilia*, responded best to the presence of a mechanical stimulus in a solution containing both proline and reduced glutathione. Either compound alone was also effective, but only at unnaturally high concentrations. The most effective concentrations for these compounds acting synergistically were 5 x $10^{-5}$M proline and $10^{-6}$M reduced gluthathione (Reimer, 1971b).

Biphasic responses to glutathione and asparagine. Lindstedt (1971b) describes an unusual case in which two phases of the feeding response of the sea anemone *Anthopleura elegantissima* are controlled by different chemical activators. Asparagine controls the contraction and bending of tentacles which brings food to the mouth; reduced glutathione controls the ingestion of food once it has contacted the mouth. A complete feeding response occurs only when both chemical activators are present.

Glutathione and tyrosine activation of "neck" response. Neck formation was discovered by Blanquet & Lenhoff (1968) using hydra (mostly *Chlorohydra viridissima* and *H. pirardi*) whose gastrovascular cavity was swollen with fluid and food particles 1-6 hours following ingestion of food. Such hydra, when presented with *Artemia* extract or a solution of reduced glutathione, formed a tight constriction in the region just below the hypostome and sometimes extending over the adjacent one-third of the body tube. If, instead of a glutathione solution, the swollen hydra were presented with a live *Artemia* nauplius, the neck constriction formed, the mouth opened, and the hydra swallowed the nauplius. During ingestion, the nauplius was carried down through the constriction, apparently by peristaltic contractions, and into the fluids of the swollen gastrovascular cavity. These neck constrictions apparently allow hydra to retain previously ingested food in the gut while swallowing newly captured prey.

Neck formation in *H. pirardi* was shown to be caused by a combination of three factors: (a) the presence of glutathione on the exterior of the hydra, (b) distention of the wall of the hydra's body tube, and (c) the presence of L-tyrosine (*p*-hydroxyphenylalanine) within the gut. No other natural amino acid, including phenylalanine, could substitute for tyrosine. Analogs of tyrosine having either the α-amino or α-carboxyl blocked were inactive.

From these experimental results we conclude that in addition to its external glutathione receptor, hydra has an enteroreceptor specific for tyrosine. The hydroxyl, the α-amino, and the α-carboxyl groups must all be present in order for the amino acid to be active (Blanquet & Lenhoff, 1968).

The existence in hydra of two chemoreceptor systems that must act in harmony represents, to our knowledge, the first report of two integrated, chemically mediated responses in the "lower" invertebrates. This system differs from the asparagine-glutathione system in the sea anemone *Anthopleura* (Lindstedt, 1971b) in which the molecules act in two sequential steps to activate feeding.

<u>Possible non-specific activation by a wide range of amino acids and some peptides.</u> There have been several reports indicating that some cnidaria respond to a large number of compounds (Williams, 1972; Lehman & Porter, 1973; Loeb & Blanquet, 1973). I suggest, however, that the acceptance of the conclusions of these reports be held in abeyance until more work is carried out on the respective organisms investigated. Such caution seems warranted because of the sensitivity of the cnidarian chemoreceptors to extremely low concentrations of feeding activators. Hence, if perchance traces of some active amino acid or peptide were present in the experimental solution, or even released from the cnidarian itself through slight tissue damage, then one would get apparent positive results with a number of "pure" compounds. One control, therefore, which is needed to prove beyond any doubt that a certain compound is a specific feeding activator, would be for an analog of the compound in question to act either as an activator or competitive inhibitor. Such experiments have been

done with glutathione (Loomis, 1955; Cliffe & Waley, 1958; Lenhoff & Bovaird, 1961) and proline (Fulton, 1963). Furthermore, competitive analogs should even inhibit the response of the cnidarian to activators present in tissue fluids released from the prey (Lenhoff, 1961a). Nonetheless, despite these cautionary words, the results claiming that a wide number of amino acids and a few peptides "non-specifically" activate feeding responses merit a further look.

## EVOLUTION OF FEEDING RECEPTORS IN CNIDARIA

### When in Evolutionary Time did the Glutathione Receptor Evolve?

In order to approximate the relative time at which cnidaria evolved receptors for a chemically controlled feeding response, it is first necessary to recognize the precise role of the controlling chemical, that of coordinating the ingestion of the prey once it is captured. Such a coordinated feeding activity requires that the captured prey release fluids containing sufficient glutathione (or proline, etc.) that can be detected by the cnidarian predator. The fluids containing the feeding activator are presumably emitted from the prey after it is punctured by the nematocysts.

Evidence for this coordinating role was obtained by Loomis (1955) in his survey of animals that serve as prey for hydra. He showed that the diet of hydra can include worms and small crustaceans, i.e., animals having either a pseudocoelom, coelom, or vascular system. When such prey were punctured by nematocysts, the wounded animals released fluids which provide sufficient glutathione to elicit the feeding response. Although hydra have been observed to sting other hydra (e.g., Ewer, 1947), they do not normally eat one another, presumably because not enough glutathione is emitted from the puncture of a few cells. Similarly, hydra have not been observed to digest captured flatworms (Ewer, 1947; Loomis, 1955). These facts suggest, then, that the nematocyst-chemical mechanism of coordinating feeding evolved as an adaptation to the presence of organisms having ample fluids which contain glutathione. Since most animals known today to have such fluids belong to phyla higher than the coelenterates, perhaps the nematocyst-chemical mechanism developed late in evolution as a secondary adaptation, much as parasitic relationships developed between some round and flat worms and their vertebrate hosts.

This same reasoning also applied to evolution of receptor sites to feeding activators other than glutathione. As long as a molecule is widely present in prey organisms and has properties distinguishing it from closely related substances, it might serve as a feeding activator. Therefore, it is not too surprising that some cnidaria have evolved receptor sites for compounds, other than glutathione, emitted by the captured prey. About six different amino acids have been shown to affect feeding in a wide variety of cnidaria.

There remains always the possibility, however, that early in evolution cnidaria used the nematocyst-chemical mechanism to feed on some fluid-containing lower organisms such as large protozoa or even medusae. Conceivably, medusae with large gelatinous mesogleas, when wounded, may leak metabolites, one of which could stimulate feeding in the aggressor cnidaria. Little is known, however, about the composition of the mesogleal fluids. The fluids of one medusa, *Aequorea aequorea*, have been shown to contain a substance affecting another medusa, *Stomotoca atra* (Lenhoff, 1964).

It is interesting to note that a glutathione-mediated response has also been demonstrated in an arthropod and in a mollusk. For example, feeding of the tick *Ornithodros tholozani* is activated by reduced glutathione, and glutamic acid competitively inhibits this action of glutatione (Galun & Kindler, 1965). Recently, Kater*et al.* (1971), investigating the neurophysiological basis of the feeding response of the freshwater snail, *Helisoma trivolvis*, found that the response is activated by reduced glutathione (S.B. Kater, personal communication).

## Do the Glutathione and Proline Receptors have a Common Origin?

Fulton has suggested (1963) that the evolution of a receptor site for glutathione into one for the α-imino acid proline may have proceeded by means of slight structural changes in the receptor site. His postulate was based on the knowledge that one of the possible cyclized forms of glutathione in solution is close in structure to an α-imino acid. Because proline is also present in the fluids released from wounded prey organisms, the change in structure of the receptor site was not disadvantageous to *Cordylophora* but, under some circumstances, advantageous, and so persisted.

In accord with this line of reasoning, we might postulate that the earliest cnidaria responded to a wide range of amino acids and to some peptides (e.g. see Lehman & Porter, 1973; Loeb & Blanquet, 1973). From organisms having these general receptors may have evolved organisms with receptors that could respond to a mixture of proline and glutathione (e.g. Reimer, 1971b). Later a single cnidarian species may have had receptors for either proline or glutathione (see e.g. Mariscal & Lenhoff, 1968). Eventually, some cnidaria may have retained receptors for either glutathione (Loomis, 1955; Lenhoff & Schneiderman, 1959) or proline (e.g. Fulton, 1963; Pardy & Lenhoff, 1968).

Other similar routes of receptor evolution in cnidaria could be postulated, such as those from receptors to general amino acids, to one for amino acids with hydrophobic side chains, to ones for either valine (Lindstedt, Muscatine & Lenhoff, 1968) or leucine (Lindstedt, 1971a).

## EVOLUTION OF CELLULAR RECEPTOR SITES IN GENERAL

Among the earliest receptor sites to evolve were probably those associated with the induction of pinocytosis in single cells. In recent years the chemical induction of pinocysotosis has been well studied in ameba (Chapman-Andresen, 1962) and in white blood cells (Cohn, 1967). Both kinds of cells respond to a range of small charged molecules; of the amino acids, aspartate and glutamate are particularly effective. In general, it might be said that single cells depend on external chemical cues which stimulate the uptake of nutrients from their environment; hence, these cells may have evolved receptor sites with broad specificity such as might prove useful to guarantee the cell sufficient food to survive.

It thus seems reasonable to suppose that cnidarian cells utilizing pinocytosis to take up nutrients from their gastrovascular cavity also respond to a broad range of molecules. In accord with this supposition in Slautterback's finding that certain amino acids could stimulate the immediate formation of a large network of microvilli at the apical end of the endodermal digestive cells that line the gut of hydra. Among the most active amino acids were the isomers of tyrosine, with *m*-tyrosine the most active. It is interesting to note that *m*-tyrosine was more active than the other isomers in neck formation (Blanquet & Lenhoff, 1968). Also, as with neck formation, phenylalanine was ineffective. Other amino acids showing activity were cysteine and glutamate (D. Slautterback, personal communication).

Recognizing the "coincidence" that in response to tyrosine hydra display two events, microvilli and "neck" formation (a cellular one and an organismic one), a number of intriguing questions then pose themselves: Is the same receptor site used to trigger both events? If this is not the case, did the receptor for neck formation evolve from the receptor for microvilli formation? It would appear simpler for hydra to use an existing receptor for two functions rather than evolve another.

This line of reasoning may be stretched even further to postulate that there exists a direct line of evolution of receptor sites from those found on single cells inducing pinocytosis, to those coordinating feeding responses in such simple "tissue-level" organisms as the cnidaria, and finally to the receptors for neurotransmitters and peptide hormones in higher organisms. For example, because dopamine and norepinephrine are formed from tyrosine, it seems simpler and more efficient from an evolutionary standpoint for organisms to retain and utilize modifications of a primitive tyrosine receptor for structurally related compounds rather than to evolve new receptor sites for each of these "analogs".

Would not the same argument apply to the evolution of receptors for such neurotransmitters as substance P, glutamic acid or glycine? Are there similar evolutionary relationships between the glutathione receptors involved in activating the cnidarian feeding response, and the glutathione receptor associated with the γ-glutamyl transpeptidase mechanism of amino acid transport (Meister, 1973)? In any of these cases, it would seem simpler for organisms, during evolution, to have modified existing receptors to control new tasks rather than to have developed a completely new receptor-effector system.

Such speculations, like most speculations about evolution, cannot be proved, but they may help to make us aware that unifying concepts, tacitly assumed in the case of enzymes and cell organelles, also may apply to the basic aspects of chemoreception. Specifically, such speculations emphasize that the behavioral responses of lower invertebrates to a peptide or an amino acid may have many fundamental features in common with some hormonal and neurotransmitter responses in man. By focusing on the primary events of the combination of the activator with the receptor to initiate a series of coordinated activities, we may find new approaches and new insights into universal, yet little understood, chemical control mechanisms.

## ACKNOWLEDGEMENTS

I thank Dr. David Slautterback for his comments and for allowing me to quote from his unpublished material on microvillus formation. The research discussed was supported by grants from the National Institutes of Health and the National Science Foundation.

## REFERENCES

1. BEIDLER, L.M. *J. Gen. Physiol.* *38:*133, 1954.
2. BEUTLER, R. *Z. Vergl. Physiol.* *1:*1, 1924.
3. BLANQUET, R.S. & LENHOFF, H.M. *Science* *159:*633, 1968.
4. CHAPMAN-ANDRESEN, C. *C.R. Trav. Lab. Carlsberg* *33:*73, 1962.
5. CLIFFE, E.E. & WALEY, S.G. *Nature (London)* *182:*804, 1958.
6. COHN, Z.A. *J. Exp. Med.* *125:*213, 1967.
7. DIXON, J. & WEBB, E.C. "Enzymes", 1st ed., Academic Press, New York, p. 120, 1958.
8. DIXON, M. *Biochem. J.* *55:*161, 1953.
9. EWER, R.F. *Proc. Zool. Soc. London* *117:*365, 1947.

10. FULTON, C. *J. Gen. Physiol.* *46:*823, 1963.
11. GALUN, R. & KINDLER, S.H. *Science* *147:*166, 1965.
12. KATER, S.B., HEYER, C. & HEGMANN, J.P. *Z. Vergl. Physiol.* *74:*127, 1971.
13. LEHMAN, J. & PORTER, J. *Biol. Bull.* *145:*140, 1973.
14. LENHOFF, H.M. Activation of the feeding reflex in *Hydra littoralis*. In "The Biology of Hydra" (H.M. Lenhoff & W.F. Loomis, eds.), Univ. of Miami Press, Coral Gables, Florida, p. 203, 1961a.
15. LENHOFF, H.M. *J. Gen. Physiol.* *45:*331, 1961b.
16. LENHOFF, H.M. *Biol. Bull.* *126:*115, 1964.
17. LENHOFF, H.M. *Amer. Zool.* *5:*515, 1965.
18. LENHOFF, H.M. *Science* *161:*434, 1968.
19. LENHOFF, H.M. *Comp. Biochem. Physiol.* *28:*571, 1969.
20. LENHOFF, H.M. On the mechanisms of action and evolution of receptors associated with feeding and digestion. In "Biology of the Coelenterata" (L. Muscatine & H.M. Lenhoff, eds.), Academic Press, N.Y., 1974. In press.
21. LENHOFF, H.M. & BOVAIRD, J. *Science* *130:*1474, 1959.
22. LENHOFF, H.M. & BOVAIRD, J. *Nature (London)* *189:*486, 1961.
23. LENHOFF, H.M. & LINDSTEDT, K.J. Chemoreception in aquatic invertebrates with special emphasis on the feeding behavior of coelenterates. In "Marine Chemoreception" (A.M. Mackie & P.T. Grant, eds.), Academic Press, New York, 1974. In press.
24. LENHOFF, H.M. & SCHNEIDERMAN, H.A. *Biol. Bull.* *116:*452, 1959.
25. LINDSTEDT, K.J. *Comp. Biochem. Physiol. A* *39:*553, 1971a.
26. LINDSTEDT, K.J. *Science* *173:*333, 1971b.
27. LINDSTEDT, K.J., MUSCATINE, L. & LENHOFF, H.M. *Comp. Biochem. Physiol.* *26:*567, 1968.
28. LINEWEAVER, H. & BURK, D. *J. Amer. Chem. Soc.* *56:*1934.
29. LOEB, M. & BLANQUET, R. *Biol. Bull.* *145:*150, 1973.
30. LOOMIS, W.F. *Ann. N.Y. Acad. Sci.* *62:*209, 1955.
31. MACKIE, G.O. & BOAG, D.A. *Pubbl. Sta. Zool. Napoli* *33:*178, 1963.
32. MARISCAL, R.N. & LENHOFF, H.M. *J. Exp. Biol.* *49:*689, 1968.
33. MEISTER, A. *Science* *180:*33, 1973.
34. PARDY, R.L. & LENHOFF, H.M. *J. Exp. Zool.* *168:*1968.
35. REIMER, A.A. *Comp. Biochem. Physiol. A* *39:*743, 1971a.
36. REIMER, A.A. *Comp. Biochem. Physiol. A* *40:*19, 1971b.
37. RUSHFORTH, N.B. & HOFMAN, F. *Biol. Bull.* *142:*110, 1972.
38. WALEY, S.G. *Biochem. J.* *68:*189, 1958.
39. WIELAND, T. Chemistry and properties of glutathione. In "Glutathione" (S. Colwick *et al.*, eds.), Academic Press, New York, p. 45, 1954.
40. WILLIAMS, R.B. *Comp. Biochem. Physiol.* *41A:*361, 1972.

# BEHAVIORAL REGULATION OF BIOCHEMICAL AND PHYSIOLOGICAL PROPERTIES OF IDENTIFIED NEURONS

Harold Gainer
Behavioral Biology Branch
National Institute of Child Health and Human Development
National Institutes of Health
Bethesda, Maryland 20014, U.S.A.

## INTRODUCTION

It is generally accepted that behavioral changes resulting from experience (e.g., learning) will be reflected in the nervous system in the form of physiological, morphological, and biochemical modifications (Glassman, 1969; Horn *et al.*, 1973). However, there are a number of difficulties in attempting to bridge the gap between the expectation and the reality of correlating behavioral changes with physico-chemical changes in the nervous system (see Horn *et al.*, 1973; for a critical discussion of these problems). While the intrinsic heterogeneity of the vertebrate nervous system has been effectively overcome by the electrophysiologist's use of "single unit" recordings (see Hubel; Blakemore; this volume), no equivalent approach has been developed for correlative biochemical studies of the nervous system. Furthermore, since the normal adaptive behaviors of most animals are quite complex, and are associated with a wide variety of endogenous and exogenous variables (e.g., multiple sensory inputs, inhibitory and excitatory synaptic interactions, spontaneous electrical activity, and hormonal influences), it is not surprising that the biochemical analysis of behavioral modifications has been slow in its advance.

This intrinsic complexity of the vertebrate nervous system has led us to use invertebrate model systems in which electrophysiological, morphological, and biochemical data can be obtained on identifiable, single neurons, and in which the intact central nervous system can be viably maintained *in vitro* for relatively long periods of time. Such experimental preparations are therefore amenable to studies on the influences of specific synaptic inputs, neurotransmitters, and hormones on the electrophysiological and biochemical properties of specific neurons. Since these variables are probably involved in short- and long-term behavioral changes, it is of interest to determine their impact on neuronal characteristics. In our laboratory, we have focused on their regulation of specific protein synthesis and bursting pacemaker potential (BPP) activity in molluscan neurons. In addition, we have studied the effects of a dramatic change in the behavioral state of the animal (i.e., hibernation and aestivation) on the electrophysiology and specific protein synthesis of a specific neuron in the snail. These studies have been of value in the elucidation of mechanisms which underly modifications of specific neuronal properties, and it is hoped that they will provide insights into the neuronal changes which occur, *in vivo*, in the normally behaving animal.

## MODULATION OF SPECIFIC PROTEIN SYNTHESIS IN IDENTIFIED NEURONS

### Specificity of Neuronal Protein Synthesis

The demonstration that specific neurons synthesize specific proteins has greatly depended on the development of polyacrylamide gel electrophoretic procedures on the microscale (see Neuhoff, 1973; for a discussion of the history and techniques of micro-gel electrophoresis). By electrophoresing proteins extracted from individual neurons, it is possible to identify specific proteins which are found uniquely in specific cells (or cell regions; e.g., axon versus soma). The results will depend greatly upon which extraction procedures are used (e.g., type of detergents in the extraction buffers) and upon the particular gel conditions chosen (Chrambach and Rodbard, 1971). In general, because of the small quantities of proteins available in such studies, we have primarily utilized separation procedures which are also analytical, largely selecting electrophoretic systems such as sodium dodecyl sulfate (SDS) microgels (Gainer, 1971; Wilson, 1971; Loh, 1973; and Neuhoff, 1973) which separate proteins on the basis of size, and micro-isoelectric focusing gels (Gainer, 1973) which separate proteins on the basis of their isoelectric points.

In a typical experiment (Gainer, 1971; Wilson, 1971), the ganglion containing the neuron(s) of interest is dissected out of the animal, and incubated in a physiological saline solution containing a radioactive amino acid precursor (usually $^{3}$H-leucine). At the end of the incubation period, a specific neuron is dissected out of the ganglion and the neuronal proteins are extracted and then separated on polyacrylamide gels. The proteins on the gel are then stained (using Coomassie brilliant blue), the gels are sliced, and each gel slice is counted for radioactivity. Thus it is possible to determine a labeling profile on the gel which is characteristic for a specific cell.

The typical molecular weight distributions of newly-synthesized proteins in three different neurons from the abdominal ganglion of *Aplysia californica*, $R_2$, $R_{14}$ and $R_{15}$ (identified according to the system of Frazier, *et al.*, 1967), after 3 hours incubation in $^3$H-leucine media is depicted in Fig. 1. All three cells showed a prominent zone of labeled protein in the 60,000 dalton region and a minor zone around 40,000 daltons. At molecular weights less than 15,500 daltons, the labeling patterns in these cells differed greatly. A small proportion of the labeled proteins in $R_2$ was found in this region. In contrast, $R_{14}$ exhibited two major peaks of protein synthesis at 12,000 and 6,000 daltons. $R_{15}$ exhibited a prominent peak of synthesis at 12,000 daltons and a smaller peak at 6-9,000 daltons. The synthesis of all molecular weight classes of proteins in these cells was inhibited 95-98% by incubation in the presence of 30 μM anisomycin (Fig. 1 shown for $R_{15}$ only), a potent protein synthesis inhibitor in *Aplysia* neurons (Schwartz, *et al.*, 1971). Similar findings of specificity in protein synthesis patterns of identified neurons of *Aplysia* have been reported (Wilson, 1971; Arch, 1972 a, b; Gainer, 1971; Peterson & Loh, 1973; Wilson, 1974).

Utilizing isoelectric focusing methods, Gainer and Wollberg (1974) demonstrated unique labeling profiles in three cholinergic ($R_2$, $L_{11}$, $L_{10}$) and three neurosecretory ($R_{3-13}$, $R_{14}$, and Bag cells) neurons of *Aplysia*. The neurosecretory neurons synthesized large quantities of specific small proteins, which were found in a putative neurosecretory granule fraction of the cells. In addition, a unique basic protein found in $R_{3-13}$ and $R_{14}$ was also found uniquely in the branchial nerve which contains the axons of these cells. These and other data support the notion that protein metabolism of a specific neuron is as much an identifiable (phenotypic) characteristic as is its morphology, synaptic connections and electrophysiology.

Although specificity in neuronal proteins can be demonstrated by these techniques, a word of caution should be introduced. It is possible that a specific region of the gel may contain more than a single protein (this is particularly true for the SDS gels which separate protein subunits according to their size), and therefore the radioactivity in a given gel slice may not represent the label from a single protein. In some experiments, labeled proteins from $R_{3-13}$ and the Bag cells were separated on individual SDS gels. The slices of these gels which contained the highly labeled low molecular weight proteins were then extracted and the proteins in the gel slices were separated by a different gel procedure (isoelectric focusing). The results indicated that the $R_{3-13}$ low molecular weight peak was composed of at least two individual components and the Bag cell peak was separated into three components (Gainer & Wollberg,

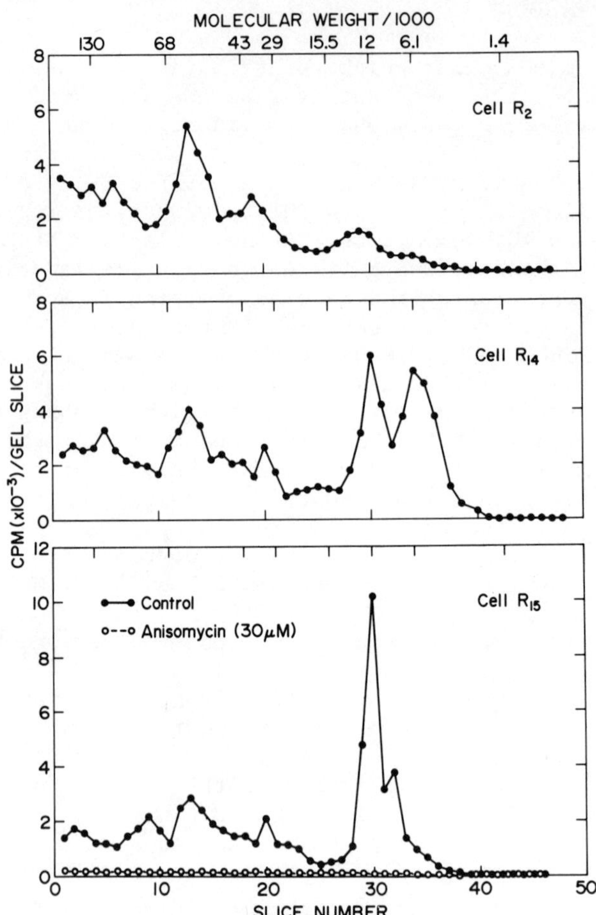


Fig. 1 Typical molecular weight distributions on 11% SDS-polyacrylamide gels of newly synthesized proteins extracted from cells $R_2$, $R_{14}$ and $R_{15}$ of *Aplysia*. Ganglia were incubated in $^3$H-leucine for three hours, after which the identified neurons were removed, and their proteins analysed. Ordinate: CPM/gel slice of $^3$H-leucine incorporated into protein of a given molecular weight (minus background). The lower abscissa represents the slice number from the gel origin (zero), and the upper abscissa represents the molecular weights of standard marker proteins corresponding to the various slice positions. Note differences in radioactive profiles between identified neurons, particularly in the low molecular weight region ( < 15,500 daltons). Anisomycin (30 μM) inhibits protein synthesis in all molecular weight regions (shown for $R_{15}$ only). (From Gainer & Barker, 1974b).

1974). Furthermore, in experiments using a gel system which separates proteins on the basis of size and charge, we have found that the Bag cells contain at least 3 low molecular weight proteins (Loh & Gainer, unpublished data), whereas SDS gel procedures showed only one prominent peak less than 12,000 daltons (Arch, 1972a; Gainer & Wollberg, 1974). With this caveat in mind, that SDS gel profiles often represent molecular weight classes and not individual proteins, we have used this system in the selective modulation studies described below.

## Synaptic Modulation of Specific Protein Metabolism in $R_{15}$

We chose to study the regulation of protein synthesis by synaptic input in cell $R_{15}$ for several reasons. First, the labeling profiles in $R_{15}$ (Fig. 1) indicated that a specific molecular weight class of proteins (i.e., 12,000 daltons) was synthesized in sufficient abundance (about 25% of the newly-synthesized proteins in $R_{15}$ appeared in this peak) so that we could easily evaluate whether this peak was selectively modified (in comparison to total cell protein synthesis) by synaptic input. Second, in contrast to $R_{14}$ which also had a favorable protein labeling profile, $R_{15}$ has a rich synaptic input (Frazier, *et al.*, 1967). Finally, some evidence for electrophysiological plasticity in $R_{15}$ had already been demonstrated (Strumwasser, 1968).

Under control conditions, $R_{15}$ neurons generated typical bursting pacemaker potential activity (Carpenter & Gunn, 1970; Frazier *et al.*, 1967; Mathieu & Roberge, 1971; Strumwasser, 1968) throughout the incubation period (see inset in Fig. 2). These cells produced a characteristic pattern of leucine incorporation into protein dominated by low molecular weight classes. The graph in Figure 2 was constructed by plotting the radioactivity in each gel slice relative to the slice having maximum radioactivity obtained in the 60,-68,000 dalton range of the gel. Such a normalization procedure permitted the comparison of the relative incorporation of $^3$H-leucine into specific molecular weight classes of proteins among different cells and under various experimental conditions, independent of absolute isotope incorporation rates, precursor permeabilities and pool sizes (Wilson, 1971; Arch, 1972a; Gainer, 1972a; Peterson & Loh, 1973).

Branchial nerve stimulation (once every five seconds) evoked inhibitory post-synaptic potentials (ipsps) in $R_{15}$, hyperpolarizing the membrane potential of the cell to about -64 mV for the entire experimental period (inset, Fig. 2). The psp evoked is actually biphasic, consisting of a rapidly decaying depolarizing component followed by a prolonged, hyperpolarizing component. The hyperpolarizing component which predominates is due primarily to an increase in the potassium conductance of the membrane, possibly mediated by dopamine (Ascher *et al*, 1967; Kerkut *et al.*, 1969). Synaptic

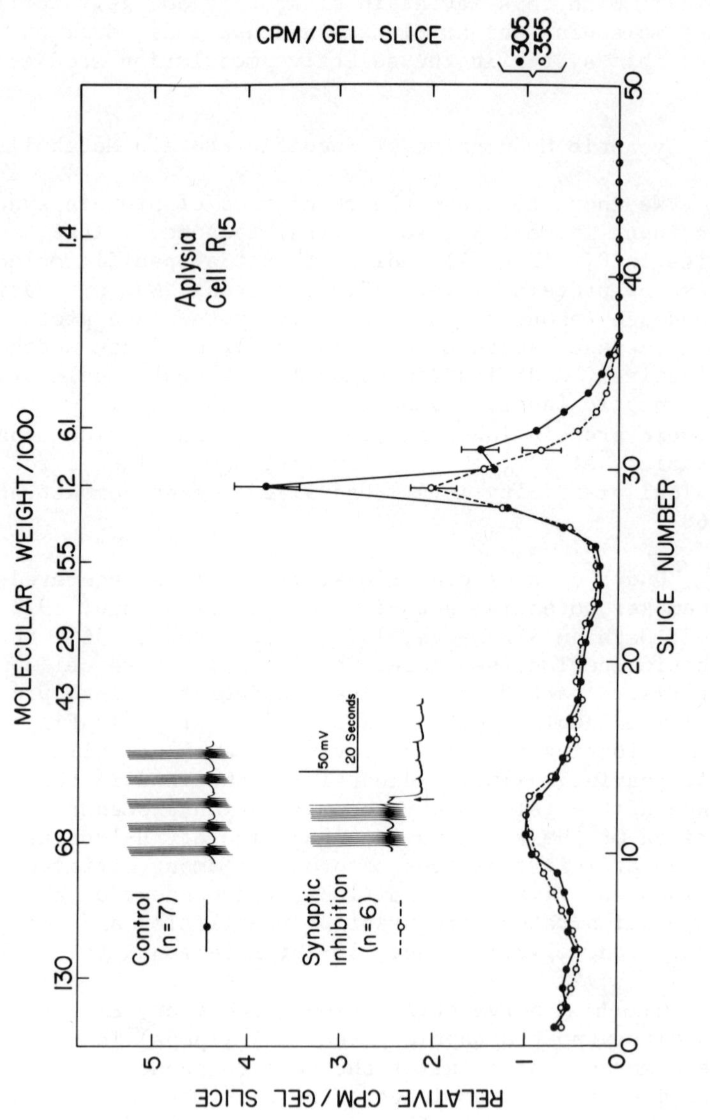

MOLECULAR WEIGHT/1000
130
68
43
29
15.5
12
6.1
1.4
CPM / GEL SLICE
•305
◦355
Aplysia
Cell $R_{15}$
Control
(n=7)
Synaptic
Inhibition
(n=6)
50 mV
20 Seconds
RELATIVE CPM / GEL SLICE
0
1
2
3
4
5
0
10
20
30
40
50
SLICE NUMBER


Fig. 2

Fig. 2

Comparison of the molecular weight distributions of newly synthesized proteins in control (unstimulated) and synaptically inhibited $R_{15}$ neurons. The inset shows the typical pattern of spontaneous bursting pacemaker potential activity in the control cells, and the abrupt inhibition of this activity upon stimulation of the branchial nerve (at arrow). Extracts of the $R_{15}$ somas incubated for 3 h under control and experimental conditions in L-$^{3}$H-leucine were separated on 11% SDS-polyacrylamide gels which were then analysed for their radioactive patterns. Left ordinate: The radioactivity (CPM/gel slice minus background) in each gel slice was plotted relative to the maximum radioactive gel slice in the 60-68,000 dalton range. Right ordinate: Average absolute CPM/gel slice found in a given condition (filled circles, control; open circles, inhibited) which corresponded to the relative CPM/gel slice of unity. The lower abscissa represents the gel slice number, and the upper abscissa shows the molecular weights of standard marker proteins corresponding to the various slice positions. Each point on the curves at a given slice number represents the average relative CPM value of 7 (control) or 6 (inhibited) cells from separate experiments. The vertical bars at the 12,000 and 6,100 dalton points reflect ±1 standard deviation. (From Gainer & Barker, 1974a.)

inhibition of $R_{15}$ did not alter the incorporation patterns of the higher molecular weight classes of proteins (> 15,500 daltons), nor the absolute incorporation rates of $^3$H-leucine into the total protein in the cell, but did produce a selective decrease in the incorporation of the 12,000 molecular weight protein species (Fig. 2). After prolonged synaptic inhibition, the relative CPM/gel slice of the 12,000 dalton peak decreased from a control value of 3.8 ± 0.4 (mean ± standard error of mean) to 2.0 ± 0.3, which represents a 47% decrease in $^3$H-leucine incorporation into the 12,000 dalton protein class (P = 0.001). The apparent decrease in the 6000 dalton peak was not statistically significant (P = 0.037). Thus, the incorporation rate of the 12,000 dalton molecular weight class of proteins in $R_{15}$ was selectively modified by this synaptic input.

Similar effects on the protein metabolism of $R_{15}$ were obtained when the ganglia were incubated in media containing $10^{-3}$ M dopamine, which hyperpolarized the membrane potential of the cell to -65 mV (Gainer & Barker, 1974a). Expressed as a percentage of the total radioactivity (CPM) on the gel, the % radioactivities (mean ± SEM) in the 12,000 dalton region of the gel for control (N = 17), synaptically inhibited (N = 6), and dopamine treated (N = 6) $R_{15}$ neurons were 26.2 ± 1.1, 20.7 ± 1.6, and 16.8 ± 0.7, respectively. No differences in the % CPM at the 60-68,000 dalton region of the gel were found for these three conditions.

Since the electrophysiological consequences of both synaptic inhibition and dopamine treatment were to hyperpolarize the membrane potential and eliminate all spontaneous spike activity, it is important to note that no changes in the incorporation patterns of $R_{15}$ were observed when the cell's spike activity was abolished by tetrodotoxin, or when the cells were hyperpolarized (to about -65 mV) throughout the incubation by replacement of the sodium ions in the media by a variety of impermeant substitutes (see Table 1 in Strumwasser, 1973; confirmed in our laboratory). These data suggest that the selective inhibition of $^3$H-leucine incorporation into the 12,000 dalton peak (Fig. 2) is probably not mediated by either membrane potential hyperpolarization or spike abolition, *per se*.

The foregoing results demonstrate that the amount of $^3$H-leucine incorporated into protein in $R_{15}$ can be selectively modulated by either the physiological synaptic input to the cell, or by direct application of the neurotransmitter dopamine. The selective decrease in incorporation of $^3$H-leucine into the 12,000 dalton peak in $R_{15}$ produced by these treatments could reflect either a decrease in the rate of incorporation of the label into this protein class and/or an increase in its "turnover" (i.e., the degradation rate of this protein and/or its transport out of the cell body). We attempted to determine whether the latter possibilities could account for the results by studying the turnover rates of proteins in $R_{15}$ cells exposed to the same experimental manipulations.

### Selective Protein Turnover in $R_{15}$

Turnover rates were determined by incubating as described above, and then post-incubating in a "chase" medium (which contained 1 mM unlabeled leucine) for various time periods (up to 20 hours). Analysis of control $R_{15}$ neurons treated in this manner showed that the newly-synthesized 12,000 dalton protein class had a very high turnover rate (ca., 2 hours half-time) in comparison to the rest of the newly-synthesized proteins in the cell (Gainer & Barker, 1974b).

These findings are depicted in Fig. 3A. There were no observable changes in the molecular weight distributions of labeled proteins at molecular weights greater than 15,000 daltons with prolonged "chases", but after only two hours of "chase", the radioactivity of the 12,000 dalton protein was profoundly decreased (Fig. 3A). The graphs of the percentage of total gel CPM found in the 12,000 dalton peak (Fig. 3B), and 60,000 dalton peak (Fig. 3C) at various times of chase, show that the 12,000 dalton peak in untreated, control cells decreased in radioactivity with a half-time of less than 2 hours, while the radioactivity of the 60,000 dalton peak increased slightly over the same time period. The increase in the 60,000 dalton peak can, in large part, be attributed to the loss of the 12,000 dalton peak and its relatively large contribution to the total activity of the cell. Similar selective rates of decay were found in $R_{15}$ neurons in which the incorporation of $^3$H-leucine into the 12,000 dalton peak had been selectively stimulated by incubation in saline solutions with elevated potassium concentrations (Fig. 3B and C, open circles). However, in the case of dopamine-treated cells, the decay rate of the 12,000 dalton peak was significantly decreased (Fig. 3B and C, filled squares). The decrease in decay rate of this peak in these cells is in the opposite direction to that which would have been expected if the altered decay rate was responsible for the selective decrease in incorporation of $^3$H-leucine into the 12,000 dalton peak in dopamine. Therefore, the regulatory effects observed with the dopamine treatments were probably not due to altered turnover (e.g., degradation) rates but most likely represent changes in synthetic rates. That the protein class which could be in its synthesis, also had a high turnover rate, is probably of significance, and this will be discussed in the CONCLUSIONS section.

## BEHAVIORAL MODIFICATIONS OF SPECIFIC NEURONAL PROPERTIES

### Aestivation (Hibernation) in the Snail

When terrestrial snails (*Helicidae*) in the laboratory are exposed to environmental conditions of low relative humidity, they enter into a state of diapause typical of their natural hibernation (and aestivation) in the field (Gainer, 1972b; Hunter, 1964; Hyman,

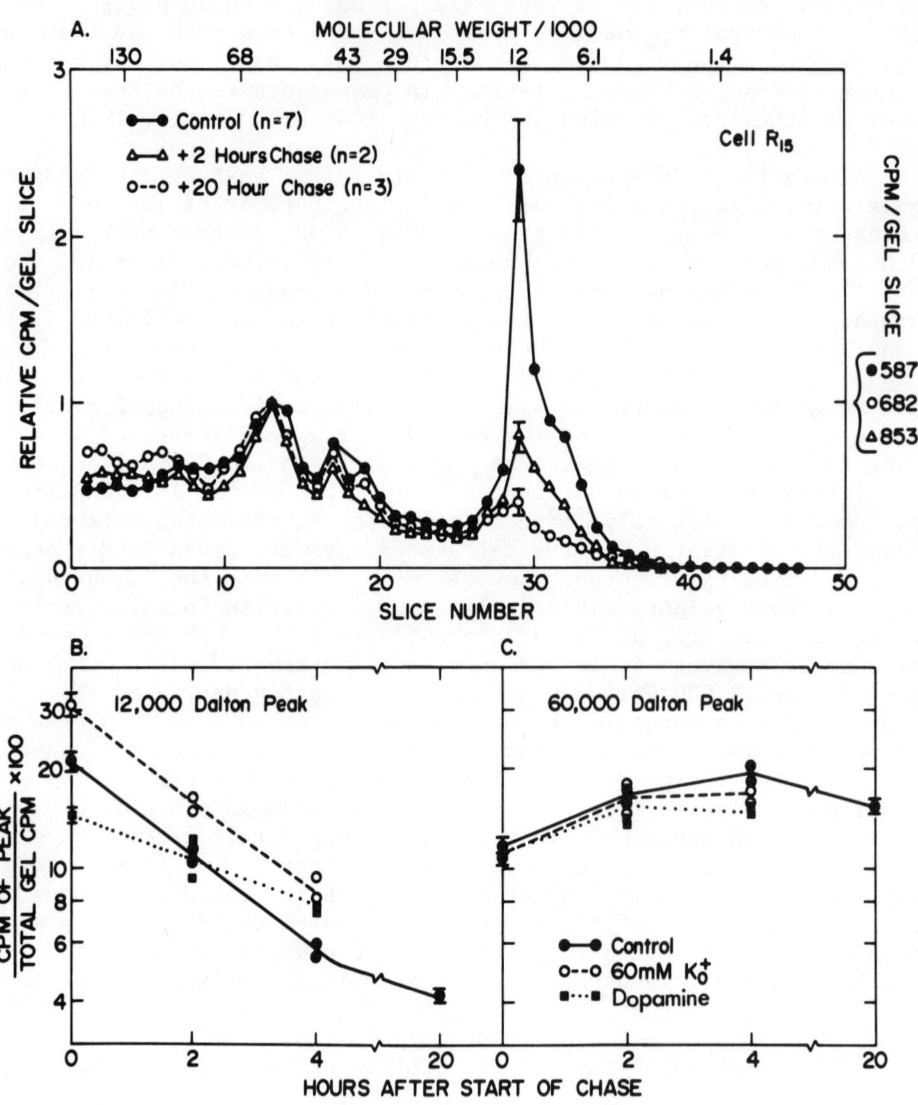
A.
MOLECULAR WEIGHT/1000
130
68
43
29
15.5
12
6.1
1.4
Control (n=7)
+2 Hours Chase (n=2)
+20 Hour Chase (n=3)
Cell $R_{15}$
RELATIVE CPM/GEL SLICE
CPM/GEL SLICE
587
682
853
SLICE NUMBER
B.
12,000 Dalton Peak
C.
60,000 Dalton Peak
CPM OF PEAK / TOTAL GEL CPM ×100
Control
60mM $K_o^+$
Dopamine
HOURS AFTER START OF CHASE

Fig. 3

Fig. 3

Comparison of the molecular weight distribtions of $^3$H-leucine-labeled proteins in $R_{15}$ after chases in media (containing 1 mM unlabeled leucine).

A. Radioactive protein profiles on SDS gels after 3 h incubation in $^3$H-leucine only (control, filled circles); after 3 h incubation plus 2 h chase (open triangles); and after 3 h incubation plus 20 h chase (open circles). Left ordinate: The radioactivity in each gel slice (CPM/gel slice minus background) is plotted relative to the maximum radioactive gel slice in the 60-68,000 dalton range. Right ordinate: Average absolute CPM/gel slice found in a given condition corresponding to the relative CPM/gel slice of unity. Upper and lower abscissae are described in Fig. 1. Each point on the curves at a given slice number represents the average relative CPM/gel slice value from separate experiments (n). The vertical bars at the 12,000 dalton point reflect ± one standard deviation. Note selective decrease in the 12,000 dalton peak.

B. Graph of the percentage of total gel CPM found in the 12,000 dalton peak (log scale) at various times of chase under control conditions (filled circles). Decrease in radioactivity of peak has a half-time value of about 2 hours. Open circles represent the % CPM on the 12,000 dalton peak in $R_{15}$ cells incubated in 60 mM $K^+$ media to increase the rate of the 12,000 dalton peak synthesis. Filled squares represent the % CPM of the 12,000 dalton peak in $R_{15}$ cells incubated in $10^{-3}$ M dopamine.

C. Similar graph as described in B, but for 60,000 dalton peak. The apparent increase in the percentage of total gel CPM is primarily due to the loss of the 12,000 dalton peak. (From Gainer & Barker, 1974b.)

1968). The most obvious difference between the active and dormant state in the snail is that the dormant snail secretes a calcareous epiphragm, composed largely of $CaCO_3$ and mucus, which closes the peristone in its shell (Fig. 4). The snail's major problem for survival is to control its body water balance, and one of the major

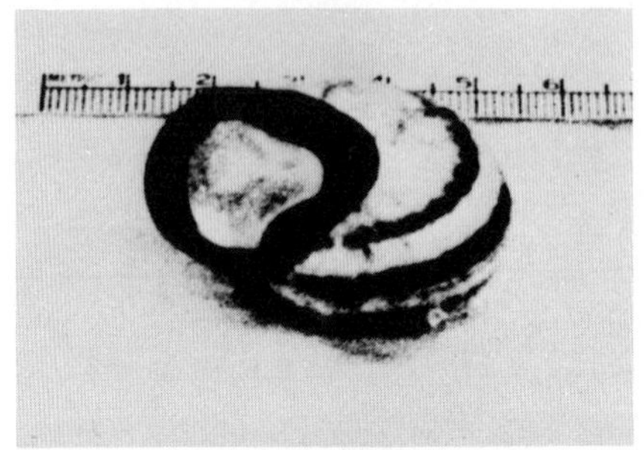

DORMANT

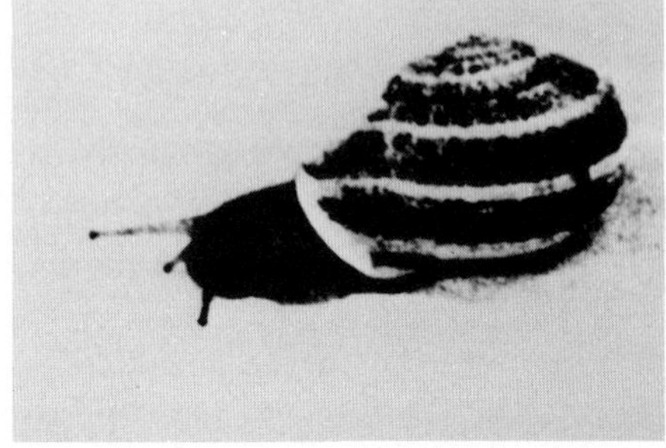

ACTIVE

Fig. 4 Dormant and active states of *Otala lactea*.

functions of diapause in this animal is to reduce water loss in periods of stress (Machin, 1972; Schmidt-Nielsen *et al*., 1971). The shell and epiphragm completely enclose the dormant animal and protect it from the evaporative effects of air currents; in addition, the snail has evolved special physiological mechanisms so that the rate of water loss through the skin of dormant animals is about 3% that in active animals (Machin, 1966). The epiphragm secreted by the dormant snails in the laboratory is of the heavy calcareous type, typical of the state of hibernation. Experimentally induced diapause is correlated with a variety of other major changes in the organism. The nitrogen metabolism of the snail is altered so that it excretes free ammonia in diapause, in contrast to the normal excretion of uric acid in the active state (Speeg and Campbell, 1968). In diapause, the oxygen consumption of the organism decreases to about one-tenth of normal (Coles, 1969), the oxidative enzyme activities in the hepatopancreas are greatly decreased, growth slows (Hyman, 1968), osmotic pressure of the blood increases (Robertson, 1964), and the heart rate at 25°C falls from 52/min to 35/min (Hyman, 1968). Hence, diapause is a total and profound change in the state of the organism, a state which may be related to the activity of specific neurons (e.g., neurosecretory cells) in the central nervous system (Krause, 1960; Van der Kloot, 1955).

Given this dramatic difference in behavioral state of the animal, an attempt was made to determine whether any correlated electrophysiological or biochemical differences in identified neurons could be found. There are a number of large, identifiable neurons in the snail brain (Fig. 5), and five of these (cells 7, 9, 10, 11 and 12) were extensively examined for changes in properties during experimental diapause (Gainer, 1972b). The effects of diapause were found to be minimal or nonspecific in 4 out of 5 of the identified neurons examined. Only cell 11 was profoundly and specifically affected by the state of diapause.

## Effects of Diapause on the Properties of Cell 11

In many respects, cell 11 (*Otala lactea*) appears to be very similar to $R_{15}$ (*Aplysia*). Both cells produce bursting pacemaker potentials (BPPs), exhibit circadian and circannual rhythms in electrical activity, receive extensive inhibitory synaptic inputs, and both contain neurosecretory granules. While the above characteristics are typical of a cell 11 from an active animal, they markedly differ from the properties of a dormant cell 11 (Gainer, 1972b, c).

Probably the most obvious electrophysiological change in cell 11 during diapause, is its loss of pacemaker (BPP) activity (see Fig. 9C). Associated with this condition, there is an increase in resting membrane potential and slope conductance of the cell (presumably due to an increase in potassium ion permeability; Gainer, 1972b); but no changes in action potential amplitude or afterpotential were observed. Furthermore, the current-voltage (I-V) relationship of the cell's membrane was qualitatively transformed by diapause (Fig. 6); the non-linear I-V relationship typical of BPP generating cells (i.e., anomalous rectification) became linear in the dormant cell. The ability to generate BPP's has been closely correlated with the presence of non-linear I-V relations over a restricted range of membrane potential (Faber & Klee, 1972; Klee *et al.*, 1973; Wachtel & Wilson, 1973; Barker & Gainer, in preparation), therefore, the loss of both these properties in the dormant cell 11 is in line with these findings.

In addition to the specific electrophysiological changes described above, cell 11 was also dramatically and specifically

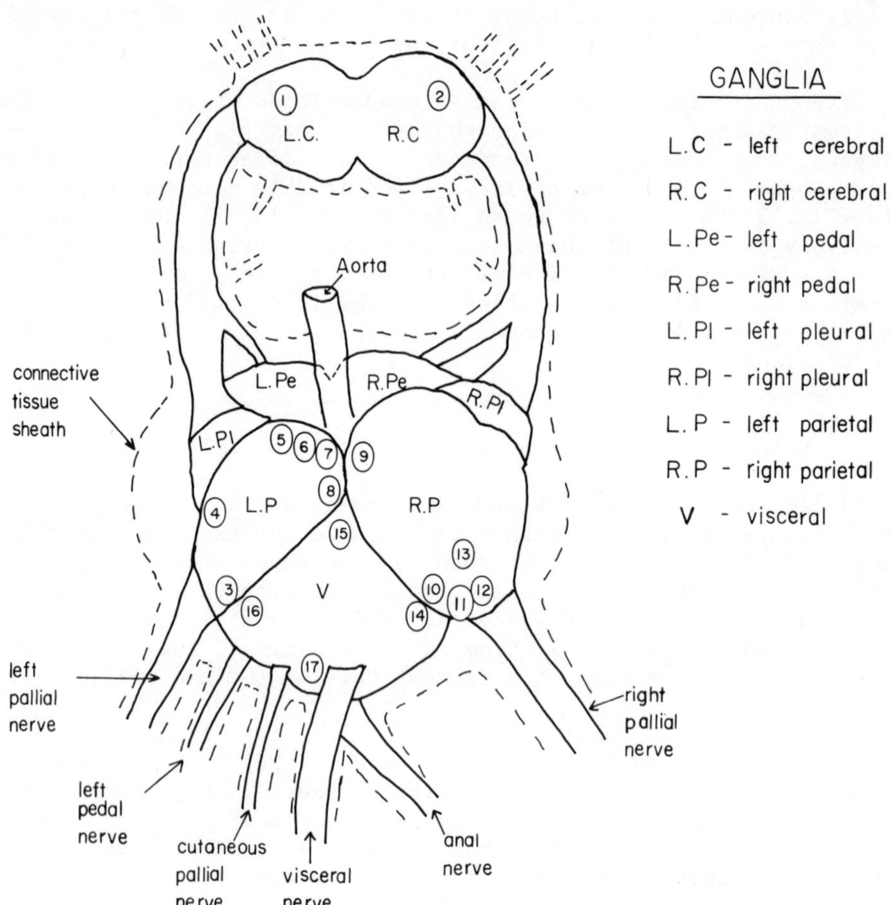


Fig. 5 Diagrammatic dorsal view of the snail brain (*Otala lactea*) which is composed of 9 fused ganglia. The positions of 17 identifiable neurons, which exceed 100 μm in diameter and can be repeatedly found in all preparations are identified by number. Cell 11 is analogous to $R_{15}$ in *Aplysia*, and is markedly affected by aestivation (from Gainer, 1972a).

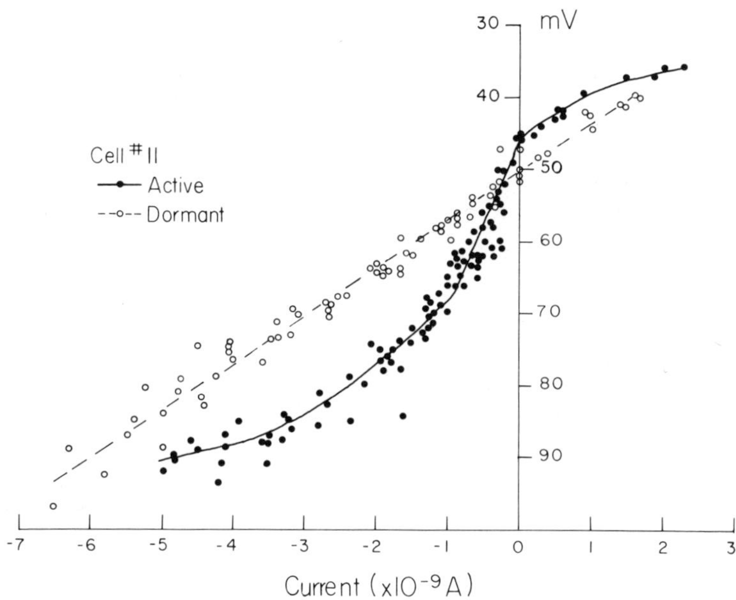


Fig. 6 Current-voltage curves from cell in active (solid line, filled circles) and dormant (broken line, open circles) animals. The points on each curve represent the combined data from cell 11 from 3 separate animals. Curves were drawn by eye, and data obtained with the use of two microelectrodes in the cell, one for passing current, and the other for recording membrane potential. Note the prominent delayed and anomalous rectification in the active cells, and their absence in the dormant cells. (From Gainer, 1972b.)

modified during diapause in its protein synthesis profile. The labeling profile of an active cell 11 depicted in Fig. 7, shows (as in the case of $R_{15}$ - Fig. 1) a preferential incorporation of $^3$H-leucine into low molecular weight proteins (i.e., less than 20,000 daltons). The peak of labeling at 4-5,000 daltons (Fig. 7) accounted for about 25% of the total label incorporated into protein in cell 11, whereas in cells 7, 9, 10 and 12 such a peak was not present at

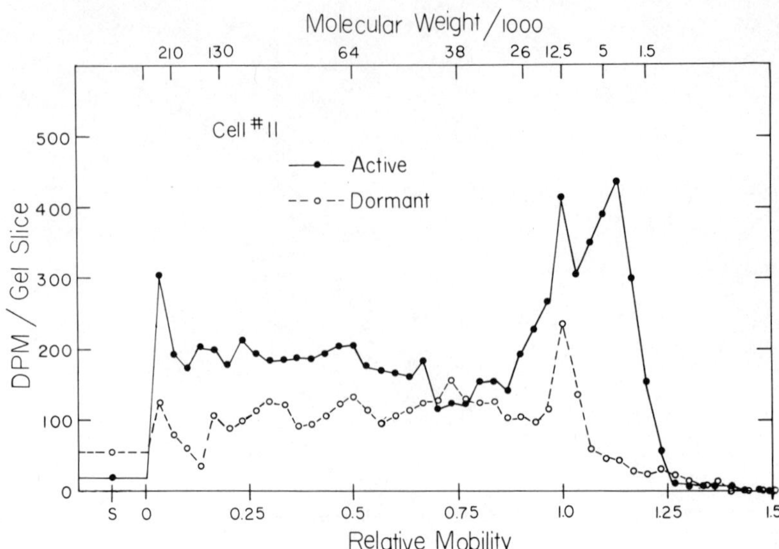


Fig. 7 Electrophoretic SDS microgel (7.5% gels) protein patterns from the extracts of the cell body of cell 11 isolated from active (filled circles, solid line) and dormant (open circles broken line) snails after 20 h incubation of the ganglion in media containing L-[$^{3}$H]leucine. Each labeling pattern in the figure is an average of 3 independent microgel patterns obtained from separate, identified neurons (i.e., each point represents the average disint./min, minus background/gel slice, of 3 separate gels at the specified relative mobilities). (From Gainer, 1972b.)

all (Gainer, 1972a). The incorporation of label into the total proteins of the dormant cell 11 was reduced to about half that found for the active cell. The labeling profile of the dormant cell was still relatively flat between 20,000-200,000 daltons, and possibly showed a slight relative increase in protein synthesis at around 38,000 daltons. There was still a prominent peak at 12,500 daltons, but the large unique 5,000 dalton peak of synthesis was completely absent. The loss during diapause of this specific molecular weight class of proteins in cell 11 is interesting for several reasons. First, this peak is only found in cell 11, and accounts for a large proportion of the cell's protein synthesis. Second, only this cell (in contrast to the other 4 identified cells), was shown to produce specific changes in electrophysiological properties as a result of diapause. Third, only cell 11 revealed neurosecretory granules upon electron microscopy (Fig. 8). Because the density of neurosecretory

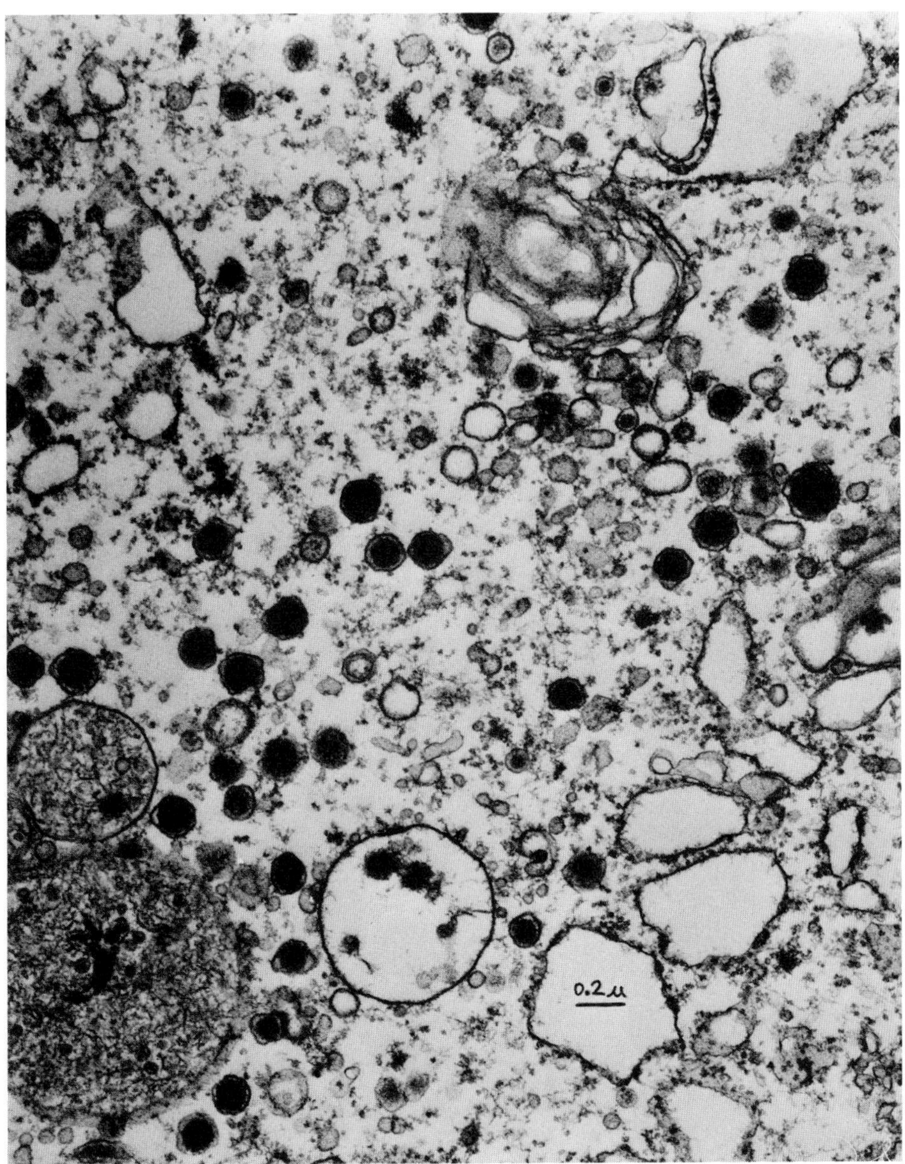


Fig. 8 Electron-micrograph of the cell body of cell 11 from an active snail. Note numerous neurosecretory granules (Reese & Gainer, unpublished).

granules in cell 11 was markedly decreased during diapause (Reese & Gainer, unpublished), it was suggested that the labeled 5,000 dalton protein lost during diapause (Fig. 7) was related to its neurosecretory role (Gainer, 1972b). As was mentioned earlier, SDS gels separate proteins on the basis of size, and the resolution of the gel for a particular molecular weight protein is dependent upon the acrylamide concentration of the gel. The data presented in Fig. 7 were obtained from a 7.5% gel. When labeled proteins from an active cell 11 was separated on 11% gels (which provide better resolution of low molecular weight proteins) the unique labeled peak ranged in molecular weight from 5-9,000 daltons, and again represented about 25% of the total labeled protein on the gel. This peak (on 11% gels) was also completely absent in the dormant cell 11 (Gainer & Barker, unpublished). Although this peak represents a particular molecular weight class, it is probably not a single protein. Recent experiments in our laboratory using other gel systems indicate that it is composed of at least 3 separate small proteins, all of which disappear during diapause (Barker & Loh, unpublished).

In summary, the effects of experimentally induced diapause, which simulated the natural conditions of hibernation and aestivation in the snail, were found to be minimal or nonspecific in 4 out of the 5 identified neurons examined. One neuron, however, cell 11, was profoundly and specifically affected by the state of diapause. The effects included a 3-fold decrease in membrane input resistance and a slight increase in resting membrane potential of the cell, both of which appear to be due to a relatively selective increase in $K^+$ permeability of this cell during diapause. In addition, the endogenous pacemaker activity of cell 11 in active animals was absent from this cell in the dormant animals. Correlated with these electrophysiological changes during diapause was a specific alteration of protein synthesis pattern in cell 11. The active cell 11 synthesized a specific molecular weight class of polypeptides which was unique to this cell and the synthesis of these specific polypeptides was completely inhibited by diapause.

Since diapause inhibited both the BPP activity and specific protein synthesis in cell 11, we next questioned whether these two events were related. Indeed, Strumwasser (1973) has suggested that the synthesis of low molecular weight proteins in $R_{15}$ was related to its BPP activity (possibly as "pacemaker proteins"). If this was the case, we reasoned that the induction of BPP activity in a dormant cell 11 should then be accompanied by an induction of synthesis of the low molecular weight proteins.

## Regulation of BPP Activity in Cell 11 by Divalent Cations

One of the most effective methods of inducing BPP activity in a dormant (aestivated) cell 11 is simply to reduce the calcium ion concentration of the physiological saline bathing the ganglion (Barker & Gainer, 1973). Such experiments are described in Fig. 9. Sustained depolarization of the membrane potential of aestivated cells by intracellular current elicited repetitive firing of spikes without BPP activity ("DEPOL", Fig. 9A). When calcium was removed from the saline, the membrane potential decreased, and the cell began to generate BPPs which could be maintained as long as magnesium remained in the medium. The appearance of BPP activity was accompanied by a change from linear to markedly non-linear current-voltage relations (not illustrated). Thus, removal of calcium from the external medium transformed the electrical properties of the aestivated cell into those of an active cell.

Cells from "transitional" snails exhibited spontaneous pacemaker activity without slow membrane potential oscillations (Fig. 9B). Injection of current of either polarity could induce the BPP rhythm under normal saline conditions. Calcium-free saline did elicit BPP activity. If the remaining divalent cation (magnesium) was removed, the membrane potential gradually depolarized, lost its ability to generate the BPP and eventually reached a high-conductance, low-potential state, characterized first by fast frequency spike activity and then by inactivity. Under these conditions, injection of hyperpolarizing current could not restore the BPP, indicating that the presence of magnesium was necessary for the generation of BPPs.

Removal of calcium from the saline bathing "active" cells spontaneously generating BPPs, led to a depolarization and increase in the frequency of bursts as well as spikes per burst (Fig. 9C). If magnesium was also removed, then the membrane potential gradually depolarized, the BPP disappeared and the cell lost its ability to generate BPPs, despite hyperpolarizing current. The latter condition was seen with cells obtained from animals in all three environmental states.

The physiological role of calcium in the regulation of BPP activity is further illustrated by Fig. 9D. A cell from a "transitional" snail spontaneously generates BPPs in calcium-free saline containing magnesium. Adding the physiological complement of calcium (10 mM) to the saline completely inhibited BPP generation. Removal of the calcium then restored the BPP activity.

To further investigate the divalent cation regulation of the BPP, we compared the BPP activity of these cells in the presence of varying concentrations (0-60 mM) of calcium, magnesium, and strontium. These experiments were conducted by washing in divalent-cation free saline until the ability to generate BPP activity disappeared, after which the appropriate divalent cation was added to the saline and BPP activity monitored by measuring the amplitude of the BPP (defined in the inset of Fig. 10). Intracellular injection of

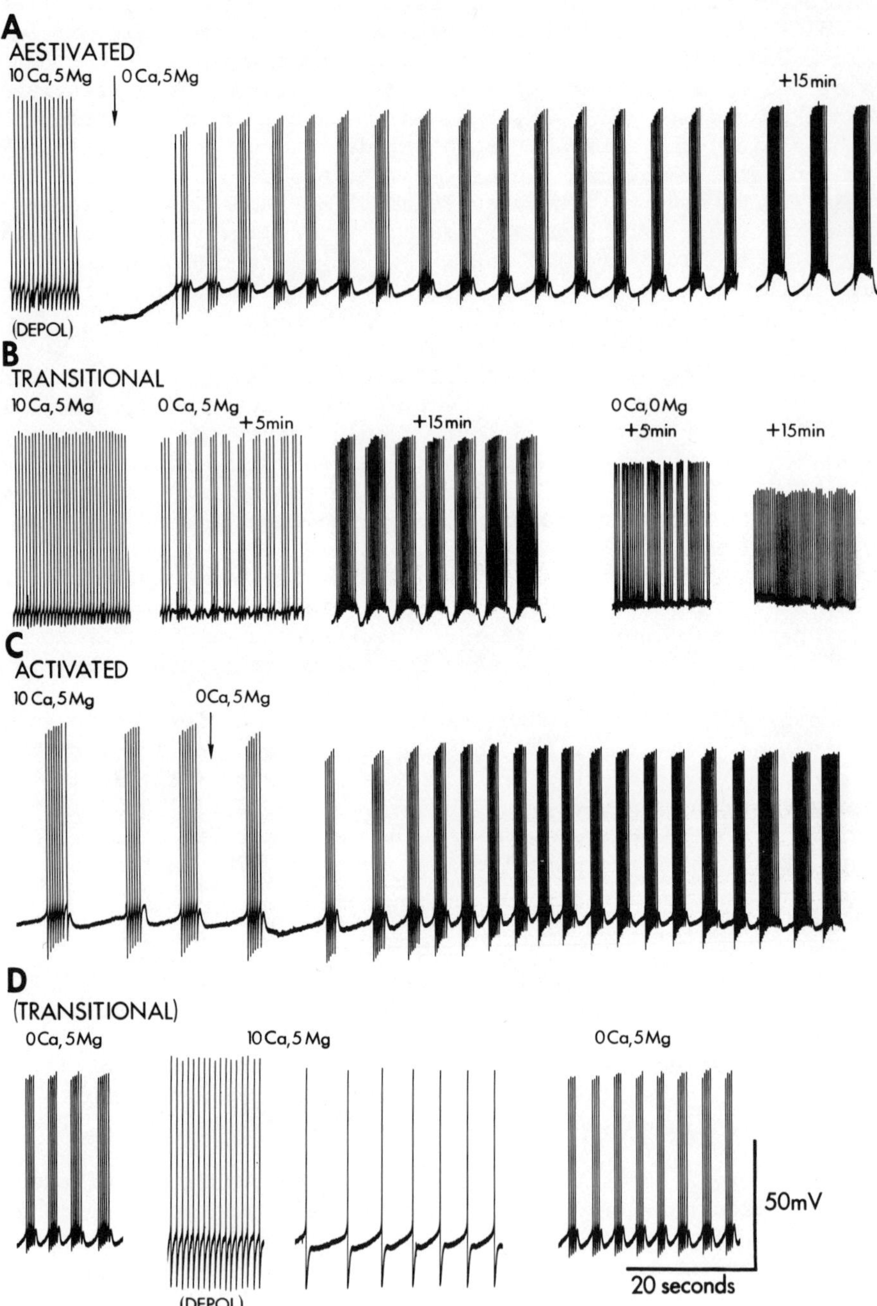
A
AESTIVATED
10 Ca, 5 Mg
0 Ca, 5 Mg
+15 min
(DEPOL)
B
TRANSITIONAL
10 Ca, 5 Mg
0 Ca, 5 Mg
+5 min
+15 min
0 Ca, 0 Mg
+5 min
+15 min
C
ACTIVATED
10 Ca, 5 Mg
0 Ca, 5 Mg
D
(TRANSITIONAL)
0 Ca, 5 Mg
10 Ca, 5 Mg
0 Ca, 5 Mg
(DEPOL)
50mV
20 seconds

Fig. 9

Fig. 9

Calcium regulates the bursting pacemaker potential (BPP) of a neurosecretory cell. Membrane potential records from the identified neurosecretory cell (#11) in specimens of the land snail *Otala lactea* at different states of activity.

A. Example from an aestivated snail. In physiological saline solutions ($[Ca^{++}]_o$ = 10 mM) the cell, which is hyperpolarized and silent, responds to sustained injection of depolarizing current with repetitive activity (DEPOL). Removal of $[Ca^{++}]_o$ from the medium leads to a depolarization and initiation of spontaneous bursting activity, which progresses and stabilizes with time.

B. Example from a snail in transition from aestivation to activation. Although the cell is spontaneously firing under control conditions, it does not burst with application of either hyper- or depolarizing transmembrane current (not shown). Removal of $[Ca^{++}]_o$ from the medium induces bursting behavior. Removal of $[Mg^{++}]_o$, resulting in a nominally divalent cation-free solution leads to a depolarization and high rate of firing of spikes with subsequent loss of the BPP.

C. Example from an active snail. The bursting rhythm is present in control saline. The frequency of bursts, as well as of spikes per burst, increases while the BPP amplitude decreases upon removal of $[Ca^{++}]_o$.

D. A transitional cell bursting in calcium-free solution stops bursting and fires repetitively when the physiological complement of $[Ca^{++}]_o$ is added to the medium (middle record) despite sustained depolarizing current (DEPOL). Return to the calcium-free condition restores the burst. (From Barker & Gainer, 1973).

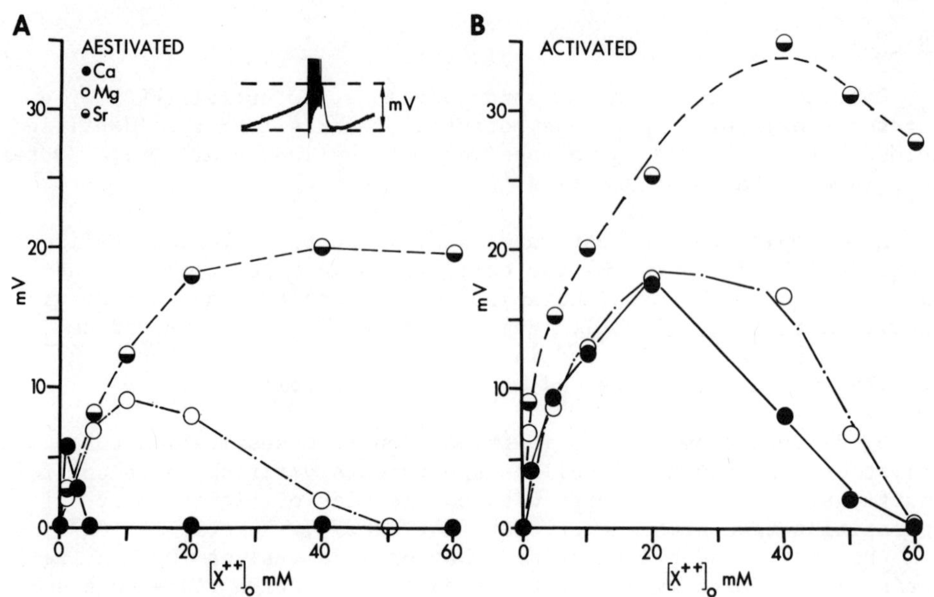


Fig. 10 Bursting pacemaker potential amplitude varies with external divalent cation concentration, type ($[X^{++}]_o$), and state of activity of the snail. BPP amplitude (mV) is defined in the inset in part A and is plotted as a function of $[Ca^{++}]_o$, $[Mg^{++}]_o$ and $[Sr^{++}]_o$ in cell #11 from an aestivated (A) and an activated snail (B). Experimental details are given in the text. BPP amplitude is parabolically dependent on $[Ca^{++}]_o$ and $[Mg^{++}]_o$ and directly dependent on $[Sr^{++}]_o$ in both cells. The range of $[Ca^{++}]_o$ over which BPP activity can be elicited is 1-5 mM in the aestivated cell and 1-60 mM in the active cell. (The interrupted line representing BPP amplitude as a function of $[Sr^{++}]_o$ indicates that the cells tended to remain depolarized at the peak of the BPP unless hyperpolarizing current was injected. The change in sensitivity of the BPP amplitude to $[Ca^{++}]_o$ appears to be the major consequence of aestivation (From Barker & Gainer, 1973).

current was always used to test the ability of the cells to generate BPP activity since the membrane potential was frequently depolarized in solutions of low divalent-cation strength and hyperpolarized in high calcium and magnesium solutions. Low strength divalent cation solutions were also associated with a decrease in the threshold for firing as well as a decrease in input resistance, while the opposite effects were seen in high strength divalent cation solutions. Since all three divalent cations produced similar changes in these parameters, their differential effects on BPP activity were compared without taking these changes into account. The amplitude of the BPP was always measured at the current just necessary to produce the BPPs.

In cells from aestivated snails, the BPP amplitude was parabolically dependent on the external calcium concentration ($[Ca^{++}]_o$) over the 1-5 mM range (Fig. 10A). In 5 mM $[Ca^{++}]_o$, the cell was hyperpolarized and could not generate BPP activity despite sustained depolarizing current. The BPP amplitude was also parabolically dependent on $[Ca^{++}]_o$ in cells from active snails, but the range over which BPP activity could be elicited was extended to 60 mM $[Ca^{++}]_o$, which is six-fold the physiological $[Ca^{++}]_o$ (Fig. 10B). Transitional cells manifested an intermediate sensitivity to calcium. BPP amplitude was also parabolically dependent on external magnesium concentration ($[Mg^{++}]_o$) in both aestivated and active cells. The range over which BPP activity could be elicited, as well as the amplitude of the BPP, was smaller in the aestivated group. BPP amplitude was found to be directly related to $[Sr^{++}]_o$ over the 1-60 mM range in both aestivated and active cells. Little, if any, inhibiting effect was observed at 60 mM $[Sr^{++}]_o$ in either group of cells. In addition, the BPP amplitudes were greater in $[Sr^{++}]_o$ than in either $[Ca^{++}]_o$ or $[Mg^{++}]_o$, although those in aestivated cells were generally smaller than those in the active group. Higher concentrations of $[Sr^{++}]_o$ (20-60 mM) frequently resulted in a depolarization of the membrane potential, with continual repetitive spiking activity (unlike similar concentrations of $Ca^{++}$ and $Mg^{++}$, which tended to hyperpolarize the membrane potentials of both groups of cells). Under these conditions, the BPP cycle could be initiated by a brief pulse of hyperpolarizing current and BPP activity maintained by proper adjustment of a sustained hyperpolarizing current.

The foregoing data show that divalent cations are required for BPP activity, but also have an inhibitory effect at higher concentrations. The dormant cell 11 appears to have increased its sensitivity ten-fold to the inhibitory effects of divalent cations (particularly $Ca^{++}$). Hence, the absence of BPP activity in the dormant cell 11 (and the accompanying linear I-V curve) can be attributed to inhibitory modulation by physiological (active) concentrations of calcium ion. The calcium ion concentration in the hemolymph of snails is actually increased during diapause (Meenakshi, 1956; Raghupathiramireddy, 1967), and therefore cell 11 would, under

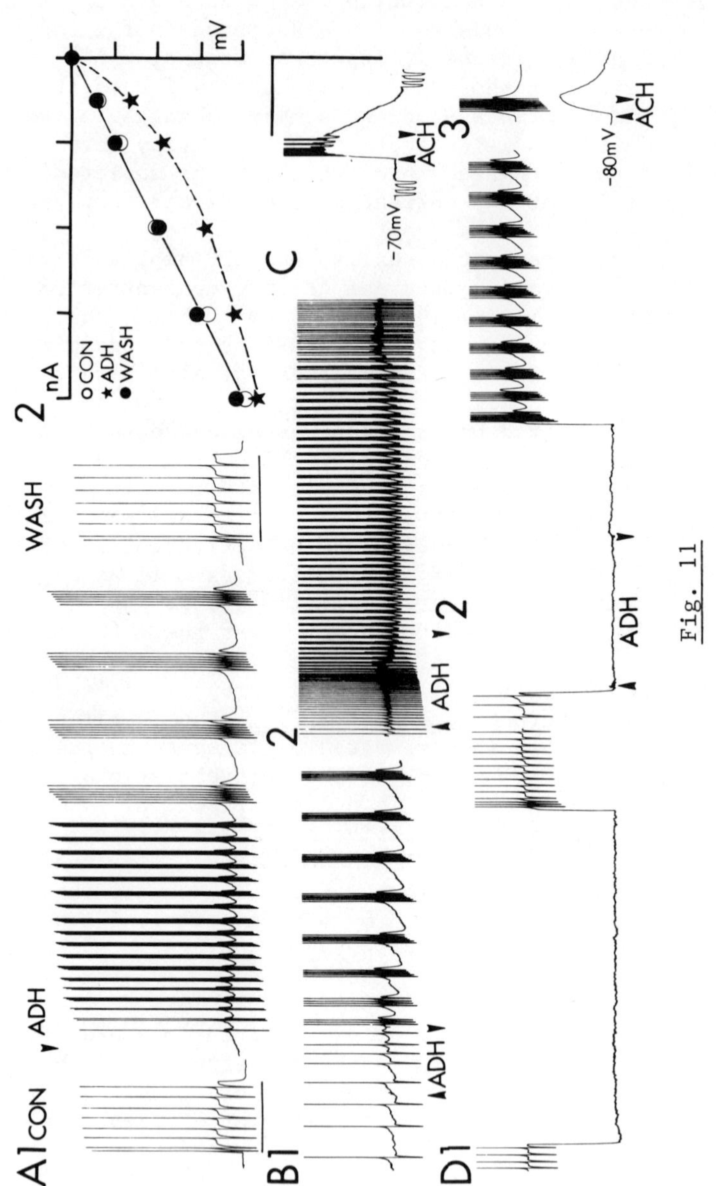
A1 CON
ADH
WASH
2
nA
CON
ADH
WASH
mV
B1
ADH
ADH
2
ADH
C
-70mV
ACH
D1
ADH
2
3
-80mV
ACH

Fig. 11

Fig. 11

Effects of ADH (vasopressin) on the membrane properties of cell 11. Membrane potential traces of cell 11 taken from aestivated and semi-aestivated snails.

A1. (Resting membrane potential: -48 mV). Control. Injection of depolarizing current (during period marked by bar beneath trace) does not produce BPP activity. Bath application of $10^{-9}$ M ADH (at arrow) induced BPP rhythm. (First half of trace is recorded at 1/4 speed of last half of trace.) Wash. Washing in ADH-free saline for 1 h restores the cell's membrane properties.

A2. Current-voltage relations of the cell before, during and after treatment with ADH. Marks on axes represent 1 nA and 10 mV intervals. Origin is threshold for firing (-42 mV). ADH reversibly induces marked non-linearity in the curve.

B1. Iontophoresis of ADH leads to BPP activity. ADH ejected between arrows using 4 nA cationic current. (Resting membrane potential: -46 mV.)

B2. Effects of ADH (iontophoresed between arrows) long outlast the application period.

C. Bath application of $10^{-5}$ M ACh depolarizes the membrane potential and increases membrane conductance. Downward deflections are voltage responses to constant current pulses (1 nA).

D1. Sustained hyperpolarization of a cell does not induce BPP activity once the hyperpolarizing current is removed. (Resting membrane potential: -48 mV.)

D2. Iontophoresis of ADH (between the arrows) when the cell is hyperpolarized does not cause an observable voltage response, but upon removal of the hyperpolarizing current well-developed BPP activity is evident.

D3. Similar hyperpolarization of the cell increases the size of the depolarizing ACh response.

Calibration: 40 mV, 12 sec in A1, B1, D1-3, 48 sec in A2, B2, 6 min in C. (From Barker & Gainer, 1974.)

natural conditions, be exposed to an "overkill" dose for inhibition of the BPP.

The rapid onset of BPP activity in the dormant cell 11 on manipulation of the divalent cation concentrations in the medium (Fig. 9) strongly suggested that synthesis of the low molecular weight proteins were not necessary for this electrophysiological behavior. Indeed, long-term inhibition of protein synthesis did not eliminate BPP activity in $R_{15}$ (Schwartz, *et al.*, 1971) and induced BPP activity in $R_2$ (Chalazonitis & Takeuchi, 1968; Klee *et al.*, 1973; Morales & Chalazonitis, 1970). Although the small proteins synthesized by cell 11 do not appear to control BPP activity directly, it is likely that the concurrent absence of both from cell 11 during diapause is significant. If the small proteins represent neurosecretory material, then the closely spaced spikes during the BPP would be particularly efficacious for secretion (Gainer, 1972b). During diapause, when the neurosecretory material is not being synthesized, it would then be parsimonious for the spontaneous BPP activity of cell 11 to be inhibited.

In addition to inhibition of BPP activity by divalent cations, it was found that steroid hormones could inhibit BPP (Barker & Gainer, in preparation). Aldosterone and hydrocortisone ($10^{-6}$ M) increased the membrane potential, transformed the non-linear to a linear I-V curve, and abolished the BPP in cell 11's from active snails. This effect was only observed in saline solutions containing $Ca^{++}$, and was reversed if the cells were perfused with media containing the steroid hormones, but with $Mg^{++}$ replacing the $Ca^{++}$. Similar results were obtained with ouabain (which has a steroid structure). Although these are simply interesting pharmacological observations, they may be of physiological significance since the sterol content of hibernating snail brains is ten-fold that of active snails (Raghypathiramireddy, 1967). Because of these considerations we were led to do other studies involving vertebrate hormones (i.e., peptides).

## Regulatory Effects of Peptides on BPP Activity

Since the properties of cell 11 appeared to be intimately associated with the water content of the snail's environment, we were prompted to examine the effects of vertebrate neurohypophysical peptide hormones (e.g., antidiuretic hormone) on this cell (Barker & Gainer, 1974).

Cell 11 from aestivated (or semi-aestivated) snails was either electrically inactive (Fig. 11 A1), or exhibited spontaneous activity, characterized by a beating pattern of spikes at a fairly constant frequency (Figs. 11 B1, 11 B2 and 11 D). The membrane current-voltage relationships of these cells were linear (Fig. 11 A2), and changes in membrane potential by injections of transmembrane current could not produce bursting pacemaker potential (BPP) activity (e.g., Fig. 11 A1 - "Control"). Bath application of $10^{-9}$ M lysine-ADH (lysine-vasopressin) rapidly induced BPP activity (Fig. 11 A1), and altered the current-voltage relationships of the membrane from linear to non-linear (Fig. 11 A2). Identical results were obtained with various similar peptides at $10^{-6}$ - $10^{-9}$ M concentrations, including arginine-vasopressin, homolysine-vasopressin, 8-L-homonorleucine-vasopressin and oxytocin. The effects of these peptides were dose-dependent and long-lasting, and required prolonged (ca. 1-4 h) washing in peptide-free saline to restore the cell's membrane properties to control values (Figs. 11 A1 and 11 A2). Higher concentrations of lysine-vasopressin (and related peptides) caused sustained depolarization of the membrane potential (and high frequency spike activity). Under these conditions, injection of hyperpolarizing current was necessary to reveal the augmented underlying BPP activity. The response of cell 11 to the active peptides was remarkably specific, since these peptides were without effect on a number of other identified neurons studied (including cells 9, 10 and 12 in *Otala*, and $R_2$, $R_{14}$, $R_{3-13}$, $L_{2-6}$, $L_7$, $L_{11}$ and LPG in *Aplysia*). Only $R_{15}$, which is analogous to cell 11 in its electrophysiological properties, was affected by the active peptides in a manner similar to that described for cell 11 (Fig. 11). Furthermore, bath application of a variety of other peptides did not change the membrane properties of cell 11. Other substances tested (in 1 mM concentration) included: angiotensin II, bradykinin-triacetate, adrenocorticotrophic hormone, various fragments of ACTH, growth-hormone releasing factor, melanocyte-stimulating hormone releasing factor, lutenizing hormone releasing factor and physalaemin. In addition, neither pressinamide, the cyclic disulfide pentapeptide ring of vasopressin nor lysine-vasopressin without the terminal glycinamide moiety could induce BPP activity in cell 11. (These agents also did not antagonize the effects of the active peptides.)

BPP activity was induced by the iontophoresis of vasopressin directly onto the surface of cell 11. This response, which developed within seconds of initiating the iontophoresis of vasopressin (Fig. 11 B1), far outlasted the period of application of the iontophoretic current (Fig. 11 B2). The activating effect of vasopressin on the cell was also present in solutions containing five times the normal $Mg^{++}$ concentration, reducing the likelihood that the vasopressin effect was pre-synaptically mediated. Iontophoresis of vasopressin onto various parts of cell 11 revealed that the sensitivity to this peptide was located primarily on the external surface of the axon hillock (Fig. 12). Of fifteen cells tested, thirteen responded exclusively to application of vasopressin in the axonal region, while in two cells the soma was also sensitive to ADH. Intracellular injection of vasopressin by iontophoresis or pressure-injection

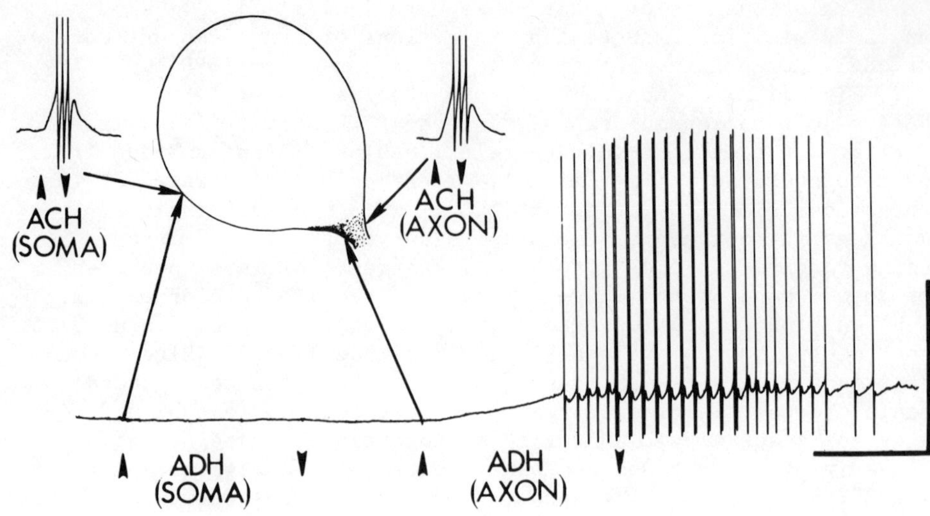


Fig. 12 Iontophoresis of lysine-vasopressin (ADH) onto the surface of cell 11 from an aestivated snail induces bursting pacemaker potential activity only when the pipette is positioned at the "axon hillock" region (Iontophoretic current was applied at upward arrowhead and stopped at downward arrowhead). In contrast, iontophoretic application of acetylcholine causes depolarization over the entire cell surface. Calibrations: 40 mV; 48 sec for lysine-vasopressin responses, and 12 sec for acetylcholine responses. (From Barker, Ifshin & Gainer, in preparation.)

techniques was without effect. In contrast, acetylcholine (ACh) responses were always elicited from both soma and axonal regions.

The membrane mechanisms underlying the vasopressin effect are unlike those associated with responses to conventional neurotransmitters. For example, in cell 11, ACh produces a transient depolarization of the membrane (Figs. 11C, 11 D3), associated with an increase in membrane conductance (Fig. 11 C). As expected from theoretical considerations, this potential change increased as the cell's membrane was hyperpolarized (Fig. 11 D3); the reversal potential of this response was estimated to be +10 mV by extrapolation. In contrast, iontophoresis of vasopressin onto a cell, the membrane potential of which was hyperpolarized (by current injection) to potentials beyond -70 mV, did not produce an observable potential (or conductance) change (Fig. 11 D2). However, after removal of the hyperpolarizing current (thus returning the cell to the membrane potential range over which the BPP could be expressed, i.e., between -35 to -65 mV), it was clear that BPP activity had in fact been induced by the vasopressin (Fig. 11 D2). It should be noted that hyperpolarization of the membrane potential alone did not induce BPP activity (Fig. 11 D1). Thus, in contrast to the transient membrane conductance changes produced by ACh and other conventional transmitters (e.g., glutamate, dopamine, octopamine, and serotonin, which all produced transient changes in conductance), the peptide interaction with this cell (at relatively lower concentration) induced a prolonged regulatory effect on specific membrane properties (e.g., the BPP).

These results demonstrate that vertebrate neurohypophysical peptides have specific effects on the BPP activity of cell 11 at concentrations comparable to those in mammalian plasma (Berde, 1968). It is possible that either these or similar peptides may exist in the snail. In recent experiments in our laboratory (Ifshin, Gainer & Barker, in preparation), we have isolated a peptide fraction from the snail brain which is similar to vasopressin in its effect on cell 11 (Fig. 13), and is eluted in the same fraction as lysine-vasopressin after chromatography on G-25 Sephadex. We are currently doing radioimmunoassays to determine if this extract contains vasopressin.

Since lysine-vasopressin effectively induced massive BPP activity in the aestivated cell 11, we checked whether this induction was accompanied by an induction of synthesis of the low molecular weight proteins typically absent in the dormant cell 11. Exposure of dormant cells to BPP-inducing levels of lysine-vasopressin for as long as 12 hours did not induce the synthesis of the small proteins (Gainer & Barker, unpublished). Thus, neither the BPP activity nor the exposure of cell 11 to the peptide hormone was sufficient to induce small protein synthesis. In some respects, this finding was not unexpected. If cell 11 is under hormonal regulation, one would not expect the signal to increase secretion (i.e., the lysine-vasopressin induction of BPP activity) to occur simultaneously with (or precede) the signal to induce synthesis of the material to be secreted. Clearly, the induction of the BPP should follow in time (by some "delayed gate" mechanism) the biochemical preparation of the cell for secretion. Possibly by extraction and isolation of various hormonal factors from the snail brain, we may be able to determine which, if any, of these factors is the signal for synthesis.

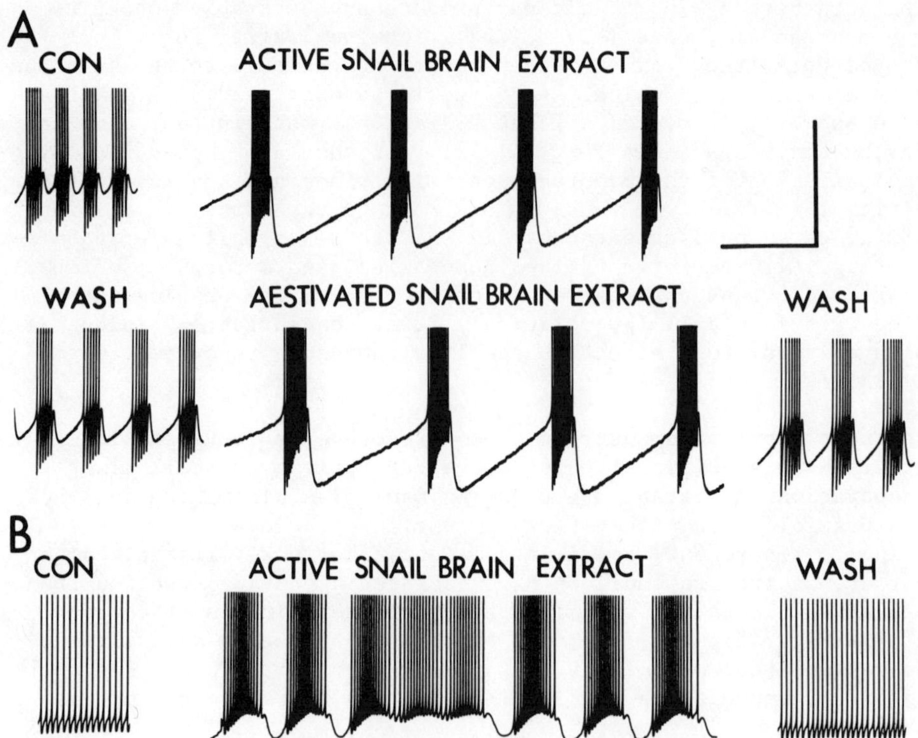


Fig. 13 Effects of whole snail brain extracts on BPP activity of cell 11.

A. Membrane potential traces of an active cell 11 exposed to the aqueous phase of a $CHCl_3$: $CH_3OH$ extract of whole brain from an active snail. Washing for 1 h restores the activity to approximately its control value (Wash, 2nd row). Addition of the aqueous fraction from an extract of aestivated snail brains produced a similar enhancement of BPP activity which is reversible.

B. Addition of the aqueous phase of active snail brain extract leads to BPP activity in a cell from an aestivated snail. Washing restores the membrane potential behavior to its control state.

Calibration: 40 mV, 12 sec (2 min. during initial application of extract in B). (Ifshin, Gainer & Barker, in preparation.)

## CONCLUSIONS

### Modulation of Specific Protein Synthesis

The data presented demonstrated that neuronal protein synthesis can be selectively modulated by synaptic input (Fig. 2). This modulation appeared to be independent of the effects of the synaptic inhibition on the spike and BPP activities of $R_{15}$, since abolition of the spike by tetrodotoxin, and abolition of the BPP by cobalt ions (unpublished data) did not modify $^3$H-leucine incorporation into the 12,000 dalton peak. However, application of dopamine, which mimics the action of the natural neurotransmitter, produced a similar modulatory effect to that of synaptic inhibition. We were not successful in selectively modulating protein synthesis in $R_{15}$ by experimental manipulations of membrane potentials and conductances (i.e., by hyperpolarization in media containing $Na^+$ substitutes; nor did inhibition or augmentation of the BPP by application of cobalt or vasopressin, respectively, influence protein synthesis). Incubations of $R_{15}$ in media containing high potassium ion concentrations did not appear to selectively increase $^3$H-leucine incorporation into the 12,000 dalton peak (see Fig. 3), but we do not know if this is due to the prolonged depolarization caused by the $K^+$, or to another action of the ion. In short, the regulation mechanism does not seem to be tightly coupled to the neuron membrane's electrical properties, and may involve a direct effect of the transmitter (or some secondary "messenger"). In this regard, it is interesting to note that dopamine also reduced the decay rate of the labeled 12,000 dalton protein in $R_{15}$ (Fig. 3).

The high turnover rate of the 12,000 dalton protein in $R_{15}$ seems to be a key factor. It is possible that proteins with high turnover rates may be more vulnerable to modulation (Schimke, 1974), and that in such short-term (3-4 hour) experiments as these, only changes in proteins that are in a highly dynamic state will be sufficiently affected by experimentally produced perturbations as to be detected by current methods. The fact that none of the protein classes in the giant neuron, $R_2$, had high turnover rates correlates with our findings that no changes in protein synthesis profiles were found in $R_2$ when it was subjected to dopamine or high $K^+$ treatment (Gainer & Barker, unpublished), or to relatively prolonged stimulation of its excitatory synaptic input (Wilson & Berry, 1972). Even the 5-9,000 dalton protein class in cell 11, which is susceptible to behavioral regulation (Fig. 7), has a slow turnover and was not affected by either dopamine or $K^+$ treatment (unpublished data).

The rapid rate of loss of the 12,000 dalton protein in $R_{15}$ raises obvious questions about its function and disposition. Unfortunately we do not know the physiological function of $R_{15}$. This neuron appears white in reflected light, and contains numerous neurosecretory granules (Frazier *et al.*, 1967). Preliminary data from recent experiments in our laboratory, using electron microscopic autoradiography, indicate that the low molecular weight proteins in $R_{15}$ reside in neurosecretory granules (E. Neale, personal communication). It is, therefore, conceivable that the 12,000 dalton protein is related to the neurosecretory material in $R_{15}$. If this is the case, then why does it disappear from the soma so rapidly? Several mechanisms which might account for this disappearance are: 1) degradation in the soma, 2) transport out of the soma into the axon, 3) secretion from the soma, and 4) conversion to another smaller peptide which is then subjected to one of the aforementioned processes (1-3).

Selective degradation of proteins has been recognized as one way in which the specific protein content of a cell can be regulated. In the liver, the turnover times of specific enzymes range from 11 minutes to 16 days (Schimke, 1974); it has been proposed that in nerve cells, protein degradation must be intimately related to such processes as axoplasmic flow, assembly and disassembly of membranes, and processes associated with neuronal plasticity (Goldberg, 1974). Apart from these normal roles of degradation, it is possible that degradation could be increased (in a selective manner) by the *in vitro* incubation condition itself. Indeed, when diaphragm or soleus muscles are incubated *in vitro* a net protein breakdown has been reported, although the muscles synthesize proteins at a linear rate (Goldberg, *et al.*, 1974). We cannot discount that one of the conditions of our incubation procedure (e.g., ion composition, temperature, absence of normal blood constituents, etc.) may be the cause of an increased rate of selective degradation in $R_{15}$. We attempted to test the degradation hypothesis by incubating cell $R_{15}$ in $^3$H-leucine in the usual manner, but afterwards removing the soma of $R_{15}$ from the ganglion, and "chasing" in the isolated cell without its axon for 4 hours in a 10 microliter droplet of medium. There were no significant changes in the labeling profile of proteins between the $R_{15}$ cells incubated for 3 hours in the ganglion *in vitro* and the isolated cells chased *in vitro* (Gainer & Barker, unpublished). Since we had shown that such isolated cells were capable of protein synthesis, we assumed that degradative processes, if any, would also be conserved in this condition. If this is the case, then it would appear that the protein is not being broken down in the soma, but rather is being rapidly transported (or secreted) out of the soma. When we attempted to block transport by "chasing" at 0°C, we found that not only were the labeled low molecular weight proteins in $R_{15}$ conserved, but that there appeared to be conversion of the labeled 12,000 dalton protein to a smaller (approximately 6,000 dalton) protein. Therefore, there appears to be processing of this protein in $R_{15}$, as has been reported for neurosecretory proteins in the bag cells of *Aplysia* (Arch, 1972a), and this processing could be revealed at the low temperature. None of the above experiments are adequate to distinguish between the alternative mechanisms of degradation and transport (or secretion), and further work is necessary before a definite conclusion can be drawn. Low temperatures would conserve the labeled protein in either case. If transport of the protein (presumably in granules) into the axon is taking place, then the processing of the protein (which we observe at 0°C) would occur, at higher temperatures, in the axon. Such a phenomenon has been proposed for the neurohypophysial hormones (Ginsburg, 1968).

In the case of the snail, the normal adaptive behavior of the animal allowed us to observe the results of a "long-term modulation experiment". Here, a dramatic change in the protein synthesis of a single neuron could be demonstrated (Fig. 7). However, the relevant variables (signals) which transformed cell 11 from a dormant to an active state (and vice versa) in these "experiments" were under the control of the animals' own behavioral mechanisms, and are still unknown to us. Thus far, in our relatively short-term, *in vitro* experiments, we have not succeeded in modifying the biochemical properties of cell 11, and it is expected (in view of the low turnover rates in this cell) that long-term, *in vitro* experiments (i.e., over days on organ-cultured ganglia) will be necessary to pursue this issue.

## Modulation of the BPP

At least two forms of inhibitory modulation of the BPP can be demonstrated. One is the conventional inhibitory post-synaptic potential mechanism which represents a ubiquitous and powerful input in cell 11 (Gainer, 1972c), and which probably is frequently utilized in the intact animal (Kater & Kaneko, 1972). The influence of the ipsp can last from seconds to minutes and in the case of $R_{15}$ may last for many minutes (see Parnas, this volume). The second form of inhibitory modulation represents a change of state of the BPP mechanism, as we have demonstrated for the aestivated land snail. In this case, the natural inhibitory influences of the divalent cations (i.e., $Ca^{++}$) are amplified by an increase in the cell's sensitivity to the inhibitory effects of $Ca^{++}$ on the BPP (see Fig. 10). Such a mechanism would be particularly appropriate for the seasonal (long-term) regulation of BPP activity, and suggests the resetting of some "allosteric gate" for the oscillator mechanism driving the BPP. The fact that application of steroid hormones such as aldosterone and hydrocortisone can mimic the aestivated state, causes us to wonder whether the active biosynthesis of sterols and steroids in gastropod molluscs (Raghupathiramireddy, 1967; Van der Horst & Voogt, 1972; Prisco *et al.*, 1973; Van der Horst, 1974) is involved in these regulatory processes.

Probably the most interesting modulation effect we have observed is the induction and augmentation of the BPP by the neurohypophysial peptides (see Figs. 11 and 12). The dramatic specificity of this effect, in terms of chemical structure, specific cell receptivity (i.e., cell 11 and $R_{15}$), and specific locus of receptivity (Fig. 12), suggests that a specific receptor to these or similar peptides in the snail brain (Fig. 13) exists on the cell's surface. The mechanism of action of these peptides appears not to involve a specific conductance change (as in the case of conventional neurotransmitters - see Gershenfeld, 1973), but rather the modulation of an existing conductance mechanism (i.e., the BPP). That the cell's receptivity to the peptide resides in a region close to the suggested site of the oscillatory mechanism (i.e., near the "axon hillock" - see Gainer, 1972C) lends credence to this view. While we do not fully understand the mechanisms of action of these peptides, they too appear to be acting on some "allosteric gating" sites for the BPP. The existence of such "modulator substances" had been proposed by Florey (1967), who defined them as "compounds of cellular and nonsynaptic origin that affect the excitability of nerve cells, and represent a normal link in the regulatory mechanisms that govern the performance of the nervous system." Florey mentions eleven neural parameters which could be affected by modulator substances (amongst these, the spontaneous activity of neurons), and points out that such modulations would resemble hormonal influences in their long duration of action. The concept that there are macromolecular entities in frog muscle which are involved in the regulation of ionic conductances in post-synaptic membrane (independent of the cholinergic receptor) has been termed the "ionic conductance modulator" (Kuba, *et al.*, 1973). What is being suggested here is that such "modulator entities" may be common in the nervous system and that they may be under the regulatory control of "modulator substances" (e.g., neurohormones).

Considering anatomic studies, various neuroendocrinologists have pondered whether there were a wide variety of communication systems in the nervous system. Scharrer (1969, 1972) has proposed that in addition to the conventional synaptic mechanism (the structures of which she refers to as "synaptoids"), there are neurohormonal mechanisms represented by type A neurosecretory cells (which are termed "peptidergic", i.e., those which store proteinaceous or peptidergic products - see Bergmann *et al.*, 1967), and type B (aminergic) cells. In the hypothalamic-hypophysial system, type B cells appear to regulate the type A cells (Scharrer, 1972), which in turn release their products into the circulation (e.g., the releasing factors). However, a more direct action of the peptidergic cells has been proposed (Zetler, 1970; Scharrer, 1972), via "neurosecretomotor junctions", particularly in the invertebrates which do not usually contain capillaries (e.g., peptidergic neurons terminate directly onto endocrine receptor cells in the corpus allatum of insects). The question whether peptidergic neurons in other parts of the nervous system exert influences via the release of such modulator substances (releasing or regulatory factors) has been raised (Zetler, 1970).

The wider question, whether specific modulator substances can provoke or inhibit specific behavior provides an attractive notion. Considerable evidence exists that peptide and steroid hormones can elicit specific types of behavior. For example, vasopressin induces spawning behavior in gonadectomized *Fundulus* (Morrel & Jard, 1968), luteinizing releasing factor induces mating behavior in hypophysectomized-ovarectimized female rats (Moss & McCann, 1973; Pfaff, 1973), estradiol and dihydrotestosterone causes copulation in castrated male rats (Baum & Vreeburg, 1973), drinking behavior is induced in rats by angiotensin II (Simpson & Routtenberg, 1973), lysine-vasopressin directly causes release of ACTH from the pituitary (Dunn & Critchlow, 1971), and seasonal changes of the hormone levels which govern spawning in the goldfish also appear to influence its learning and activity patterns (Shashoua, 1973). It is very tempting to speculate that there are ensembles of neurons associated with discrete behaviors (e.g., fixed action patterns) which are specifically modulated by specific neurohormones.

## ACKNOWLEDGEMENTS

The author wishes to thank his colleagues Drs. J.L. Barker, Z. Wollberg, Y. Peng Loh, and Y. Sarne for their very active collaboration and discussions.

## REFERENCES

1. ARCH, S. *J. Gen. Physiol. 60:*102, 1972a.
2. ARCH, S. *J. Gen. Physiol. 59:*47, 1972b.
3. ASCHER, P., KEHOE, J.S. & TAUC, L. *J. Physiol., Paris 59:* 331, 1967.
4. BARGMANN, W., LINDNER, E. & ANDRES, K.H. *Zschr. Zellforsch 77:*282, 1967.
5. BARKER, J.L. & GAINER, H. *Nature 245:*462, 1973.
6. BARKER, J.L. & GAINER, H. *Science*, in press, 1974.
7. BAUM, M.J. & VREEBURG, J.T.M. *Science 182:*283, 1973.
8. BERDE, B. Neurophypophysial Hormones and Similar Peptides. Handbook of Experimental Pharmacology XXIII, Springer-Verlag, Berlin, 1968.
9. CARPENTER, D.O. & GUNN, R. *J. Cell Physiol. 75:*121, 1970.
10. CHALAZONITIS, N. & TAKEUCHI, H. *C.R. Soc. Biol. (Paris) 162:* 1552, 1968.
11. CHRAMBACH, A. & RODBARD, D. *Science 172:*440, 1971.
12. COLES, G.C. *Comp. Biochem. Physiol. 25:*517, 1969.
13. DUNN, J. & CRITCHLOW, V. *Proc. Soc. Exp. Biol. Med. 136:*1284, 1971.
14. FABER, D.S. & KLEE, M.R. *Nature NB 240:*29, 1972.
15. FLOREY, E. *Fed. Proc. 26:*1164, 1967.
16. FRAZIER, W.T., KANDEL, E.R., KUPFERMAN, I., WAZIRI, R. & COGGESHALL, R.E. *J. Neurophysiol. 30:*1288, 1967.
17. GAINER, H. *Anal. Biochem. 44:*589, 1971.
18. GAINER, H. *Brain Res. 39:*369, 1972a.
19. GAINER, H. *Brain Res. 39:*387, 1972b.
20. GAINER, H. *Brain Res. 39:*403, 1972c.
21. GAINER, H. *Anal. Biochem. 51:*646, 1973.
22. GAINER, H. & WOLLBERG, Z. *J. Neurobiol.*, in press, 1974.
23. GAINER, H. & BARKER, J.L. *Brain Res.*, in press, 1974b.
24. GAINER, H. & BARKER, J.L. *Comp. Biochem. Physiol.*, in press, 1974.
25. GERSHENFELD, H.M. *Physiol. Rev. 53:*1, 1973
26. GINSBURG, M. In: Handbook of Experimental Pharmacology XXIII, B. Berde, Ed., Springer-Verlag, Berlin, p. 286, 1968.
27. GLASSMAN, E. *Ann. Rev. Biochem. 38:*605, 1969.
28. GOLDBERG, A.L. In: The Neurosciences, Third Study Program. F.O. Schmitt & F.G. Worden, Eds., MIT Press, Cambridge, p. 827, 1974.
29. GOLDBERG, A.L., HOWELL, E.M., LI, J.B., MARTEL, S.B. & PROUTY, W.F. *Fed. Proc. 33:*1112, 1974.
30. HORN, G., ROSE, S.P.R., BATESON, P.P.G. *Science 181:*506, 1973.
31. HUNTER, W.R. In: Physiology of Mollusca, K.M. Wilbur & C.M. Yonge, Eds., Vol. I, Academic Press, New York, p. 83, 1964.
32. HYMAN, L.H. The Invertebrates, Vol. VI, Mollusca I, McGraw-Hill, New York, p. 792, 1968.

32. KATER, S.B. & KANEKO, C.R.S. *J. Comp. Physiol.* *79:*1, 1972.
33. KERKUT, G.A., HORN, N. & WALKER, R.J. *Comp. Biochem. Physiol.* *30:*1061, 1969.
34. KLEE, M.R., FABER, D.S. & HEISS, W-D. *Science* *179:*1133, 1973.
35. KRAUSE, E. *Z. Zellforsch.* *51:*748, 1960.
36. KUBA, K., ALBUQUERQUE, E.X. & BARNARD, E.A. *Science* *181:*853, 1973.
37. LOH, Y.P. Ph.D. dissertation in mol. biol., Univ. of Pennsylvania, 1973, 82 pp.
38. MACHIN, J. *J. Exp. Biol.* *45:*269, 1966.
39. MACHIN, J. *J. Exp. Biol.* *57:*103, 1972.
40. MATHIEU, P.A. & ROBERGE, F.A. *Can. J. Physiol. Pharmacol.* *49:*787, 1971.
41. MEENAKSHI, V.R. *Current Sci.* *25:*321, 1956.
42. MORALES, T. & CHALAZONITIS, N. *Soc. Biol. Marseille*, 1792, 1970.
43. MORREL, F. & JARD, S. In: Handbook of Experimental Pharmacology XXIII, B. Berde, Ed., Springer-Verlag, Berlin, p. 655, 1968.
44. MOSS, R.L. & MC CANN, S.M. *Science* *181:*177, 1973.
45. NEUHOFF, V. *Micromethods in Molecular Biology*, Springer Verlag, Berlin, 428 pp., 1973.
46. PETERSON, R.P. & LOH, Y.P. *Prog. Neurobiol.* *2:*179, 1973.
47. PFAFF, D.W. *Science* *182:*1148, 1973.
48. PRISCO, C.L., FULGHEFI, F.D. & TOMASUCCI, M. *Comp. Biochem. Physiol.* *45B:*303, 1973.
49. RAGHUPATHIRAMIREDDY, S. *Life Sci.* *6:*341, 1967.
50. ROBERTSON, J.D. In: Physiology of Mollusca, K.M. Wilbur & C.M. Yonge, Eds., Vol. I, Academic Press, New York, p. 283, 1964.
51. SCHARRER, B. *J. Neuro-Visceral Relations, Suppl.* *IX:*1, 1969.
52. SCHARRER, B. *Prog. in Brain Res.* *38:*7, 1972.
53. SCHIMKE, R.T. In: The Neurosciences, Third Study Program, F.O. Schmitt & F.G. Worden, Eds., MIT Press, Cambridge, p. 813, 1974.
54. SCHMIDT-NIELSEN, K., TAYLOR, C.R. & SHKOLNIK, E. *J. Exp. Biol.* *55:*385, 1971.
55. SCHWARTZ, J.H., CASTELLUCHI, V.F. & KANDEL, E.R. *J. Neurophysiol.* *34:*939, 1971.
56. SHASHOUA, V.E. *Science* *181:*572, 1973.
57. SIMPSON, J.B. & ROUTTENBERG, A. *Science* *181:*1172, 1973.
58. SPEEG, K.V. & CAMPBELL, T.W. *Amer. J. Physiol.* *214:*1392, 1968.
59. STRUMWASSER, F. In: Physiological and Biochemical Aspects of Nervous Integration, F.D. Carlson, Ed., Prentice-Hall, New Jersey, p. 329, 1968.
60. STRUMWASSER, F. *The Physiologist* *16:*9, 1973.
61. VAN DER HORST, D.J. *Comp. Biochem. Physiol.* *47B:*181, 1974.
62. VAN DER HORST, D.J. & VOOGT, P.A. *Comp. Biochem. Physiol.* *42B:*1, 1972.
63. VAN DER KLOOT, V.G. *Biol. Bull.* *109:*276, 1955.

64. WACHTEL, H. & WILSON, W.A. In: Neurobiology of Invertebrates, Tihany, p. 59, 1973.
65. WILSON, D.W. *J. Gen. Physiol.* *57:*26, 1971.
66. WILSON, D.W. & BERRY, R.W. *J. Neurobiol.* *3:*369, 1972.
67. WILSON, D.W. *J. Neurochem.* *22:*465, 1974.
68. ZETLER, G. In: Aspects of Neuroendocrinology. V. International Symposium on Neurosecretion, W. Bargmann & B. Scharrer, Eds., Springer-Verlag, Berlin, p. 287, 1970.

# LONG-LASTING CHANGES IN THE ACTIVITY OF A BURSTING NEURONE PRODUCED BY SPECIFIC SYNAPTIC INPUTS

I. Parnas
Division of Neurobiology
Institute of Life Sciences
The Hebrew University
Jerusalem, Israel

Long-lasting modifications of behavior are believed to be associated with long-lasting changes at the neuronal level. Comparisons have been made between various behavioral parameters before and after direct or synaptic stimulation of a single neuron (Castellucci *et al.*, 1970; Berry & Cohen, 1972; Cedar *et al.*, 1972). Similarly, long term changes have been demonstrated in the activity of a group of neurons (Lippold, 1970; Pettigrew *et al.*, 1973) or in single neurons after inducing changes in behavior (Strumwasser, 1965; 1971; Kupfermann *et al.*, 1970; for review see Horn & Hinde, 1970). Chemical as well as electrical changes have been found, but a clear cut correlation between the behavioral and the neuronal changes has not been demonstrated.

Kandel and his associates (reviewed in Kandel & Kupfermann, 1970; Blankenship *et al.*, 1971; Wachtel & Kandel, 1971) have demonstrated a wide range of synaptic mechanisms in *Aplysia*. They found many orders of complexity, including a case where different synaptic potentials (epsp's or ipsp's) are produced by the same transmitter substance, interaction with different receptors on the same cell producing different ionic changes. They also found similar synaptic potentials produced by different ionic mechanisms in the same cell. Kehoe (1972b) distinguished three kinds of acetylcholine receptors in *Aplysia*, their activation resulting either in an epsp, a short inhibitory response or long-lasting inhibition. Gerschenfeld and his associates (Gerschenfeld & Stefani, 1968; Gerschenfeld, 1971; 1973; Paupardin-Tritsch & Gerschenfeld, 1973) have demonstrated in *Aplysia* and snail a variety of receptors and responses to 5-hydroxytriptamine (5HT); such a variety of responses at the synaptic level considerably extends the possible diversity of control mechanisms in the nervous system.

The finding that, in a given cell, similar synaptic potentials can be induced by different ionic mechanisms raises the possibility that a post-synaptic cell "recognizes" an input by means other than the induced electrical signal. It is possible that in addition to, or even instead of, the electrical signal, changes produced in the specific conductance at the post-synaptic cell and/or the movement of specific ions are involved in the transfer of information between cells, thereby inducing long-lasting changes.

It is this last point that I would like to emphasize; I would like to demonstrate a case of long-lasting synaptic modulation of the electrical activity of an identifiable neuron ($R_{15}$, the "parabolic burster", in the abdominal ganglion of *Aplysia*, Strumwasser, 1965, Fraizer *et al.*, 1967) and to show that the synaptic potential in itself is not a parameter sufficient to produce the long-lasting change. $R_{15}$ is known to receive several synaptic inputs. The electrical signals produced by the different synapses may appear quite similar (at least when recorded from an electrode in the soma) and yet only two of these synapses produce changes which outlast the stimulus for periods of up to many hours.

$R_{15}$ is a neuron that produces bursts of endogenous spikes (Strumwasser, 1965; Alving, 1968; Strumwasser & Kim, 1969; Strumwasser, 1971). In the isolated abdominal ganglion, $R_{15}$ shows a circadian rhythm of impulse activity; this rhythm can be entrained in the intact animal to different light-dark cycles (Strumwasser, 1965). It was recently confirmed that the eyes are essential for such an entrainment (Audesirk, personal communication).

The finding that lasting changes in the firing pattern of such a bursting neuron can be induced simply by the control of the light-dark cycle makes $R_{15}$ a convenient model to study mechanisms involved in long-lasting changes in neuronal activity. At present, neither the physiological role of $R_{15}$ nor the physiological significance of the changes in the circadian rhythm are understood. Nor is it known whether the circadian rhythm entrainment is achieved by synaptic, hormonal or neurohumoral control.

In spite of the sparcity of information, we were interested to see whether we could induce long-lasting changes in the bursting activity of $R_{15}$ by synaptic inputs, especially those from axons in the connectives, since these axons come from the ganglionic ring to which the optic nerves are connected.

Several inputs to $R_{15}$ were described in the detailed work of Frazier *et al.* (1967). One major input from the right connective produces a large epsp which is blocked by d-tubocurarine (dTc) (Gerschenfeld, 1973). Another input which is of interest comes from interneuron II, located in the abdominal ganglion, and producing inhibition of long duration (ILD - Stinnakre & Tauc, 1969; Tauc, 1969). In addition, an input from Neuron $L_{10}$ (Frazier *et al.*, 1967) produces a large epsp.

While looking for the effects of the excitatory input from the right connective, we found that at least three axons in the right connective innervate $R_{15}$. One is the "classical" excitatory dTc-sensitive input. The other two produce biphasic postsynaptic potentials (bpsp). The evidence for the presence of these three axons can be found in an article which appeared recently by Parnas, Armstrong & Strumwasser (1974). We found that stimulation of the excitatory axon for a few minutes leads to an increase in the number of spikes per burst which persists for hours. This effect is not produced solely by the electrical signal; other concommitants of transmitter release are required as well.

An opposite effect is achieved by stimulation of one of the inhibitory axons (input III, Parnas *et al.*, 1974). After only a few impulses, all spiking is blocked for several hours. We showed that stimulation of this inhibitory synapse could cancel the effects induced by the excitatory axon; but, whenever the long-lasting inhibition was induced, activation of excitatory synapses (either input I of Parnas *et al.*, 1974 or that from $L_{10}$) could not "release" the cell from inhibition. Under these conditions, the cell did not fire, in spite of intense activation of the excitatory inputs.

I will not describe in detail how we established that at least three axons in the right connective innervate $R_{15}$ nor discuss whether they innervate it directly of through interneurons. In Fig. 1 the connectivity of these three axons to $R_{15}$ is illustrated. Input I, which is excitatory, innervates $R_{15}$ directly. The epsp induced by it is blocked by dTc and is thought to be cholingeric. From the magnitude of the epsp (after facilitation it reaches an amplitude of 45 mv, Parnas *et al.*, 1974) and its shape, we concluded that this input is electrically quite close to the soma. This input produces long-lasting excitatory effects.

Axon II produces a bpsp which affects the bursting activity of $R_{15}$ only during the stimulation period. There are no long-lasting effects even after prolonged periods of stimulation.

The third axon, III, innervates $R_{15}$, probably through interneuron II. It is not clear at this stage whether axon III is actually a collateral of interneuron II, or whether it activates interneuron II via a chemical or electrical synapse. It is possible to induce the response of input III by stimulation of the branchial

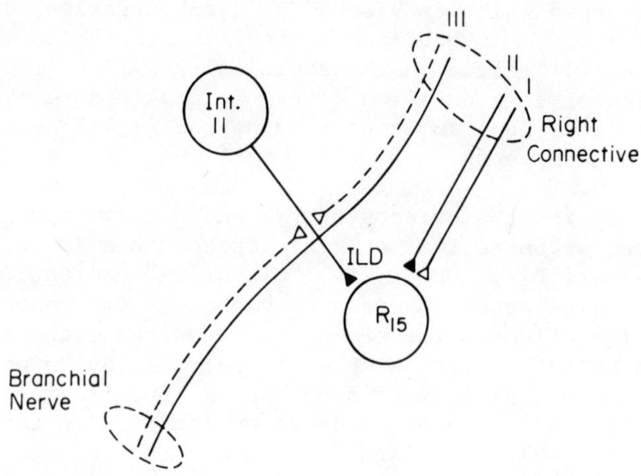


Fig. 1 Schema of the connectivity of the three inputs to neuron $R_{15}$. Open triangles - excitatory synapses. Filled triangles - inhibitory synapses. See text. (From Parnas *et al.*, 1974).

nerve. Neither the response induced by axon II nor that induced by axon III are blocked by dTc. Thus it is possible to activate each of the three synapses separately. Axon I is recruited by stimulation of the right connective at the lowest stimulus voltage, axon II can be recruited alone after blocking input I with dTc and the input III response can be induced alone by stimulating the branchial nerve.

## LONG-LASTING EFFECTS INDUCED BY INPUT I

Fig. 2 demonstrates the long-lasting effects of input I. In Fig. 2A, the activity of $R_{15}$ during a control period is shown. The bursting is regular; that is, the number of spikes per burst (burst size), the duration of the burst and the interburst interval are all more or less constant. In Fig. 2B, axon I was stimulated at a rate of 10/sec for three minutes. During the stimulation period, bursting was disrupted and the cell fired regularly every third epsp. After cessation of stimulation, bursting resumed, but at this time there was a clear increase in burst size, from 17-18 (Fig. 2A) to 27-29 (Fig. 2C), which built up slowly over a number of bursts (Figs. 3, 4). Such an effect of activation of axon I at frequencies between 6-10/sec was observed in many experiments. These frequencies are well within the physiological range (Audesirk, personal communication). The increase in burst size persisted at its

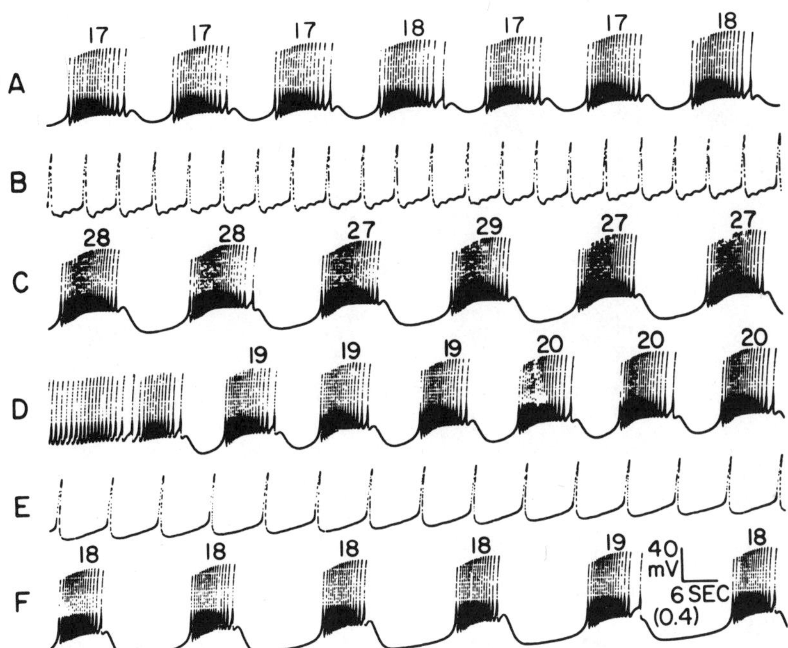


Fig. 2 Long-lasting excitatory effects of input I. A. Control, a section from a 25 min period. B. Stimulation of input I at 10/sec for a 4 min period. C. 8 min after the stimulation was over. D. After 4 min of hyperpolarization. E. Depolarization producing continuous spiking for 4 min did not alter the burst size, afterwards in F. Numbers above bursts indicate burst size. Calibration, traces B and E 0. 4 sec. (From Parnas *et al.*, 1974).

maximal value for several hours (Fig. 3). In some experiments the effect lasted for shorter periods. It may be noted that the increase in burst size produced by stimulation of axon I was not always an all or none effect. At times, repeated periods of stimulation were required in order to induce the change. In general, the longer the stimulation period, the stronger the effect of stimulation of axon I. Also, at higher frequencies of stimulation, the effect of increase in burst size was achieved sooner and usually was more pronounced. There was, however, a limit beyond which the burst size could not be increased (35-37 spikes/burst); even with very long periods of stimulation, further increase was not induced.

Fig. 2D shows the bursting of the same neuron after a three minute period of hyperpolarization, sufficient in degree to stop all spiking. After the injection of inward current was stopped,

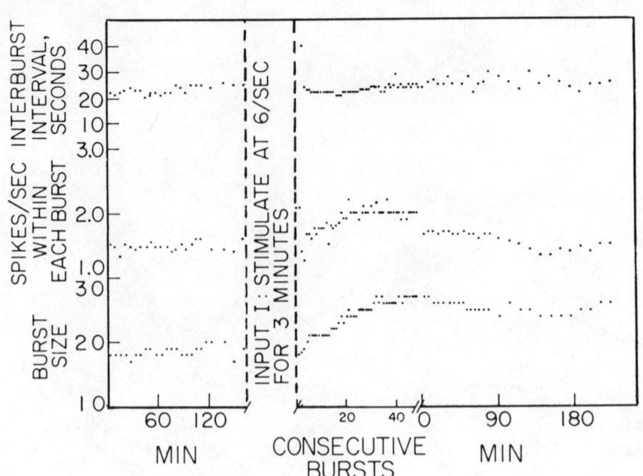


Fig. 3 Effect of input I (3 min stimulation at 6/sec) on the burst size, spike frequency within a burst and interburst interval. Left (abscissa in minutes) control. After the stimulation period the abcissa is expressed as consecutive bursts. Right - the abscissa is again expressed in minutes to show that the effect lasted for at least three more hours. (From Parnas *et al.*, 1974.)

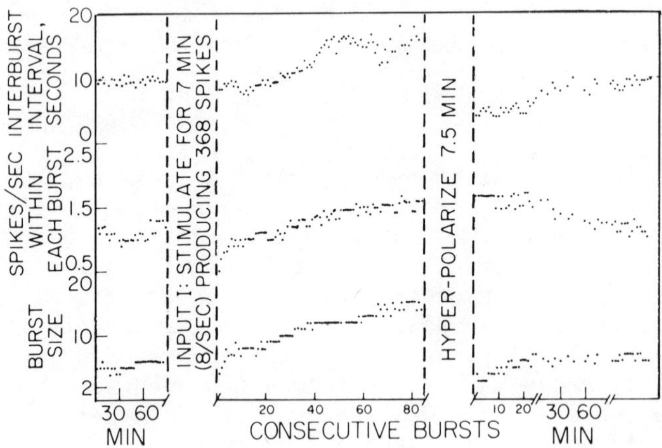


Fig. 4 Burst parameters as in Fig. 3. Note that hyperpolarization for 7.5 min abolished the excitatory effect. (From Parnas *et al.*, 1974).

there was a rebound and a short period of continuous spiking (Fig. 2D, left) but soon bursting was resumed, this time at about the control level (compare 2D and 2A). Evidently the hyperpolarization reversed the effect induced by stimulation of axon I. Again, the effect of the hyperpolarization was not all or none - at times repeated periods of hyperpolarization were required to abolish the excitatory effect. We also found that the longer the period after the excitatory effect was established, the more difficult it was to produce abolition by hyperpolarization. Once hyperpolarization did cancel the excitatory effect, however, the burst size remained constant at the new level (Fig. 4). I should like to emphasize that we were never able to reduce the burst size below that found in the control period even with very long periods of hyperpolarization. We could abolish only the excitatory effects induced by the epsp and even these could be abolished only after relatively short periods at the excited level. Obviously it would be of great interest to conduct careful experiments to establish the time periods after which, if the cell is set in the new state of increased burst size, it is impossible to produce cancellation by hyperpolarization. Abolishment of the excitatory effect could be also achieved by the activation of the inhibitory axon (axon III) that caused prolonged hyperpolarization.

In spite of the finding that hyperpolarization could cancel the effect induced by the excitatory axon, steady depolarization (Fig. 2E), sufficient to produce about the same rate of firing as in Fig. 2B, did not induce the increase in burst size. Neither was it possible to induce the effect by injection of outward current impulses which mimicked the membrane potential changes of the epsp's. Even much stronger depolarization could not mimic the long-lasting effects of input I. It appears that *synaptic activation* by axon I is required to produce this long-lasting change. In some experiments, when neuron $L_{10}$ fired spontaneously for several minutes, acceleration of the bursting was observed, but no long-lasting effects were seen that outlasted $L_{10}$ firing.

From these experiments it is clear that the important factor in inducing the long-lasting changes is the synaptic activity of input I. Furthermore, if input I and II are activated together and spiking is blocked, the long-lasting effect is still observed. Thus, the spiking activity of $R_{15}$ is not an important factor since direct stimulation does not mimic the effect.

## LONG-LASTING EFFECTS OF INPUT III

Stimulation of input III (either from the right connective or from the branchial nerve) at 1/sec for a few seconds resulted in long-lasting inhibition. The membrane potential was hyperpolarized to approximately -70 mv and was followed by a delayed hyperpolarization (DH) which may last for many minutes (Fig. 5). The hyperpolarization was associated with a marked membrane conductance increase. The duration of the inhibition and the increase in conductance depend on the number of impulses given to axon III (Fig. 6).

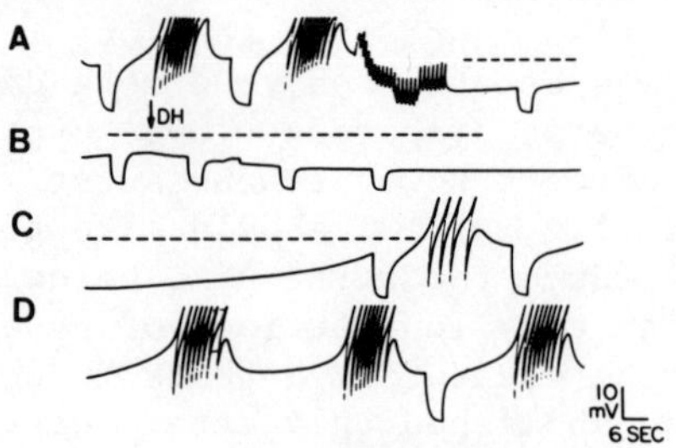


Fig. 5 Long-lasting inhibitory effect caused by input III. A and B are continuous records. A, Control and stimulation at 1/sec. Note the marked increase in membrane conductance during stimulation as reflected by the decrease in membrane potential change in response to constant current pulses. B. A delayed hyperpolarization developed. C. Thirty minutes after B, the membrane conductances return to the control value. D. After 15 more minutes bursting recovered. The interrupted line represents the pre-stimulation resting potential. (From Parnas *et al.*, 1974.)

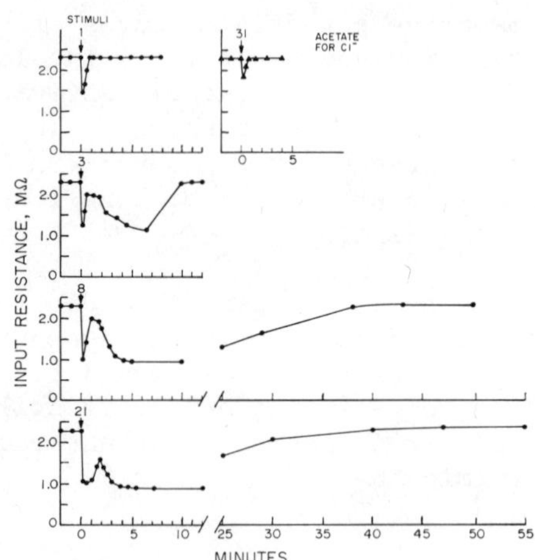


Fig. 6 Effects of increasing number of impulses of input III on membrane conductance. Number of stimuli is given above arrows. Note that when acetate replaces chloride (top right) the long-lasting effect is missing. (From Parnas & Strumwasser, 1974.)

The prolonged increase in conductance does not depend on the activity of a sensitive electrogenic pump, neither does it depend on activity in reverberating circuits (Parnas & Strumwasser, 1974). Removal of chloride from the medium abolishes hyperpolarization (Fig. 7). The reversal potential of the early hyperpolarization (about -70 mv) is more negative than the chloride equilibrium potential (Kunze *et al.*, 1971). The delayed hyperpolarization shifts the membrane potential to a value close to the $K^+$ equilibrium potential and is reversibly blocked by intracellularly injected tetraethylammonium (TEA, Fig. 8). After the injection of TEA the reversal potential of the early hyperpolarization is shifted to about -57 mv (Fig. 9). These

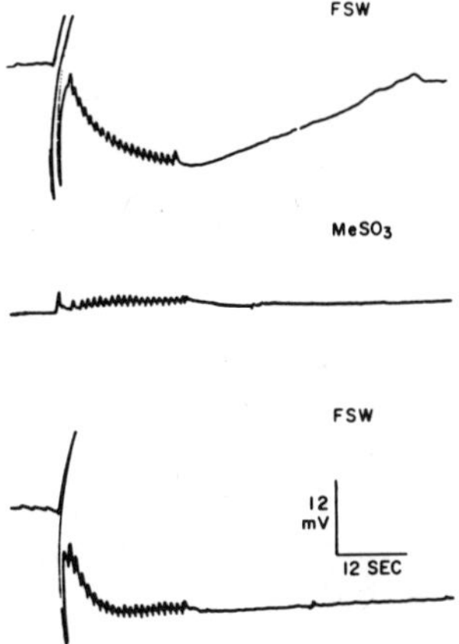


Fig. 7 Effects of input III in normal and chloride free medium. Top - in filtered sea water (FSW). Middle - chloride replaced by methanesulfunate, no pH is observed. Bottom - recovery after washing with FSW. (From Parnas & Strumwasser, 1974.)

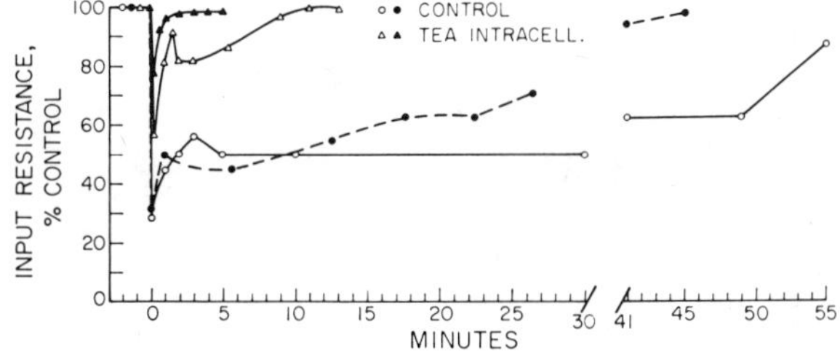


Fig. 8 Membrane resistance changes after stimuli to input III in control (open circles). After first injection (30 min, 4nA) of TEA (open triangles) and after second injection of TEA (filled triangles). Filled circles - 24 hours after the withdrawal of the TEA electrode there was a recovery of the long-lasting response. (From Parnas & Strumwaser, 1974.)

results indicate that the early hyperpolarization is produced by an increase in membrane conductance to both chloride and potassium ions, while the delayed hyperpolarization results from an increase in conductance to potassium ions. Since Meech (1972) suggested that $Ca^{++}$ does control $K^{+}$ conductance, we lowered intracellular $Ca^{++}$ concentration by the injection of EGTA. Under these conditions, activation of input III did not produce the long-lasting response (Fig. 10).

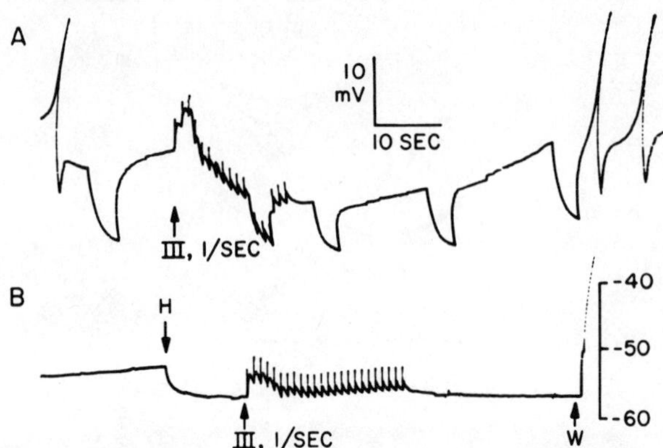


Fig. 9 Reversal potential of the hyperpolarizing phase of the bpsp of input III after intracellular injection of TEA. A. Note that after stimulation of input III the DH is missing. B. The reversal potential is -57 mv as measured by the withdrawal (W) of the microelectrode. (From Parnas & Strumwasser, 1974).

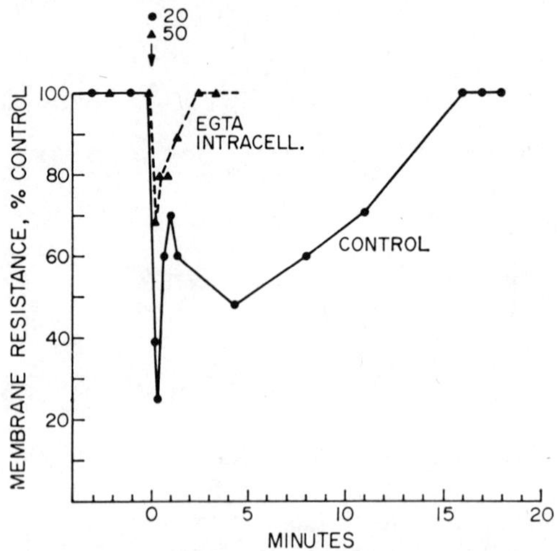


Fig. 10 Membrane conductance changes produced by input III before (filled circles) and after (filled triangles) injection of EGTA. (From Parnas & Strumwasser, 1974.)

## DISCUSSION

We have thus demonstrated two synaptic inputs to $R_{15}$ which can produce long-lasting effects in opposite directions - input I produces long-lasting excitation, while input III evokes long-lasting inhibition. At this stage, little is known as to the molecular mechanisms responsible for the increase in burst size, especially in that the mechanism of bursting generation is not completely understood (see Strumwasser, 1968, 1973; Strumwasser & Kim, 1969; Carpenter, 1973; Junge & Stephens, 1973 for different views). Various experimental manipulations that we have tried, such as oubain, changes in ionic concentrations, injection of different ions ($Na^+$, $Cl^-$, $Ca^{++}$), disrupted the bursting to such a degree that measurement of the only reliable parameter (burst size) was no longer possible.

We can speculate, however, on the specific synaptic mechanism which produces the long-lasting excitatory effect. We cannot exclude at this stage the release of another compound from axon I, in addition to the transmitter responsible for the long-lasting effect in itself or producing the prolonged excitation in combination with the transmitter. If the effect is produced by the transmitter alone, we must assume that the long-lasting excitation results from a highly specialized activity of the transmitter other than its depolarizing action or from activation of specialized receptors, since another presumably cholinergic depolarizing input to this neuron (from $L_{10}$) does not produce the effect.

It is interesting to note that hyperpolarization which is produced either by injection of inward current or by the activation of input III is sufficient to cancel the excitatory effect, while the weaker hyperpolarization produced by axon II is not. It is possible that the magnitude of hyperpolarization is an important factor in the abolition of long-lasting excitation.

The ionic mechanisms associated with long-lasting inhibition are better identified. As other investigators (Tauc, 1968; 1969; Kehoe, 1972a; Ascher, 1972) have found in studying inhibition of long duration, the long-lasting inhibition produced by input III is also associated with an increase in potassium conductance (gK). The requirement for the presence of external chloride ions for the development of DH is not yet understood. It also appears that intracellular $Ca^{++}$ ions are required for the increase in gK.

It is not known as yet whether or not the two inputs, I and III, are involved in the entrainment of the circadian rhythm activity of $R_{15}$. Long-term experiments with isolated nervous systems and *in vitro* entrainment of $R_{15}$ are technically feasible and should clarify this point. Strumwasser (1973) has succeeded in keeping a functional isolated ganglion in an organ culture for many weeks. Until the long-term studies are done, we must be satisfied with the ability to produce specific long-lasting changes in the activity of this single neuron by the action of specific synaptic inputs. Indeed, if the inputs are not responsible for the entrainment of circadian rhythm, they must have other long-lasting effects of functional significance.

## REFERENCES

1. ALVING, B.O. *J. Gen. Physiol.* *51:*29, 1968.
2. ASCHER, P. *J. Physiol., London* *225:*173, 1972.
3. BERRY, R.W. & COHEN, M.J. *J. Neurobiol.* *3:*209, 1972.
4. BLANKENSHIP, J., WACHTEL, H. & KANDEL, E.R. *J. Neurophysiol.* *34:*76, 1971.
5. CARPENTER, D.O. Ionic mechanisms and models of endogenous discharge of *Aplysia* neurones. Neurobiology of Invertebrates. Tihany, p. 35, 1973.
6. CASTELLUCCI, V., PINSKER, H., KUPFERMANN, I. & KANDEL, E.R. *Science* *167:*1745, 1970.
7. CEDAR, H., KANDEL, E.R. & SCHWARTZ, J.H. *J. Gen. Phys.* *60:* 558, 1972.
8. FRAIZER, W.T., KANDEL, E.R., KUPFERMANN, I., WAZIRI, R. & COGESHALL, R.E. *J. Neurophysiol.* *30:*1288, 1967.
9. GERSCHENFELD, H.M. *Science* *171:*1252, 1971.
10. GERSCHENFELD, H.M. *Physiol. Rev.* *53:*1, 1973.
11. GERSCHENFELD, H.M. & STEFANI, E. *Adv. Pharmacol.* *6A:*360, 1968.
12. HORN, G. & HINDE, R.A. (Eds.) Short-term changes in neuronal activity and behaviour. Cambridge Univ. Press, 1970.
13. JUNGE, O. & STEPHENS, C.L. *J. Physiol., London* *235:*155, 1973.
14. KANDEL, E.R. & KUPFERMANN, I. *Ann. Rev. of Physiol.* *32:*193, 1970.
15. KEHOE, J.S. *J. Physiol., London* *225:*85, 1972a.
16. KEHOE, J.S. *J. Physiol., London* *225:*115, 1972b.
17. KUNZE, D.L., WALKER, J.L. & BROWN, H.M. *Fed. Proc.* *30:*255, 1971.
18. KUPFERMANN, I., CASTELLUCCI, V., PINSKER, H. & KANDEL, E. *Science* *167:*1743, 1970.
19. LIPPOLD, O.C.J. Long-lasting changes in activity of cortical neurons. In: Short term changes in neural activity and behaviour. (G. Horn & R.A. Hinde, eds.) Cambridge Univ. Press, p. 405, 1970.
20. MEECH, R.W. *Comp. Biochem. Physiol.* *42:*493, 1972.
21. PARNAS, I., ARMSTRONG, O. & STRUMWASSER, F. *J. Neurophysiol.* *37:*594, 1974.
22. PARNAS, I. & STRUMWASSER, F. *J. Neurophysiol.* *37:*609, 1974.
23. PAUPARDIN-TRITSCH, O. & GERSCHENFELD, H.M. *Brain Research* *58:*529, 1973.

24. PETTIGREW, J., OLSON, C. & BARLOW, H.B. *Science 180:*1202, 1973.
25. STINNAKRE, J. & TAUC, L. *J. Exp. Biol. 51:*347, 1969.
26. STRUMWASSER, F. Demonstration and manipulation of a circadian rhythm in a single neuron. In: Circadian Clocks. (J. Aschoff, ed.) Amsterdam, North Holland Publishing, p. 442, 1965.
27. STRUMWASSER, F. Membrane and intracellular mechanisms governing endogenous activity in neurons. In: Physiological and biochemical aspects of nervous integration. (F.D. Carlson, ed.) Englewood Cliffs, N.J., Prentice-Hall, p. 329, 1968.
28. STRUMWASSER, F. & KIM, M. *Physiologist 12:*367, 1969.
29. STRUMWASSER, F. *J. Psychiat. Res. 8:*237, 1971.
30. STRUMWASSER, F. *Physiologist 16:*9, 1973.
31. TAUC, L. Some aspects of post-synaptic inhibition in *Aplysia*. In: Structure and function of neuronal inhibitory mechanism. (C. Von-Euler, S. Skoglund and U. Soderberg, eds.) Oxford, Pergamon, p. 377, 1968.
32. TAUC, L. Polyphasic synaptic activity. In: Progress in brain research. (A. Akert & P.G. Waser, eds.) Amsterdam, Elsevier, Vol. 31. p. 247, 1969.
33. WACHTEL, H. & KANDEL, E.R. *J. Neurophysiol. 34:*56, 1971.

MECHANISMS AND FUNCTIONS OF ELECTRICALLY MEDIATED INHIBITION IN THE VERTEBRATE CENTRAL NERVOUS SYSTEM

H. Korn[1] and D.S. Faber[2]
Laboratoire de Physiologie, C.H.U. Pitie-Salpetriere
Paris, France
[1]Maitre de Recherches (I.N.S.E.R.M.)
[2]Present address: Research Institute on Alcoholism
Buffalo, New York, U.S.A.

Although electrophysiologists have come to accept the concept that excitatory interactions between neurons can be mediated both electrically and chemically, it is generally assumed that inhibition is best carried out chemically (Bennett, 1972). Since inhibition generally results in a sign inversion, that is, depolarization of the presynaptic neuron leads to hyperpolarization of the postsynaptic element, it cannot commonly be mediated by electrotonic junctions. Exceptions under special conditions involve the preferential transmission of the spike after-hyperpolarization relative to the depolarizing phase of the action potential itself. In addition, this particular form of inhibition, which can be due to either a summation of after-hyperpolarizations during presynaptic firing (Tauc, 1969) or to a rectifying junction (Arvanitaki & Chalazonitis, 1959), results in a complex biphasic postsynaptic potential rather than in a pure hyperpolarization. Finally, it has been pointed out that these electrotonic junctions would favor excitatory transmission in the opposite direction (Arvanitaki & Chalazonitis, 1959).

A second type of electrical interaction between neurons may be considered rather as a "field effect"; it does not involve electrotonic junctions and is dependent on the orientation and electrical properties of the neurons involved as well as the properties of the surrounding tissue. Theoretically, such effects could result in a sign inversion. In fact, from the only three clear demonstrations of field effects in the vertebrate central nervous system (Faber & Korn, 1973; Korn & Faber, 1973; Furukawa & Furshpan, 1963; Nelson, 1966) two are in the goldfish medulla, and apparently result in a reciprocal negative feedback (Korn & Faber, 1975). Since the demonstration of such a system could be important for analysis of the behavior of complex neuronal networks, we review here the evidence for these particular types of electrically mediated phenomena and their underlying mechanisms.

## ELECTRICAL INHIBITION OF THE MAUTHNER CELL

The two examples of field effect inhibitions both involve the goldfish Mauthner cell (M-cell), which has been the subject of extensive electrophysiological as well as morphological studies (Bartelmez, 1915; Bodian, 1937; Furshpan & Furukawa, 1962; Furukawa & Furshpan, 1963; Furukawa, 1966; Diamond, 1968; see Diamond, 1971 for a comprehensive review; Nakajima, 1974; Robertson, 1963; Robertson *et al.*, 1963). Furukawa & Furshpan (1963) first demonstrated an electrical inhibition of the M-cell which can be evoked by its activation either antidromically or synaptically by stimulation of the contralateral eighth nerve; it is correlated with a positive extrinsic hyperpolarizing potential (EHP) which can be recorded extracellularly in the axon cap, that is, in the vicinity of the cell's axon hillock (Fig. 1). This positive potential is not observed during intracellular recording from the neuron itself, but when the true transmembrane potential change - the difference between the intra- and extra-cellularly recorded potentials - is calculated, one sees that this potential change is associated with a 15 - 20 mV membrane hyperpolarization. These observations demonstrated that the M-cell is not the EHP generator, and that the source for the hyperpolarization is external to this neuron.

The inhibitory nature of the EHP was also clearly shown by Furukawa and Furshpan (1963). The EHP is able to block both antidromic and orthodromic activation of the M-cell (Fig. 2A-C). These authors further demonstrated that the action of the EHP can be mimicked using an external anode located in the vicinity of the axon hillock (Fig. 2D, E), and postulated that it can thus be compared to such an external anodal source.

As far as the generation of the EHP is concerned, Furukawa and Furshpan's hypothesis was that impulse conduction failed in fibers invading the axon cap, with the inactive terminals of these fibers serving as passive current sources for the more distal sinks, thereby creating this external positivity. Presumably, some of the current is drawn by the M-cell and enters into the region of the axon hillock, while it excites the neuron at some more distal points, as was confirmed experimentally (Furukawa & Furshpan, 1963). This illustrates a basic property of field effect interactions: an external source which hyperpolarizes one region of the "post-synaptic" neuron should depolarize another more remote region while leaving it. Therefore, the functional nature of the field effect depends upon the relative orientation of the neurons involved; in the present case, the inward

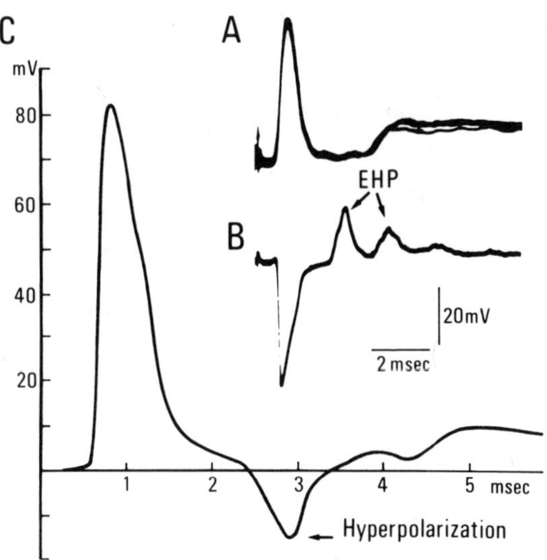


Fig. 1 Hyperpolarization of the Mauthner cell during the EHP. The recordings were made with the microelectrode tip very close to the axon hillock of a Mauthner cell (negative spike, 38 mV); response B was obtained immediately before entering the cell; the electrode was advanced slightly and entered the cell at which time response A was recorded. The stimuli were applied to the spinal cord. To determine the actual change in membrane potential, B was subtracted algebraically from A. The result is shown in C; at the peak of the EHP, the patch of membrane is hyperpolarized by 15 mV. The antidromic spike in A is followed by an IPSP, the polarity of which is inverted by $Cl^-$ ions. Note that the second component of the EHP in B is also part of this collateral inhibition (from Furukawa & Furshpan, 1963). The record in A has been retouched to remove several superimposed testing spikes.

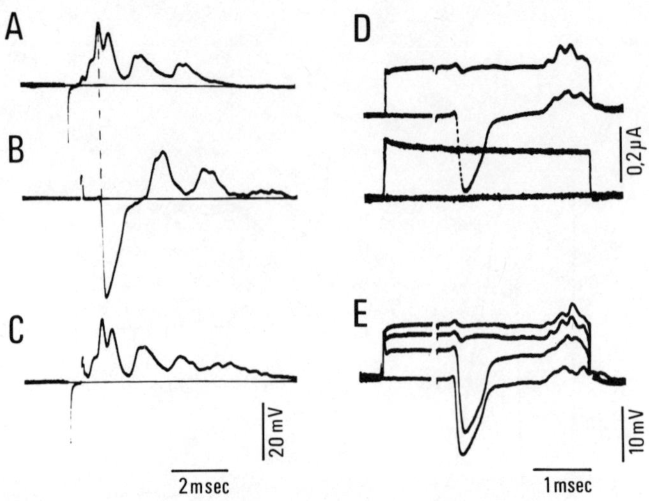


Fig. 2 Inhibitory effect of the EHP. A-C: the EHP, evoked by contralateral eighth-nerve stimulation, blocks the antidromic spike. Extracellular recording near the M-cell axon hillock. When a contralateral eighth-nerve shock (A) and a spinal-cord stimulus (B) are delivered during the same sweep (C), timed so that the antidromic spike arrives at the peak of the EHP, the spike fails to appear. Both of the first two peaks of this EHP can block the spike. D-E: blocking of the antidromic spike with artificial extrinsic potentials. Two extracellular microelectrodes were placed in the vicinity of an M-cell, one for passing current, the other to record potential. The current-passing microelectrode was close to the axon hillock (when it was used to monitor potential, a negative spike of 28 mV was recorded) while the recording electrode was at a greater distance (negative spike, 15 mV). D: a double exposure; upper trace, potential; lower trace, current; stimuli applied to spinal cord; during one of the sweeps a pulse of anodic current (ca. 0.17 μ A) is passed (outward) through the microelectrode. E: a multiple exposure; same conditions as in D (but current records not shown). Three pulses of anodic current are delivered with intensities less than, equal to, and greater than necessary to block the main part of the negative spike (from Fig. 7 and Fig. 14 of Furukawa and Furshpan, 1963).

current is inhibitory because it hyperpolarizes the M-cell axon hillock, which is the site of impulse initiation (Furshpan & Furukawa, 1962; Diamond, 1968) and the outward current depolarizes the distant, electrically inexcitable, soma and dendrite.

## ELECTRICAL INHIBITION MEDIATED BY THE M-CELL

The M-cell action currents generate an extracellular negative field (Fig. 1B; Fig. 3A) which can be as large as 35 mV in magnitude at its focus in the axon cap and which falls off steeply from that point (Furshpan & Furukawa, 1962). We recently reported (Korn & Faber, 1973; Faber & Korn, 1973) that these extracellular currents generate a hyperpolarizing potential in some of the medullary neurons located within 50 to 300 μ of the maximum negative spike focus (Fig. 3, B, C). We have named these hyperpolarizations "passive hyperpolarizing potentials" or PHPs. They are intracellularly recorded hyperpolarizations which are larger than the corresponding extracellular field potentials monitored in the immediate vicinity of the neurons being investigated. For each neuron the net PHP, or transmembrane hyperpolarizaiton, is the difference between these intra- and extra-cellularly recorded potentials; it averaged 2.02 mV in the 229 cells that were studied. The conclusion that the PHP is passively generated was primarily based on the findings that it has the same latency, threshold, time course and all-or-none character as the M-cell antidromic spike. Furthermore, the PHP amplitude and time course are independent of the membrane potential (Fig. 4), a finding which is consistent with the hypothesis that its generation does not involve alterations in membrane conductance associated with chemically mediated transmission (see Eccles, 1964).

The inhibitory nature of the PHP has been clearly established: when adequately timed, it blocks or delays spikes initiated either directly by transmembrane current pulses or transsynaptically, following eighth nerve stimulation (Fig. 3, D, E); this suppression of spike initiation is a consequence of the fact that when it is paired with a depolarizing PSP, the two summate algebraically.

Our observations are consistent with the hypothesis that the PHP is an example of a field effect inhibition, and is generated by an intracellular channeling of the M-cell action current flowing back to the axon hillock. One implication of this concept, however, is that neurons exhibiting PHPs issue processes which lie parallel to lines of return current flow, and more specifically, that these processes should run into the axon cap toward the axon hillock. This has been confirmed with the use of Procion Yellow, which was injected according to the method described by Stretton and Kravitz (1968). Dye-injected PHP neurons (Korn & Faber, 1975; and Fig. 5) have small somata (12 - 35 μ diam.) with relatively large axons (3 - 9 μ diam.)

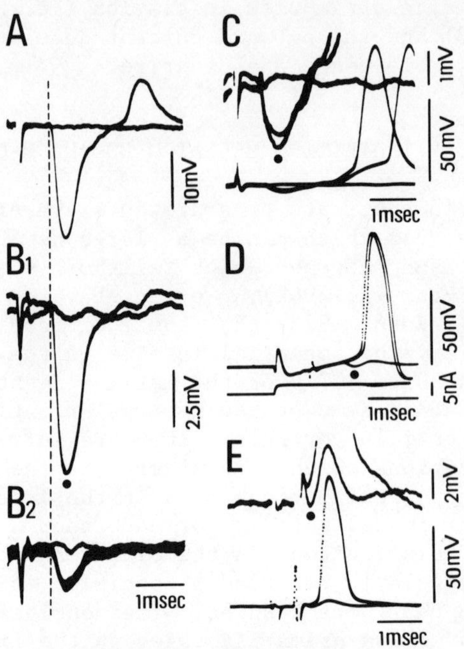


Fig. 3 Evidence that impulses evoked in the M-cell can generate inhibitory PHPs in adjacent neurons and inhibitory effect of the PHPs. A-C: the spinal cord is stimulated at strengths straddling the threshold for M-cell antidromic activation; several sweeps are superimposed on each record. A: antidromic field potential extracellularly recorded in the axon cap. $B_1$: intracellular recording obtained during the same experiment as in A from a neuron located 75 μm caudal to the axon cap; the spinal stimulus evokes a PHP. $B_2$: field potential recorded outside that cell. The vertical dashed line indicates that the potentials in A and B have the same latency. C: another example of an intracellular PHP, followed in this case by an EPSP which fires the cell. The records in D and E are from two different neurons; in each record, sweeps are superimposed without and with spinal stimulation. D: a spike evoked by a depolarizing current pulse (lower trace) is blocked by an adequately paired PHP. E: a spike synaptically evoked by stimulation of the ipsilateral eighth nerve is similarly blocked; its failure unmasks a now subthreshold EPSP (the upper and lower traces in C and E are recordings at high a-c and low d-c gain, respectively). In all records, positivity is upward, and the PHP is indicated by a filled circle in this and subsequent figures (from Faber & Korn, 1973).

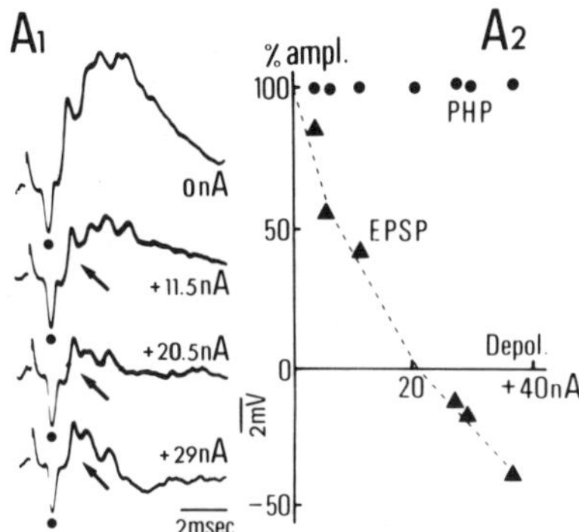


Fig. 4 PHP independence of membrane potential. $A_1$: intracellular recordings from a PHP-exhibiting neuron using a double barreled electrode, one for potential measurements and one for current injections. A spinal stimulus produces a PHP followed by an EPSP. Steady depolarizing currents sufficient to cause a polarity reversal of the EPSP leaves the PHP unaffected. Note that the early part of the depolarizing potential (indicated by arrows) is reduced in amplitude but is not inverted; it is presumably a consequence of the "pick-up" of the EHP by the axon of the neuron within the axon cap (The current amplitude is indicated on each record). $A_2$: graph of the PHP and EPSP amplitudes versus current magnitude. *Ordinate:* EPSP and PHP amplitudes in percentages of their control values in the absence of applied current. *Abscissa:* depolarizing (Depol.) current magnitude: (nA). ●: PHP amplitude. ▲: EPSP amplitude (from Faber & Korn, 1973).

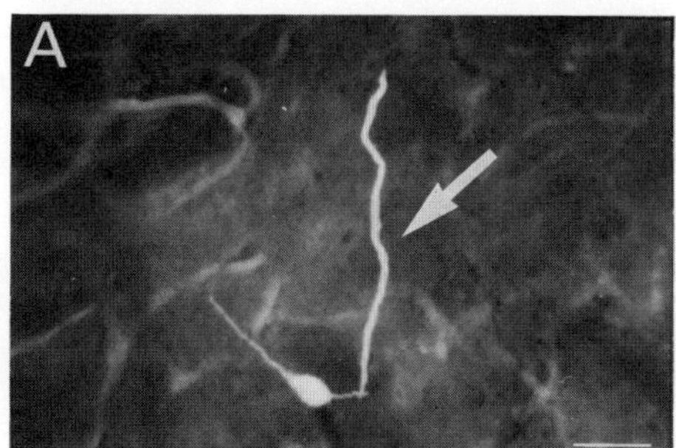


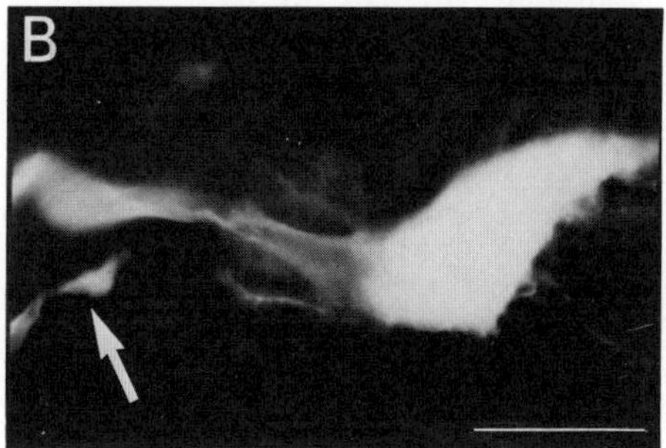


Fig. 5 Photomicrographs of Procion Yellow dye-filled PHP-exhibiting neurons and Mauthner cell. A: typical PHP-exhibiting neuron; the arrow indicates the enlargement of a process, presumably the axon, in the direction of the area of the ipsilateral M-cell axon cap. B: terminal of a PHP-exhibiting neuron and a Mauthner cell filled with dye. The terminal which is signalled by an arrow, ends in the area of the axon cap. Calibrations: 40 μ in A; 100 μ in B (from Korn & Faber, 1975).

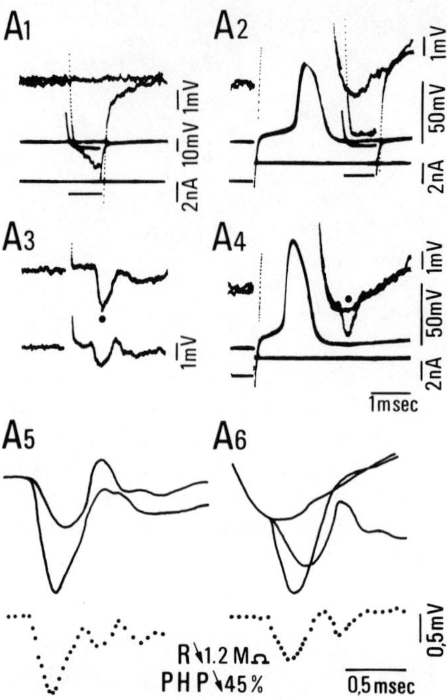


Fig. 6 Reduction of the PHP during increased membrane conductance. $A_1$ - $A_2$ - $A_4$: upper and middle traces, high gain a-c and low gain d-c intracellular recordings, respectively; lower traces: intracellularly applied current. $A_1$: transmembrane potential change produced by a brief hyperpolarizing square pulse. $A_2$ illustrates the responses of the neuron to double current pulses: the same hyperpolarizing one as in $A_1$ is applied during a directly evoked spike. The reduction in the electrotonic potential demonstrates an increased membrane conductance during the after-hyperpolarization. $A_3$, upper trace: superimposed records of the all-or-none PHP produced by a threshold spinal cord stimulation; lower trace: corresponding extracellular field potential. $A_4$: adequate timing of the direct stimulation of the cell and the spinal stimulus results in the occurrence of the PHP during the spike hyperpolarization and it is thereby reduced. $A_5$: expanded superimposed tracings of the intracellularly recorded PHP and extracellular field in $A_3$. The lower dotted line is the net PHP calculated (the difference between the upper two traces). $A_6$: superimposed tracings of the after-hyperpolarization alone, of the PHP recorded throughout, and of the extracellular field potential, after spinal cord stimulation. The lower dotted line is the net PHP, reduced by 45% during the after-hyperpolarization; correspondingly, the conductance is increased by 1.2 MΩ, as calculated from $A_1$ - $A_2$. (unpublished data).

which do indeed project to the axon cap region. Possibly only specific medullary neurons exhibit PHPs, that is, other neurons in the vicinity of the M-cell do not, and these cells do not send processes towards the M-cell axon hillock.

Final confirmation of the hypothesis that the PHP results from an intracellular channeling of the current flowing back to the M-cell axon hillock has been provided by evidence that it is shunted by increased membrane conductance (Fig. 6) and from experiments in which PHPs have been mimicked using an "external cathode" situated in the axon cap (Korn & Faber, 1975). Cathodal current pulses (current flowing to an axon cap electrode from a distant reference electrode) produce passive hyperpolarizations of neurons exhibiting PHPs (Fig. 7, $A_1$, $A_2$). In contrast, no transmembrane hyperpolarizations are produced when the cathode is raised above the axon cap (Fig. 7, $A_3$, $A_4$) or, as expected, in those neurons which do not exhibit PHPs after spinal cord stimulation. These simulated PHPs are also functionally inhibitory, for example they can block the orthodromic activation evoked by spinal cord stimulation (Fig. 8).

## GENERATION OF PASSIVE HYPERPOLARIZATIONS

Our initial studies resulted in an electrical analog (Fig. 9) which served as the conceptual basis for analyzing the mechanisms underlying the generation of the PHP as well as that of the previously studied EHP. The basic assumption of this model is that PHP exhibiting neurons draw some of the M-cell current flowing back to the axon cap; such a current flow distribution could be due to either a low specific membrane resistance of the neurons, or a relatively high extracellular convergence resistance in the axon cap ($R'_2$ in Fig. 9). Both hypotheses have been tested.

1) The input resistance of the PHP-exhibiting neurons is in the range of 1.9 - 10 MΩ (ave. = 4.03 mΩ, n = 60). Correlation of input resistance and the geometry of the dye-injected cells suggests a minimal value for specific membrane resistance in the range of 900 - 2000Ω $cm^2$, which is somewhat low compared to recent estimates of 2000 - 4000Ω $cm^2$ for cat spinal motoneurons (Barrett & Crill, 1971; Lux *et al.*, 1970; Rall, 1959). However, arguments have been presented that due to possible axonal dominance of the conductance measurements, we have significantly underestimated the magnitude of this parameter (Korn & Faber, 1975). In any case, it may be concluded that PHP generation is not due merely to a relatively low specific membrane resistance.

2) On the other hand, preliminary results of two different experimental approaches designed to determine the extracellular resistivity in the axon cap region indicate that it is at least 2.5 times

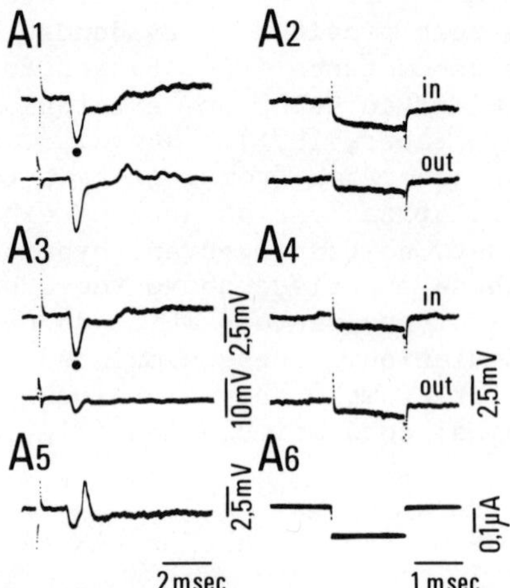


Fig. 7 Simulation of the PHP with an external cathode in the axon cap. Two microelectrodes were used, one for intracellular recording from a PHP-exhibiting neuron and the other for both recording in or above the axon cap and for passing cathodal current pulses. $A_1$: simultaneous recordings from a medullary neuron (upper trace) and from the axon cap (lower trace). A spinal stimulus evokes a PHP in the neuron and a large M-cell spike in the axon cap. $A_2$: upper and lower traces, intra- and extra- cellular recordings, respectively, of the electrotonic potential produced by a constant cathodal current pulse delivered through the current electrode in the axon cap. The pulse hyperpolarizes the cell by 1.5 mV, thus producing an artificial PHP. $A_3$ and $A_4$: same conditions as in $A_1$, $A_2$, respectively, but the current electrode is now withdrawn above the axon cap and the M-cell spike is reduced ($A_3$, lower trace). Note that the cathodal current now produces no transmembrane hyperpolarization. $A_5$: extracellular field potential recorded outside the neuron after a spinal stimulation. $A_6$: hyperpolarizing pulse used in $A_2$ and $A_4$ (unpublished data).

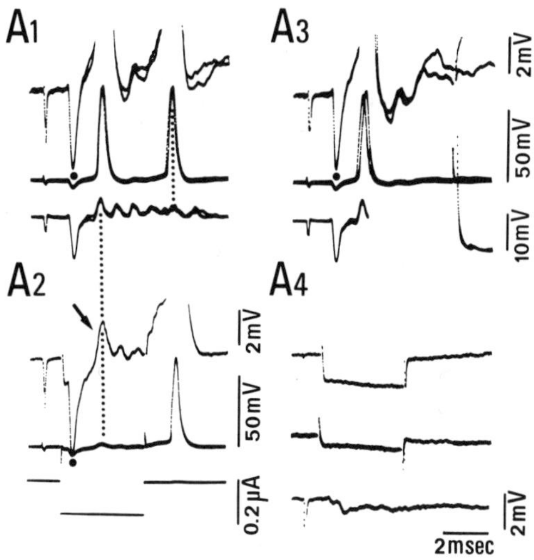


Fig. 8 Inhibitory nature of the simulated PHPs. Two microelectrodes were used, the first to monitor intracellular potentials from a PHP-exhibiting neuron. The second (current passing electrode) was placed in the axon cap for all records. $A_1$ - $A_3$, upper and middle traces: high and low gain intracellular recordings, respectively, from the PHP-exhibiting cell; lower traces: extracellular recordings from the axon cap in $A_1$ - $A_3$ and current record in $A_2$. $A_1$: a spinal stimulation produces a PHP followed by two spikes in the neuron, and a large negative M-spike followed by an EHP in the cap. $A_2$: a cathodal current pulse blocks the first spike and unmasks a now subthreshold depolarization (arrow) with the same peak time and waveform as the EHP recorded in the axon cap (first dotted vertical line). $A_3$: when the current pulse is delayed, it blocks the second spike. $A_4$, upper and middle trace: intra- and extra-cellular records, respectively, from the same neuron. The same pulse as that used in $A_2$ - $A_3$ hyperpolarizes this cell by about 1 mV; lower trace, extracellular field produced by spinal cord stimulation. Voltage calibrations in $A_3$ pertain to $A_1$ as well; time scale in $A_4$ is for all records (from Korn & Faber, 1975).

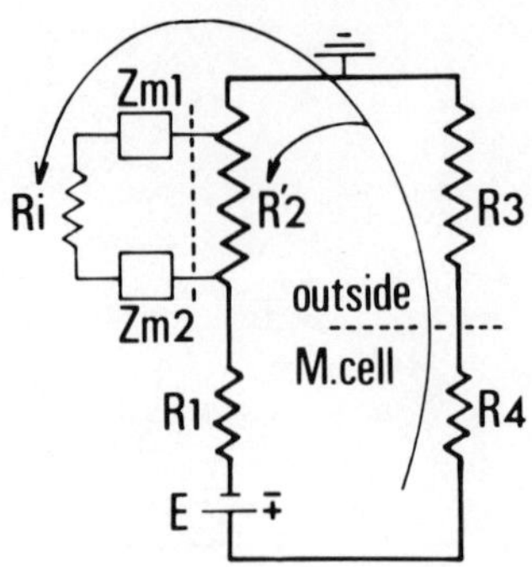


Fig. 9 A model for PHP generation. The schematic is an expansion of that proposed to explain the extracellular fields associated with the M-cell spike. The lower half represents the M-cell, $R_1$ and E being, respectively, the membrane resistance and the driving electromotive force of the activated portion of the cell, and $R_4$ the passive resistance of the inactivated membrane. $R'_2$ and $R_3$ are the extracellular resistances associated with these two parts of the M-cell. In parallel with $R'_2$ is a simplified model of a cell exhibiting a PHP. Some of the current generated by the M-cell spike flows inward across one membrane of the cell, producing a hyperpolarizing potential, or PHP, across this membrane and exits from the cell at a point presumably within the axon cap. $Z_{m1}$ and $Z_{m2}$ are the effective impedances of these two portions of the cell, the PHP being generated across $Z_{m1}$, and $R_i$ is the internal resistance of the cell (from Faber & Korn, 1973).

greater than that of the surrounding tissue. The records illustrated in Fig. 10 are typical of the findings in one of these experimental series. Potential recordings were obtained at different depths within the medulla from one barrel of a double-barreled microelectrode while constant current pulses were passed between the second barrel and a reference electrode on the tail. The amplitude of the electrotonic potentials induced by the applied currents is a measure of the resistance between the electrode and the reference point. The extracellular M-cell spike serves as a marker, being maximal within the axon cap. The depth profiles of the two potentials are qualitatively the same; the increase in the pulse potential within the axon cap (Fig. 10 $A_2$) indicates that the tissue resistance in this region is greater than that in the surrounding areas (Fig. 10 $A_1$).

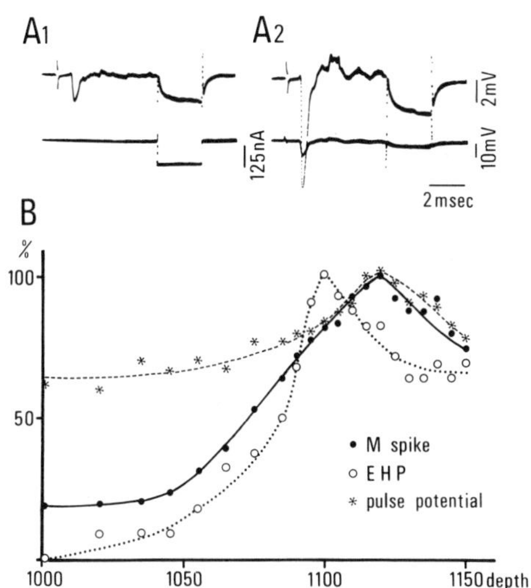


Fig. 10 Higher resistivity of the axon cap relative to that of surrounding tissue. A double-barreled microelectrode was used in this experiment, one barrel for recording extracellular potentials and the other for passing current. Recordings of the M-spike, of the EHP, and of the potential produced by passing a constant current pulse are made at different depths below the medullary surface. This electrotonic potential is a direct measure of the resistance between the recording electrode and the reference point. $A_1$, upper trace: sample record obtained at a depth of 1040 μ below the surface of the medulla. Spinal stimulation is followed by the current pulse. Lower trace: current used throughout the experiment. $A_2$: upper and lower traces, high and low gain recordings, respectively, obtained when the microelectrode is moved 100 μ deeper into the axon cap. B: plots of the depth profiles of the M-cell spike (•), of the EHP (O) and of the pulse potential (*). The amplitude of each is expressed relative to its maximum (100%). Note that the resistance increases within the axon cap (unpublished data).

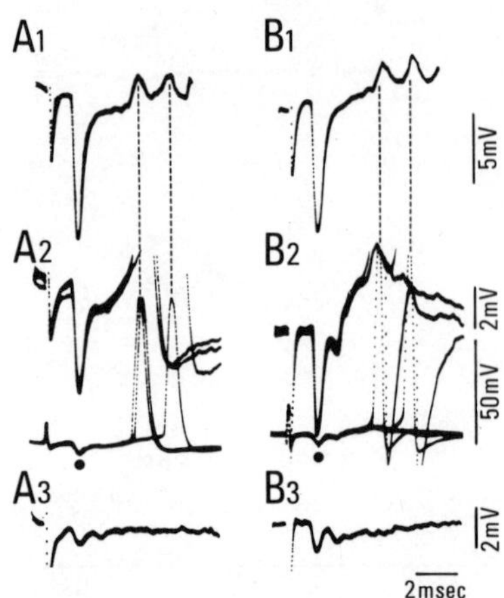


Fig. 11 Correlation between the discharges of the PHP-exhibiting neuron and the EHP. Responses $A_1$ - $A_3$ and $B_1$ - $B_3$ were obtained from two different experiments; for all records the spinal cord is activated above threshold for the antidromic activation of the M-cell. $A_1$ - $B_1$: the spinal stimulus evokes a large negativity which is followed by a biphasic positive EHP. $A_2$ - $B_2$, upper and lower traces: high a-c and low d-c intracellular recordings from two PHP-exhibiting neurons which were respectively located 75 and 110 μ from the axon cap. The PHP is followed by a short latency depolarization which generates an action potential. The latency is shifting, but in all cases, the peak of the spikes is time-locked with one of the EHP components as indicated by the vertical dashed lines. $A_3$ - $B_3$: corresponding extracellular field potentials (unpublished data).

The high extracellular resistivity in the axon cap is presumably sufficient to produce the intracellular channeling of the M-cell current which brings about the PHP. While the specific cause of this high extracellular resistivity is not yet established, certain potential contributing factors have been identified. They include the presence of densely packed glia surrounding the cap which could present a barrier to current flow (Furshpan & Furukawa, 1962), and of a large number of cytoplasmic membranes within small extracellular spaces (Nakajima, 1974), together with conspicuously electron-dense material in these spaces (Robertson *et al.*, 1963) which might well be of low conductivity.

### Relationship Between the EHP and the PHP

The model used for the analysis of PHP generation (Fig. 9) suggests that action potentials generated by PHP exhibiting neurons could generate passive hyperpolarizations (i.e. EHPs) in the M-cell if these action potentials do not actively invade the terminals of the cells. Such a prediction obviously followed the considerations that these cells send processes into the axon cap and that the extracellular resistance in the latter ($R'_2$ in Fig. 9) is relatively high; two conditions which were confirmed by our experiments. Under these conditions, the M-cell would draw an appreciable portion of the current generated by these axons. The validity of this postulate is already indicated by the strict correlation which is consistently observed between the firing of the PHP exhibiting neurons and the extracellularly recorded EHP (Fig. 11); clearly, the generation of the latter is time-locked with the action potentials intracellularly recorded in the neurons. Further confirmation of this postulate has been obtained (Korn & Faber, 1975) with simultaneous intracellular recordings from PHP exhibiting neurons and the M-cell: action potentials in the former produce unitary EHPs in the axon cap of about 200 - 400 μV magnitude (while, as expected, during intracellular recording from the M-cell the corresponding potential change is negligible).

## FUNCTIONS OF ELECTRICAL INHIBITION IN THE CENTRAL NERVOUS SYSTEM

The M-cell is the medullary output neuron responsible for the goldfish tail flip or startle reflex (Wilson, 1959; Diamond, 1971). This reflex is initiated by the eighth nerve input to the ipsilateral M-cell, which in turn excites the spinal motoneurons innervating the contralateral tail musculature. As mentioned, excitation of either M-cell subsequently activates a powerful collateral inhibition of both of them, the EHP being the earliest component of this rather complex negative feedback. Furukawa and Furshpan (1963) suggested that the function of the collateral system, including that of the

EHP, is to prevent repetitive firing of the M-cell as well as successive activation of the two cells, presumably in order to allow more meaningful orientation and swimming movements following the occurrence of one tail flip. Following this reasoning, there are two functions which the PHP might well serve, the first of which is a consequence of the reciprocal electrical inhibitory coupling between the M-cell and the PHP exhibiting neurons.

First, neurons with PHPs do not form a homogenous population. Some of them are activated by the recurrent collaterals of the M-cells' axons (Fig. 3 and Fig. 11) and, in turn, at least a fraction of these are capable of generating EHPs. Thus they belong to the above-described network and are interneurons which produce the electrically and, possibly, the chemically mediated collateral inhibition. Since unitary EHPs are quite small, the maximal EHP recorded in the axon cap must involve the synchronous activity of about 50 - 70 neurons. Clearly, the PHP contributes significantly to this synchronization, that is, it functions to reset the activity of the inhibitory interneurons and to increase the probability that they will be excited by the collaterals. This concept has been supported by observations that in some of the neurons the PHP is followed by a depolarizing pick up of the EHP (indicated by arrows in Fig. 4) such that the PHP-EHP sequence aids in the recruitment of the less excitable cells which otherwise would not be brought to the firing level by the collateral input alone (Korn & Faber, 1975). This synchronizing system, which guarantees maximal short-latency inhibition of the M-cell, could not operate so quickly with a longer latency chemically-mediated transmission alone.

Other PHP exhibiting neurons are activated monosynaptically by low-intensity stimulation of the ipsilateral eighth nerve and are presumably vestibulo-spinal neurons. Excitation of such descending neurons by the eighth nerve input which on the other hand triggers the M-cell spike could degrade the startle reflex by activating at the same time antagonistic motoneurons; therefore, it can be expected that the M-cell will exert an inhibitory control over them without delay, that is electrically.

Although potentials comparable to the PHP and EHP have not yet been clearly recorded elsewhere in the central nervous system, it is conceivable that the goldfish medulla is an ideal preparation for demonstrating them but that they do in fact exist in other systems. PHPs are quite large, probably in part as a result of the uniquely large extracellular current generated by the M-cell. Similar field effects occurring in other systems might be smaller in magnitude and therefore difficult to detect. However, if present, they still would have subtle synchronizing or modulating effects which could become more pronounced under conditions associated with large extracellular field potentials, such as can occur in many structures or situations - in the CNS, for example, during seizures which involve the synchronous activity of a large number of neurons.

## REFERENCES


1. ARVANITAKI, A. & CHALAZONITIS, N. *Bull. Inst. Oceanogr. Monaco 1143:*1, 1959.
2. BARRETT, J.N. & CRILL, W.D. *Brain Res. 28:*556, 1971.
3. BARTELMEZ, G.W. *J. Comp. Neurol. 25:*87, 1915.
4. BENNETT, M.V.L. A comparison of electrically and chemically mediated transmission. In: Structure and Function of Synapses. (G.D. Pappas & D.P. Purpura, eds.) New York, Raven Press Publ., p. 221, 1972.
5. BODIAN, D. *J. Comp. Neurol. 68:*117, 1937.
6. DIAMOND, J. *J. Physiol. (London) 194:*669, 1968.
7. DIAMOND, J. The Mauthner cell. In: Fish Physiology. Vol. V. (W.S. Hoar & D.J. Randall, eds.) New York, Academic Press, p. 265, 1971.
8. ECCLES, J.C. The Physiology of Synapses. Berlin: Springer Verlag, 1964.
9. FABER, D.S. & KORN, H. *Science 179:*577, 1973.
10. FURSHPAN, E.J. & FURUKAWA, T. *J. Neurophysiol. 25:*732, 1962.
11. FURUKAWA, T. *Prog. Brain Res. 21A:*44, 1966.
12. FURUKAWA, T. & FURSHPAN, E.J. *J. Neurophysiol. 26:*140, 1963.
13. KORN, H. & FABER, D.S. *J. Gen. Physiol. 61:*261, 1973.
14. KORN, H. & FABER, D.S. *J. Neurophysiol. 38:*452, 1975.
15. LUX, H.D., SCHUBERT, P. & KREUTZBERG, G.W. Direct matching of morphological and electrophysiological data in cat spinal motoneurons. In: Excitatory Synaptic Mechanisms. (P. Anderson & J.K.S. Jansen, eds.) Oslo, Universitetsforlaget, p. 189, 1970.
16. NAKAJIMA, Y. *J. Cell Biol.* In press.
17. NELSON, P.G. *J. Neurophysiol. 29:*275, 1966.
18. RALL, W. *Exp. Neurol. 1:*491, 1959.
19. ROBERTSON, J.D. *J. Cell Biol. 19:*201, 1963.
20. ROBERTSON, J.D., BODENHEIMER, T.S. & STAGE, D.E. *J. Cell Biol. 19:*159, 1963.
21. STRETTON, A.O.W. & KRAVITZ, E.A. *Science 162:*132, 1968.
22. TAUC, L. Polyphasic synaptic activity. In: Mechanisms of Synaptic Transmission. (K. Akert & P.G. Waser, eds.) Elsevier, Amsterdam, p. 247, 1969.
23. WILSON, D.M. *Science 129:*841, 1959.

# THE ROLE OF ELECTROTONIC SYNAPSES IN THE CONTROL OF BEHAVIOUR

M.E. Spira
Institute of Life Sciences
The Hebrew University
Jerusalem, Israel

Chemical synapses are considered to be the tool whereby information is transmitted in a manner which allows integration and fine processing. The graded excitatory and inhibitory actions of chemical synapses, changes in their transmission potency as a result of their activity (facilitation and fatigue), temporal summation and unidirectional conduction are well documented. These properties are considered the major processes for handling and integration of information in neuronal networks. Therefore, when we study information processing or when we design neuronal models to fit some known behaviour, we search for or introduce into the model system chemical synapses or their operational properties.

A second type of synapse, the electrotonic synapse, is usually not considered to play a major role in fine information processing (Furshpan & Potter, 1958; for recent reviews see Bennett, 1966; 1972a; b; 1973). Until recently, investigators ascribed to this type of synapse only rigid properties. Unlike the chemical synapse, transmission across the electrotonic synapse was not altered by the previous history of activity. Furthermore, inhibition by electrotonic synapses is generally less effective than by chemical synapses (Effective inhibition by current flow from one neuronal element to another via the extracellular space, and therefore not an electrotonic synapse, has been demonstrated in one system, cf., Furukawa and Furshpan, 1963; Faber and Korn, 1973). In these chemical synapses where the transmitter release process is long compared to the duration of the presynaptic spike, temporal summation is more effective than in electrical synapses (for comparisons, see Bennett 1972a; b). Even though unidirectional conductance is also found in some electrotonic synapses (for example, see Furshpan & Potter, 1958;

Auerbach and Bennett, 1969), in most cases it is not complete.

Two related functional advantages are usually ascribed to electrotonic synapses. The first is speed of transmission: the delay in electrical transmission is less than the delay of 0.4 - 1.0 msec at chemical synapses*. Indeed, electrotonic synapses occur in neuronal networks in which the saving of time has a behavioral advantage - for example in the lateral giant septae and the lateral giant to motor giant synapses in the crayfish, which are specialized for escape responses (cf., Furshpan & Potter, 1958; Watanabe & Grundfest, 1961).

A second and more widely distributed functional advantage of electrotonic synapses over chemical lies in synchronization of activity within a group of neurons. In such an electrotonically coupled group, a more depolarized cell depolarizes the other cells, or a less depolarized cell inhibits the other neurons within the group. The reciprocal synchronizing effect within the electrotonically coupled group of neurons is more effective than would be possible using chemical synapses. In the latter case, both inhibitory and excitatory elements are needed and subsequent long delays would be introduced.

Most of the available information based on electrophysiological experiments correlated with behavioural studies show that electrotonic synapses are involved in neuronal circuits in which speed of conduction or synchronization of the motor output is important. It is probable that the concept of electrotonic synapses as rigid circuit elements was a consequence of concentration of such studies on those systems where synchronization played the dominant functional role. The study to be discussed in this paper will demonstrate the possibility of a more flexible role for electrotonically coupled neurons. In addition, recent findings in a variety of nonexcitable as well as excitable tissues indicate that electrotonic synapses are capable of plastic changes; that is, the degree of coupling can be altered under different physiological conditions or as the result of past activity (Asada & Bennett, 1971; Rose & Loewenstein, 1971; Socolar & Politoff, 1971; Spira & Bennett, 1972; Getting & Willows, 1973; also see review by Bennett, 1973). In addition to these observations, the accumulating documentation of the frequent presence of the morphological counterpart of electrotonic synapses, the gap junction (Bennett, 1973), in the central nervous systems of both invertebrates and vertebrates (Dowling & Boycott, 1966; Hinrichsen &

*The Ia synapse in cat spinal motoneurons has been reported to be as brief as 0.2 to 0.3 msec. There has been some doubt placed on the chemical nature of transmission at this synapse (Carlen & Werman, personal communication).

Larramendi, 1968; Sotelo & Palay, 1970; Sotelo & Taxi, 1970; Pinching & Powell, 1971; Sloper, 1972; Sotelo & Llinas, 1972; Pappas & Waxman, 1972; Bennett, 1973), raises the possibility that electrotonic synapses are found all too frequently to be involved only in the synchronization of activity. Therefore, the possibility of other, more flexible roles for electrotonic synapses should be considered.

I will now discuss one system which demonstrates that the degree of coupling among a group of neurons can be altered under physiological control, and describe how this phenomenon may be related to a rather complex motor repertoire.

*Navanax inermis* (Gastropoda) is a slow-moving mollusc. It locates its prey by following the mucus trail left by other molluscs (Paine, 1965; Murray, 1971). When proper mechanical contact and chemical stimulation to the phalliform sense organs is applied, the prey is sucked into the pharynx. The intake of the prey is extremely rapid and takes less than 0.5 sec (Murray, 1971; Wollacott, 1972) (Fig. 1). The rapid sucking in of the prey is accompanied by a sudden expansion of the pharynx which results from the simultaneous contraction of the radial muscles in the pharynx wall. The suction is produced by the expansion of the pharynx together with contraction of the sphincter muscle at the caudal end of the pharynx. The act of pharyngeal expansion is followed immediately by a series of peristaltic-like movements of the pharyngeal wall which push the prey into the mid-gut. The expansion and the peristaltic action of the pharynx can also be observed when the pharynx together with the buccal ganglion is isolated from the animal.

In the experiment illustrated in Fig. 2, using the isolated pharyngeal preparation, we inserted a deflated balloon into the pharynx (Fig. 2A). Sudden inflation of the balloon is depicted in Fig. 2B. This act was followed by a series of contractions of the wall of the pharynx which pushed the inflated balloon back, through the caudal sphincter (Fig. 2C, D) and into the mid-gut (Fig. 2E, F).

When the buccal ganglion was disconnected from the pharynx and the experiment repeated, the response to stretching of the wall of the pharynx was abolished. Spontaneous expansion of the pharynx can be observed when the ganglion is connected to the pharynx and this was also abolished by removal of the buccal ganglion.

The neurons that control pharyngeal expansion and the subsequent peristaltic contractions are located in the buccal ganglion (Spira & Bennett, 1972; Woollacott, 1972). We have identified some of the neurons that control pharyngeal expansion (Spira & Bennett, 1972) as the electrotonically coupled neurons G, M and S that were first described and studied by Levitan, Tauc and Segundo (1970). When the pharynx was isolated together with the buccal ganglion and one of

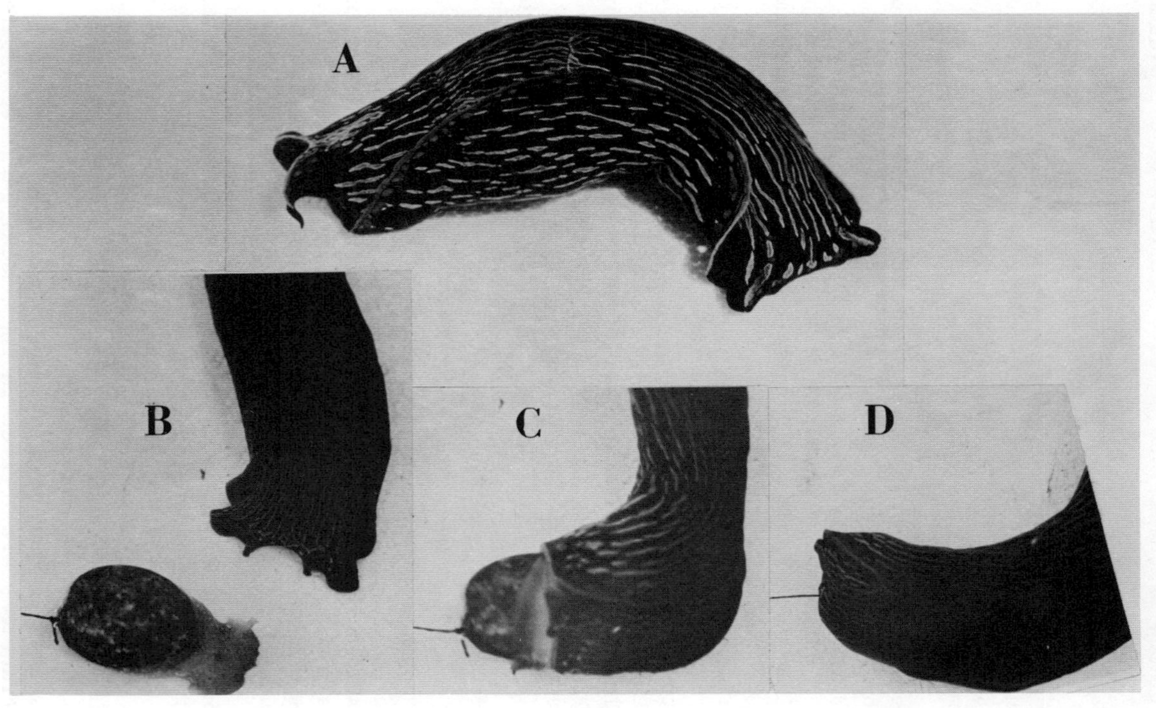


Fig. 1 Capturing of prey by *Navanax*. A. The whole animal, rostral end to the right. The length of the animal is about 20 cm. B. *Navanax* follows the mucus trail left by a small gastropod. Notice the extended, medially located, phalliform organs. After appropriate contact with the prey, the latter is sucked into the pharyngeal cavity. In C the prey is halfway into the pharynx. The entire action of swallowing is over in 0.3 sec. In D, capture of the prey is complete. From Spira and Bennett (unpublished).

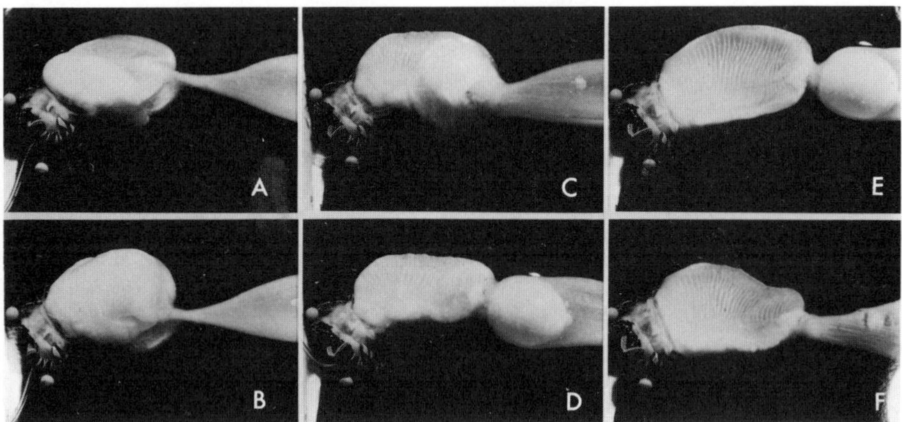


Fig. 2 Pharyngeal peristalsis controlled by the buccal ganglion. In A, a deflated balloon has been inserted into the pharynx. The balloon is inflated in B. In C, D, E and F, the balloon is driven into the mid-gut by peristaltic-like contractions of the pharyngeal wall. From unpublished results of Spira and Bennett, which were quoted in a review (Bennett, 1974).

the cells of this group was stimulated by an intracellular microelectrode, pharyngeal expansion was elicited. (Fig. 3; compare A and B representing the situation before and during stimulation of a G cell, respectively). Further evidence that G, M and S neurons are motoneurons was obtained by antidromic activation of the neurons on stimulating the nerve innervating the pharyngeal muscles. Although the electrical coupling among these motoneurons is rather weak, it is sufficient to synchronize the contraction of the pharyngeal muscles which is necessary for the rapid expansion of the pharynx. The coupling between two neurons in this group (G, M) and their synchronized action is shown in Fig. 4. The synchronized motor activity during pharyngeal expansion and the finding that this

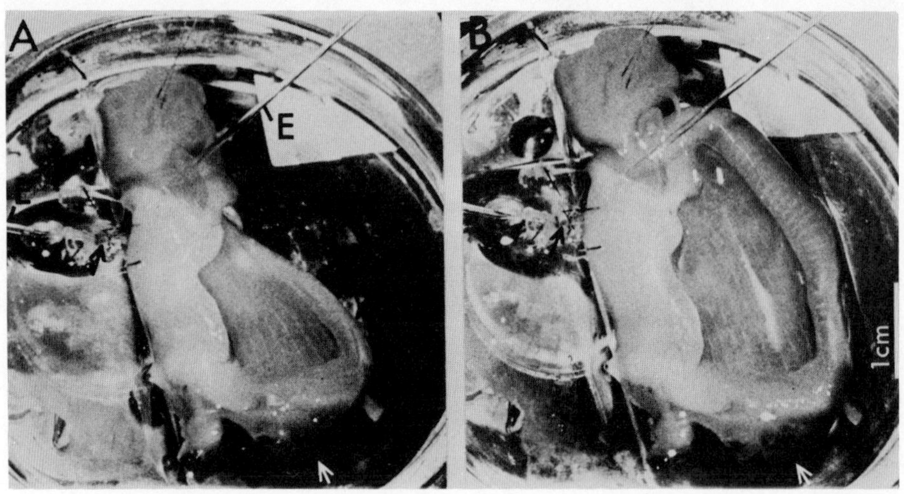


Fig. 3 Pharyngeal expansion evoked by G cell stimulation. Part of the pharyngeal wall is cut away. The pharynx lies on its right side, placed in a Petri dish, with the dorsal aspect of the pharynx to the right; the mouth is indicated by a white arrow. The buccal ganglion (black arrow) lies to the left. The pharyngeal nerve connecting the ganglion and the pharyngeal wall are intact, but not visible. Stimulation of the G cell at 10/sec produces pharyngeal expansion by contraction of radial muscles in the wall. A. Control. B. During stimulation. From Spira and Bennett (1972).

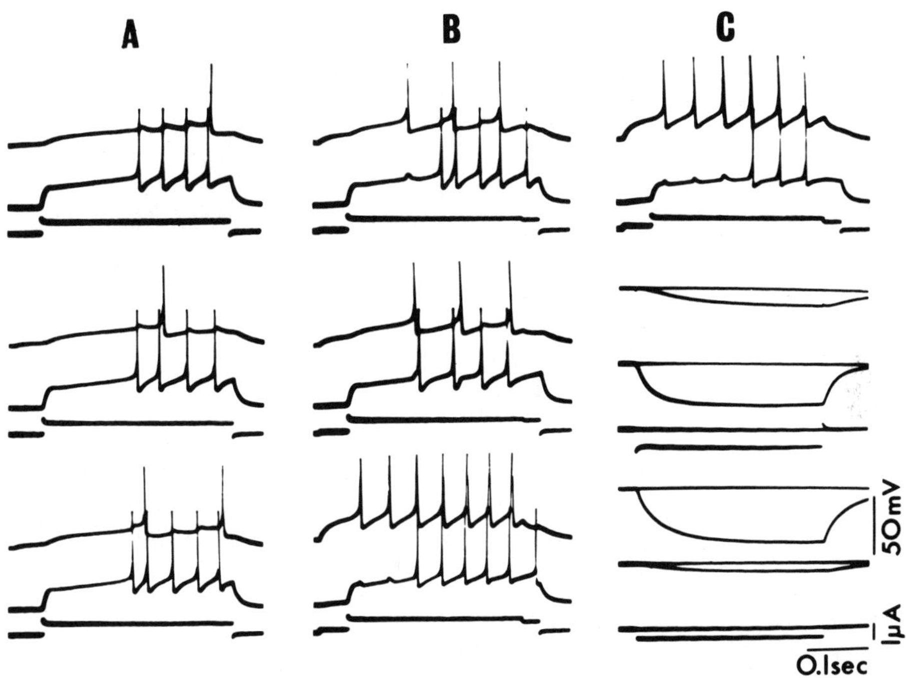


Fig. 4 Electrotonic coupling and synchronized firing of G and M cells. Upper and middle traces: voltage recordings from an M cell and the ipsilateral G cell, respectively. Lower trace, current injection into both cells. A constant current pulse was applied to the G cell (columns A, B and top of column C), while a longer pulse of current of increasing strength (up to down, left to right) was applied to the M cell. With appropriate depolarization of both cells, synchronized firing is seen (lower end of column B). In column C, hyperpolarizing currents were applied separately to each cell. In the middle record, current was applied to the G cell, and in the lower record, to the M cell. From unpublished results of Spira and Bennett quoted in a review (Bennett, 1974).

activity is mediated by a group of electrotonically coupled neurons supports the current concept that electrical synapses are usually found in neuronal circuits in which fast action and precise synchronization are needed.

As described earlier, the act of pharyngeal expansion is immediately followed by peristaltic-like contractions of the pharynx. Based on current concepts and knowledge, one would predict that this latter activity could not be mediated by the electrotonically coupled neurons. However, in the course of our investigations of the system, we discovered that the degree of electrotonic coupling among G, M and S neurons is drastically reduced when the wall of the pharynx is stretched or when the pharyngeal nerves are electrically stimulated. When this uncoupling occurs, the neurons can be fired independently. Thus, it is quite possible that the same group of electrotonically coupled neurons can fire synchronistically or asynchronously and thereby transmit different behavioural information.

The phenomenon of uncoupling described above is demonstrated in Fig. 5. The electrical coupling between the G and M cell is measured by injecting current into one cell and simultaneously recording the voltage difference between the interior of each cell and the external medium (Fig. 5A, B). The coupling coefficient from G to M (current injected into G) was 0.4 and from M to G was 0.1 (current injected into M - see Levitan *et al.*, 1970 for details of coupling coefficients among all cells of this group). The difference in coupling coefficients results from differences in the nonjunctional membrane resistances of the two cells. In *Navanax*, the G cell is much larger than the M cell and its input resistance is therefore lower. In Fig. 5C and D, is shown depolarizing current injected into G and M cells, respectively, which initiates trains of action potentials in the stimulated cell. Decremental electrotonic spread of the spikes from the polarized cell to the other cell are seen as small, somewhat slowed down components. When a short, high frequency train of electrical stimuli was applied to the ipsilateral pharyngeal nerve, the electrotonic coupling between the two cells was almost completely abolished (Fig. 5A', B', C', D'). The uncoupling by nerve stimulation is associated with a marked decrease in the nonjunctional resistance of each cell; this is probably due to a large increase in the synaptic input, as evidenced by the high frequency inhibitory synaptic potentials which are apparent during the applied hyperpolarizations as shown in Figures 5A' and B'.

Uncoupling similar to that induced by electrical stimulation can be observed during pharyngeal expansion using an inflated balloon (Fig. 6). Here, too, the uncoupling (Fig. 6 B, C) was associated with an increase in synaptic bombardment of the neurons. Both electrical stimulation and stretch induce uncoupling which can

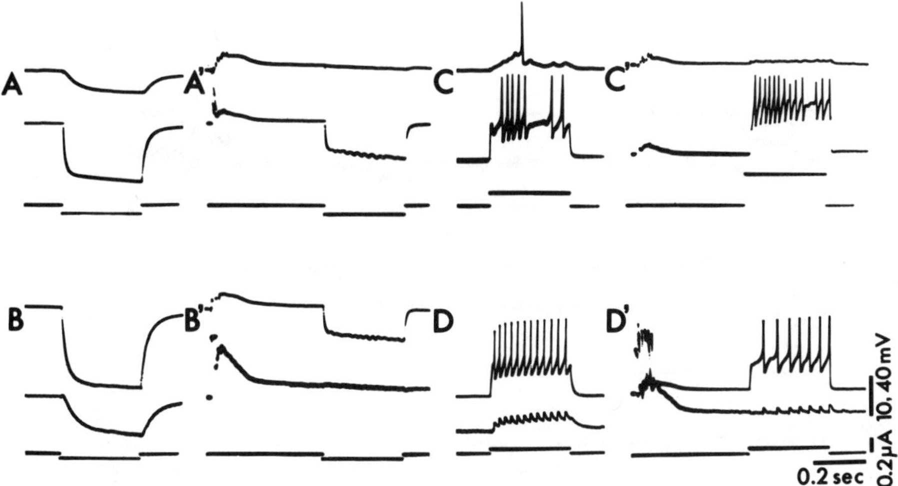


Fig. 5 Modulation of electrotonic coupling by chemical synapses. Recordings from M and G cells, upper and middle traces, respectively. Lower trace: polarizing current applied to a G cell in the upper row and to an M cell in the lower row. The electrical coupling between the two neurons is shown in A and B for hyperpolarizing currents. In C and D, spikes in the polarized cell produced small depolarizing components in the unpolarized cell. Electrotonic coupling was almost completely abolished by short trains of stimuli delivered to the pharyngeal nerve at the beginning of the sweeps in A', B', C' and D'. In C', stimulation of the G cell at a higher frequency than in C fails to initiate spikes in the M cell. The higher gain calibration refers to the middle trace in row B - D'. From Spira and Bennett (1972).

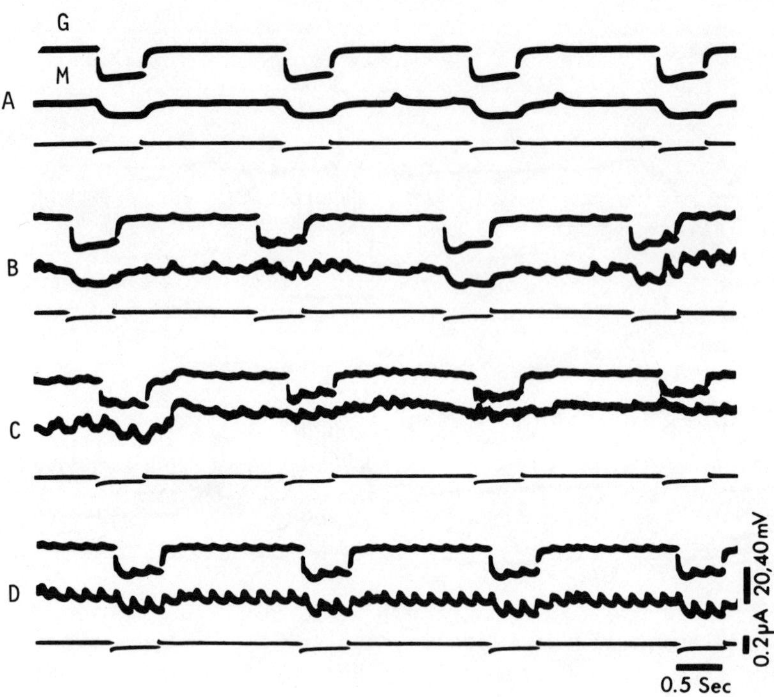


Fig. 6 Decoupling of G and M cells by stretching the pharynx. The pharynx together with the buccal ganglion was isolated and coupling between G and M cells measured before, during and after the inflation of a balloon inserted into the pharynx. Upper and middle traces, recordings from G and M cells, respectively; lower trace, current injected into the G cell. In B, the balloon was gradually inflated, and an increase in synaptic bombardment was recorded. In C, uncoupling of the cells was seen, associated with depolarization of both cells. In D, the balloon was deflated; the cells are partially recoupled, concomitant with repolarization of both cells and a change in the pattern of synaptic activity. The higher voltage gain refers to the middle trace. From Spira and Bennett (unpublished).

last for 30 - 60 seconds after cessation of stimulation and the onset of uncoupling is often followed by a burst of unsynchronized spikes in the M and S cells.

We ascribe the decoupling to a decrease in nonjunctional resistance. In a system of two electrically coupled cells, the coupling coefficient when current is injected into cell 1, denoting the voltages recorded from cells 1 and 2 by $V_1$ and $V_2$, respectively, is:

$$K_{1,2} = V_2/V_1 = r_2/r_2 + r_c$$

where $r_2$ represents the nonjunctional resistance of cell 2 and $r_c$ the junctional resistance. It is apparent that when $r_2$ decreases, the coupling coefficient in this direction will be reduced (see also Bennett, 1966; Spira & Bennett, 1972). This rather simple explanation for uncoupling due to decrease in input resistance of the nonjunctional membrane is not sufficient to account for the marked degree of uncoupling observed experimentally. It is possible, however, to assume that an important group of inhibitory synapses are located at such points along the coupling path that a more effective shunt of current is achieved than would be produced by only a homogenous decrease in nonjunctional membrane resistance. A second, less parsimonious, explanation would be that transmitter liberated by the stimulation produces an increase in the junctional membrane resistance, concomitant with its effect of reducing the nonjunctional membrane resistance. However attractive this explanation may be, it is not as yet supported by experimental evidence.

Although we have been successful in demonstrating decoupling by physiological stimulation, we have not yet unequivocally demonstrated the physiological role of the uncoupled group of neurons. Nevertheless, based on the electrophysiological evidence and the pattern of motor activity, we can now design a neuronal model in which the electrotonically coupled neurons can act flexibly, both synchronously and asynchronously through modulation by chemical synapses. A minimal model to explain the observed behavioural phenomena requires that appropriate mechanical and chemical stimulation of the sense organs excites the electrotonically coupled neurons via interneurons. Only when the intensity of input is sufficient to reach the high threshold of the group will synchronized firing occur. (Since the electrotonically coupled cells load each other down, the current threshold is elevated in the individual cells and in the group as a whole.) Successful synchronous activation of the coupled cells produces pharyngeal expansion. The presence of the prey in the pharynx and the consequent stretching of the walls of the pharynx fire stretch receptors embedded in the wall, which in turn uncouple the cells, via chemical synapses. Together with the uncoupling, the cells are again activated (probably also via interneurons) but now fire asynchronously to produce the peristaltic-like movement of the pharynx.

Recent work by Llinas, Baker and Sotelo (1974) and Sotelo, Llinas and Baker (1974) indicates that a similar mechanism for modulation of the degree of electrotonic coupling may exist in inferior olivary neurons of the cat. Electrotonic coupling between those neurons occurs most commonly at the dendritic glomeruli which are surrounded by a large number of chemical synapses. These authors suggest that the inhibitory inputs that are located close to the site of the electrotonic synapses in these neurons could shunt the coupling between the cells by a "mechanism similar to that suggested by Spira and Bennett".

The experimental evidence of synaptic modulation of electrotonic coupling, as well as other experimental demonstrations of changes in the degree of cell coupling during development, broadens the spectrum of action that can be assigned to electrotonic synapses. The current concept of a limited physiological role in integration and fine processing of information of electrotonic synapses should therefore be re-evaluated by future experiments.

## ACKNOWLEDGEMENTS

The experimental work reported here was carried out in the laboratory of Prof. M.V.L. Bennett and I am indebted to him for agreement to use unpublished figures. I thank my friend, Prof. R. Werman, for useful and stimulating discussions.

## REFERENCES

1. ASADA, Y. & BENNETT, M.V.L. *J. Cell. Biol.* *49*:159, 1971.
2. AUERBACH, A.A. & BENNETT, M.V.L. *J. Gen. Physiol.* *53*:211, 1969.
3. BENNETT, M.V.L. *Ann. N.Y. Acad. Sci.* *137*:509, 1966.
4. BENNETT, M.V.L. Electrical versus chemical neurotransmission. In: Research Publications of the A.R.N.M.D., Vol. 50, p. 58, "Neurotransmitters", Williams & Wilkins, Baltimore, 1972a.
5. BENNETT, M.V.L. A comparison of electrically and chemically mediated transmission. In: Structure and Function of Synapses (Eds. G.D. Pappas and D.P. Purpura), p. 221. Raven Press, New York, 1972b.
6. BENNETT, M.V.L. *Fed. Proc.* *32*:65, 1973.
7. BENNETT, M.V.L. Flexibility and rigidity in electrotonically coupled systems. In: Synaptic Transmission and Neuronal Interaction (Ed. M.V.L. Bennett), p. 153, Raven Press, New York, 1974.

8. DOWLING, J.E. & BOYCOTT, B.B. *Proc. Roy. Soc. Lon. Ser. B.* *166*:80, 1966.
9. FABER, D.S. & KORN, H. *Science* *179*:577, 1973.
10. FURSHPAN, J. & POTTER, D.D. *J. Physiol.* *145*:289, 1958.
11. FURUKAWA, T. & FURSHPAN, E.J. *J. Neurophysiol.* *26*:140, 1963.
12. GETTING, P.A. & WILLOWS, A.O.D. *Brain Research* *63*:424, 1973.
13. HINRICHSEN, C.F.L. & LARRAMENDI, L.M.H. *Brain Research* *7*:296, 1968.
14. LEVITAN, H., TAUC, L. & SEGUNDO, J.P. *J. Gen. Physiol.* *55*: 484, 1970.
15. LLINAS, R., BAKER, R. & SOTELO, C. *J. Neurophysiol.* *37*:560, 1974.
16. MURRAY, M.J. The biology of a carnivorous mollusc: anatomical, behavioral and electrophysiological observations on *Navanax inermis*. Ph.D. Dissertation, Univ. of Calif., Berkeley, 1971.
17. PAINE, R.T. *Veliger* *6*:1, 1963.
18. PAPPAS, G.D. & WAXMAN, S. In: Structure and Function of Synapses, (Ed. G.D. Pappas and D.P. Purpura), Raven Press, New York, 1972.
19. PINCHING, A.J. & POWELL, T.P.S. *J. Cell. Sci.* *9*:347, 1971.
20. ROSE, B. & LOEWENSTEIN, B. *J. Membrane Biol.* *50*:20, 1971.
21. SLOPER, J.J. *Brain Research* *44*:641, 1972.
22. SPIRA, M.E. & BENNETT, M.V.L. *Brain Research* *37*:294, 1972.
23. SOCOLAR, S.J. & POLITOFF, A.L. *Science* *172*:492, 1971.
24. SOTELO, C. & PALAY, S.L. *Brain Research* *18*:93, 1970.
25. SOTELO, C. & TAXI, J. *Brain Research* *17*:137, 1970.
26. SOTELO, C. & LLINAS, R. *J. Cell Biol.* *53*:271, 1972.
27. SOTELO, C., LLINAS, R. & BAKER, R. *J. Neurophysiol.* *37*:541, 1974.
28. WATANABE, A. & GRUNDFEST, H. *J. Gen. Physiol.* *45*:267, 1961.
29. WOOLLACOTT, M.H. Neuronal correlates of the prey-capture response of *Navanax inermis*. Ph.D. Dissertation, Univ. of So. Calif., Los Angeles, 1972.

# ANALYSIS OF SINGLE GENE SEX LINKED BEHAVIORAL MUTANTS IN *DROSOPHILA MELANOGASTER*

D. Dagan[1], W.D. Kaplan[2] and K. Ikeda[1]
[1]Department of Biology of Behavior, Technion School of Medicine, Haifa, Israel. [2]Departments of Biology and Neurosciences, City of Hope Medical Center, Duarte, California, U.S.A.

## INTRODUCTION

In order to study the genetic component underlying behavior, one must keep the environment constant and control the genome of the organism. The mechanisms of gene transcription have been studied very thoroughly; the behavioral output of organisms has also received great attention - the link between the two, however, is still largely an open field for research. Over the past 5 years, several hundred single gene sex-linked mutations have been generated in fruit flies with the purpose of analysing them and attempting to gain insight into the inter-relationship between gene and behavior. Although the generation of behavioral mutants has been rather proliferous, detailed analyses of the focus and mechanism of the altered genome's action are very scarce. It is in such analysis that an interdisciplinary approach is necessary. In the few cases where electrophysiological tools have been applied to analyse these mutants, much additional information was obtained (Hotta and Benzer, 1969; Ikeda and Kaplan, 1970a, 1970b; Pak *et al.*, 1969). After choosing a suitable mutant, one must first localize the focus of the mutated gene's action. This may be achieved by combined genetic mapping and electrophysiological recordings from the flies' sensory organs, CNS, peripheral nerves and muscles. After the localization of the defect, one must attempt to analyse the defective mechanism, be it in transduction, conduction, transmission or muscle contraction. Examples of defects in these fundamental mechanisms underlying behavior already exist (e.g. Kikuchi, 1973; Williamson *et al.*, 1974). However, many more are needed before one can make any generalizations about principles of genic control of behavior.

In this study, we report an analysis of a single gene, sex-linked mutant of *Drosophila melanogaster* exhibiting general inactivity under normal conditions. Our attempt is to explain this inactivity on the basis of the underlying functions of excitable tissues synthesizing this behavior.

## METHODS

### Mutant Induction, Isolation and Mosaic Generation

The mutation was induced by the mutagen, ethyl methane sulfonate (EMS). Adult males of *Canton-S* were fed a 0.025 M solution according to the protocol of Lewis and Bacher (1968). The mutation has been localized at 18.0 on the X chromosome. No screening procedures were employed since the inactive (*iav*) mutant was found by chance as an inactive stock. (For behavioral description of mutant, see results.) A detailed description of gynandromorph generation is given by Ikeda and Kaplan (1970b).

### Behavioral Quantitization

The difference between the inactive mutant and the wild-type *Canton-S* stock is exhibited in the difference in the time required for the flies to settle in their respective culture bottles after receiving a shock. A culture bottle of *Canton-S* and another of the inactive mutants, each containing 100 flies, were placed on a sponge rubber pad and the flies were allowed to settle and left undisturbed for an hour. Each bottle was then raised and brought down sharply on the rubber pad and the duration of the ensuing disturbance was measured. This is similar to the procedure used by Manning to compare the activity of *Drosophila melanogaster* and *D. simulans* (Manning, 1959).

In another method to quantitate this lack of reactivity in the mutants, 20 adult male *iav* flies were placed in a 40 cm long, straight, transparent tube and 20 *Canton-S* flies were placed in an identical adjacent tube. After introduction of the flies into the tubes, each end was closed with a cork stopper and the tubes were placed on a testing table 50 cm below a 60 W bulb. The twin tubes were agitated in a vertical position to concentrate all the flies on the lower stoppers, and then immediately brought back to a horizontal position. The number of flies in each tube that crossed a mark 3 cm from the end of the tube in a 5 sec period was scored for 90 seconds. After 5 trials in which the flies moved from left to right, the direction was reversed in order to control the possible effect of odor trails that might bias the data.

In order to compare the behavior of inactive and wild-type third instar larvae, the number of larvae of each genotype able to traverse a given distance within a measured time period was observed. Ten inactive larvae were placed in a petri dish and 20 ml of a modified Bodenstein's solution (Ikeda and Kaplan, 1970a) was added, barely covering the larvae but permitting them to crawl freely on the bottom of the dish. Ten *Canton-S* larvae were placed in a second dish and each was then positioned above a disc with concentric circles. The dish holding the *Canton-S* larvae was on the right for the first five runs and on the left for the second series. Illumination was provided by a 60 W incandescent light bulb 50 cm above the petri dishes. A small glass rod was used to position the larvae at the center of their respective dishes and the number of larvae crossing out of the inner circle (2.5 cm in diameter) in each 10 sec. period was then scored. After 3 min, the number of larvae in each circular section was also scored.

## Morphology

Whole heads were removed from etherized flies and fixed with 3% gluteraldehyde in 0.08 M cacodylic buffer and 0.5 g/100 ml $CaCl_2$. The fixed heads were dehydrated and embedded in JB-4 Embedding Media (Sorvall Inc.). Thin (2 μ) serial sections were cut on a LKB glass knife microtome. Toluidine blue stained sections were then photographed.

## Stimulation and Recording

For stimulation and recording experiments, flies were mounted in wax (Softseal tackiwax - Cenco Inst. Corp.) in a petri dish. The abdomen was cut and the open end submerged in a modified Bodenstein's solution (Ikeda and Kaplan, 1970a). Further perfusion was achieved by applying a glass capillary containing the solution to the proboscis. Tungsten electrodes electrolytically etched and insulated to the tip were used for extracellular recordings. Air puffs to antennae were delivered via a glass capillary connected to an electromagnetic relay. Recordings from third instar larvae were obtained by pinning down dissected larvae on Sylgard in a petri dish.

## Biochemistry

*D. melanogaster* heads were decapitated at 5°C and incubated in 10 mm long plastic tubes, with stainless steel EM grids as a sieve at one end while the other was connected to an Ependorf pipette. Incubation was carried out in a modified Bodentstein's solution (Ikeda and Kaplan, 1970a) with $10^{-8}$ w/v Paraoxon (American Cyanamid

Corp.) and 25 μC choline-$H^3$ (New England Nuclear Corp.) in a final volume of 50 μl. After 15 min incubation, wash out curves were obtained. Every 90 seconds, 50 μl of the solution was drawn into the chamber and then expelled into 2 ml of Bray's solution for counting. Brain extractions were carried out in a 1:9 glacial acetic acid solution for 5 h. Electrophoresis was run in a 1:3 pyridine-glacial acetic acid mixture including 31 water at pH 4.2. The counts were read on a Beckman strip scanner. Ach and choline markers were detected by iodine vapors.

## RESULTS

### Behavioral Analysis

The *iav* mutant of *D. melanogaster* exhibits general inactivity in a culture. Following mechanical stimulation of a bottle (see methods) *iav* flies remain quiet on the surface of the food. There is only a small amount of walking and wing fluttering in response to the tap. The wild-type *Canton-S* flies fly about and crawl up the side of the bottle, settling at the top, on the side of the bottle, or on the stopper. They have not returned to the original pattern of activity by the time the next shock in the series is delivered. On the other hand, inactive flies do not leave the surface of the food until after the sixth tap, when some of them crawl up the side of the bottle, the number increasing in successive trials until about 35% settle on the side of the bottle. This pattern holds for inactive flies for five days; at six days, a curious behavior sets in which we refer to as the "popcorn effect". After the bottle has been tapped on the rubber pad, a few flies take off and in so doing cause swirls of activity like dust storms on the desert floor. Landing flies trigger flights of others resting on the food, presenting a picture of flies popping up and down within the culture bottle. This popcorn behavior lasts for about ten days, starts to decrease in intensity when the flies are 15 days old and disappears when they reach day 24. Furthermore, 6 - 24 day old flies, left undisturbed in their culture bottles, do not manifest any behavior which distinguishes them from 1 - 5 day old flies. Both age groups present a picture of a quiet population with almost no activity.

The times required by two day old and seven day old *Canton-S* and inactive flies to settle after shock, determined by ten sequential measurements, are represented in Table I.

Another measure of activity was employed in which a preset number of flies was used (see methods). The number of flies that crossed a mark in a tube in a 5 sec period was scored for 90 sec.

TABLE I

DATA FROM ACTIVITY TEST OF *CANTON-S* AND INACTIVE FLIES

| Age | Trial | 1 | 2 | 3 | 4 | 5 | 6 | 7 | 8 | 9 | 10 |
|---|---|---|---|---|---|---|---|---|---|---|---|
| 2 days | *Canton-S* | 15 | 25 | 30 | 42 | 51 | 47 | 58 | 46 | 52 | 47 |
| | Inactive | 2 | 2 | 3 | 2 | 4 | 3 | 5 | 7 | 9 | 8 |
| 7 days | *Canton-S* | 18 | 25 | 35 | 46 | 49 | 52 | 51 | 55 | 58 | |
| | Inactive | 90 | 70 | 65 | 52 | 47 | 60 | 36 | 52 | 35 | |

In each experiment, the time in seconds required for flies to settle after shock is given for 2 and 7 day old flies. Note the marked differences between wild type and inactive flies at 2 days of age and also that between 2 and 7 day old inactive flies.

All scores were pooled. A significant difference between *iav* and *Canton* activity can be seen in the curves of Fig. 1, where the cumulative mean number of flies passing a 3 cm mark line is plotted for each 5 sec period. (This method is convenient for measuring relative activities of mutant lines in small populations over a short time span.)

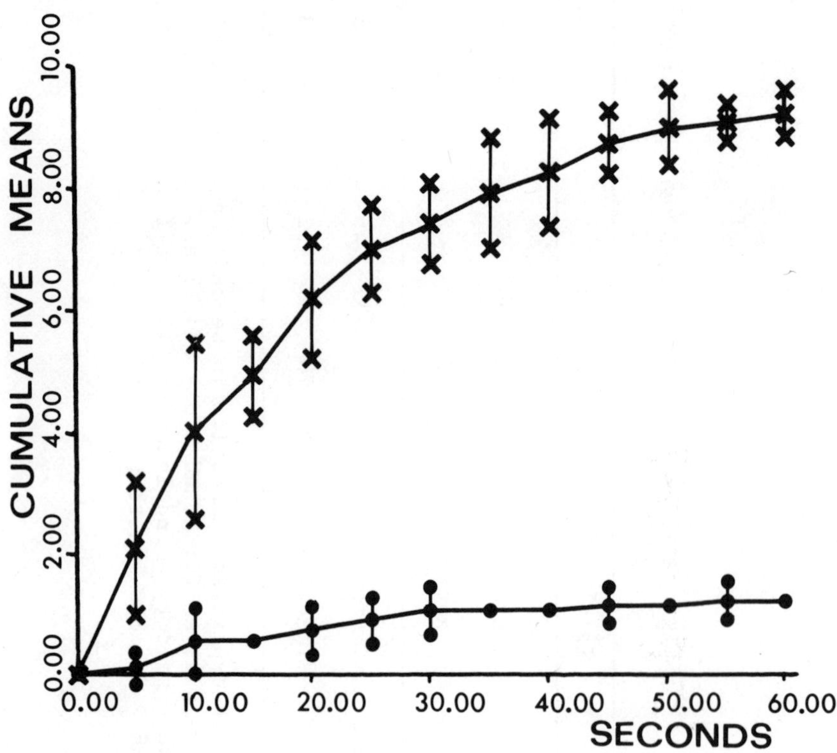


Fig. 1 Pooled data of activity measurements on 4 day old flies. Cumulative means of number of flies crossing a 3 cm mark in a tube are plotted for 5 sec periods. Circles; *inactive* flies and crosses; *Canton-S* flies. Standard deviations are shown for each point.

Although the contrast in behavior between *Canton-S* and *iav* adults is readily apparent, there is no obvious difference between the larval stages of the two strains when they are observed in culture bottles. A separate experimental method was designed to measure larval activity (see methods).

The results of 5 experiments (each of 10 runs with 10 larvae each) are summarized in Fig. 2. The curves are plotted as the cumulative mean number of larvae crossing out of the first circle in a petri dish in each 5 second period. A significantly greater activity of *Canton-S* larvae over the mutants is apparent (This

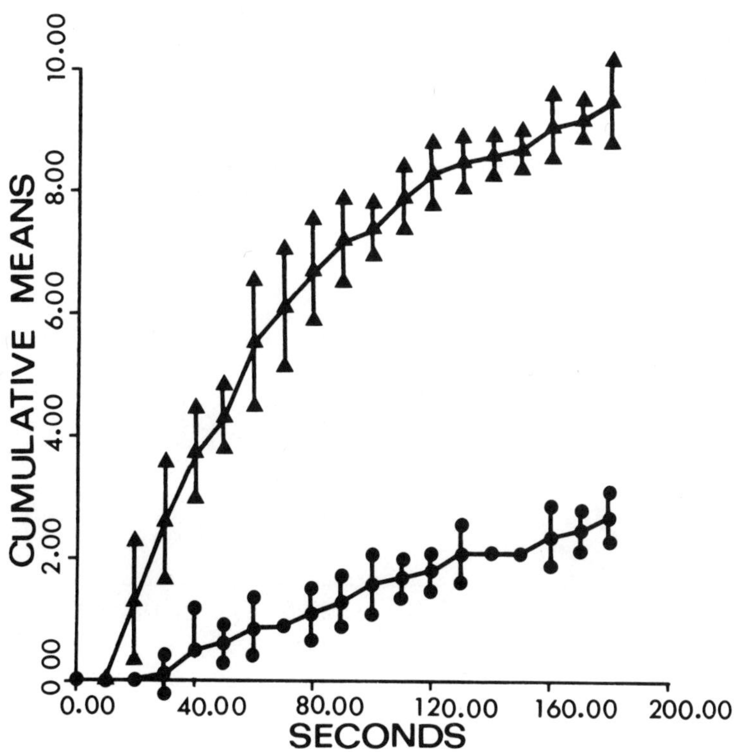


Fig. 2 Pooled data of activity measurements on 3rd instar larvae. Cumulative means of number of larvae crossing out of an inner circle in a petri dish are plotted for 10 sec periods. Dots: *iav* larvae, triangles: *Canton-S* larvae.

simple method of testing the activity of small numbers of larvae essentially to a tactile stimulus of the glass rod can easily be extended to the effect of externally applied drugs into the medium). Using the same experimental design, the dominance relationship of the *iav* gene was tested. Female larvae were used for this test because males of *Drosophila* have only one X chromosome. The behavior of homozygous *iav/iav*, and heterozygous *iav/+* third instar larvae were compared. Fig. 3 shows that *iav* is clearly recessive.

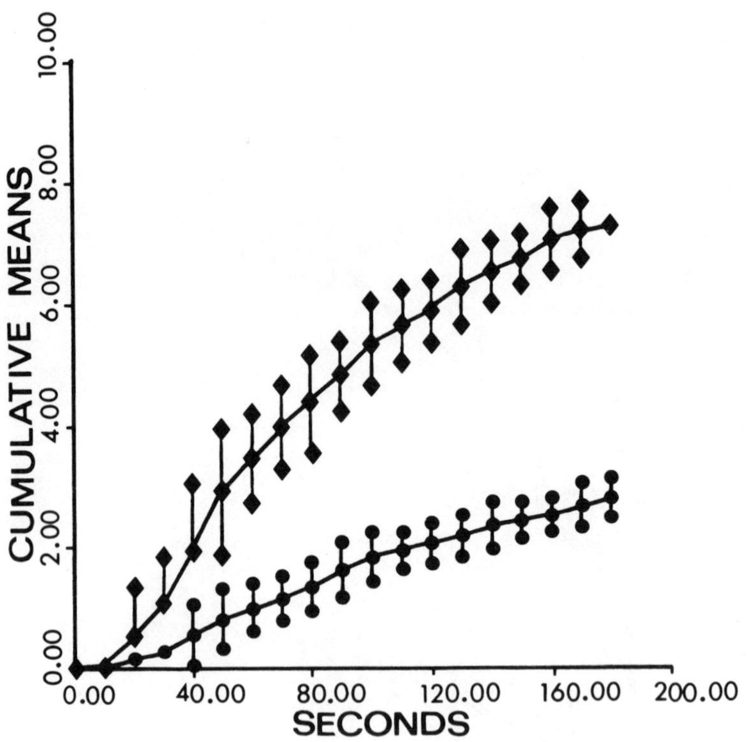


Fig. 3 Pooled data of activity measurements on 3rd instar larvae. Cumulative means of number of larvae crossing out of an inner circle in a petri dish are plotted for 10 sec periods. Dots: *iav/iav* larvae; diamonds: +/+ larvae.

## Morphology of Antennae

An obvious difference in behavior between the *iav* mutant and *Canton-S* flies is the latter's flight response to slight air movements. Although *iav* flies can be induced to fly, very strong agitation is required. One of the organs responsible for air movement sensation is the antenna with its well developed arista and high concentration of receptor hairs. Although the external morphology of the mutant, including that of its antennae, appears normal, sections of the antennae were examined by light microscopy for possible internal abnormalities. Since minor differences in tissue appearance may be caused by non-identical histological procedures on individual heads, bilaterally mosaic heads were used. Fig. 4 shows a longitudinal section through the three segments of an *iav* mutant antenna. All the components of the antenna as described by Hertweck (1931) are present in the antenna and appear identical to those of a *Canton-S* antenna. The antennal nerve was traced further into the head as far as the ventral part of the cerebral ganglion and no differences were observed between the mutant and wild-type flies at the light microscope level.

## Antennal Responses

A brief air puff directed at one antenna deflects it from its normal position; a subsequent contraction of the muscles in the second antennal segment returns the antenna to its previous position. This reaction has been reported in other dipterans and a possible monosynaptic sensory-to-motor link has been postulated (Pareto, 1972). Extracellular recordings from these muscles in *Drosophila* show a compound response following a brief air puff directed at the arista (Fig. 5). The response has an average latency period of 4 msec and shows no fatigue or adaptation even at high frequency stimulations (Fig. 5c). This is consistent with its function in detecting the direction of air currents during flight, or perceiving wing movements of up to 200 cycles/sec.

Responses of the antennal muscles (AM) to hand movements and a gentle prolonged air puff are shown in Fig. 5a, b. These responses could not be detected in AM of *iav* mutants, Fig. 6 (right hand trace).

## Genetic Autonomy of the *iav* Gene

In order to ascertain whether this lack of response in the AM of an *iav* mutant is due to a gene product freely circulating in the haemolymph and affecting one of the components involved in the AM responses, recordings were performed on mosaic flies (see methods). External recordings of both left and right AM were made simultaneously

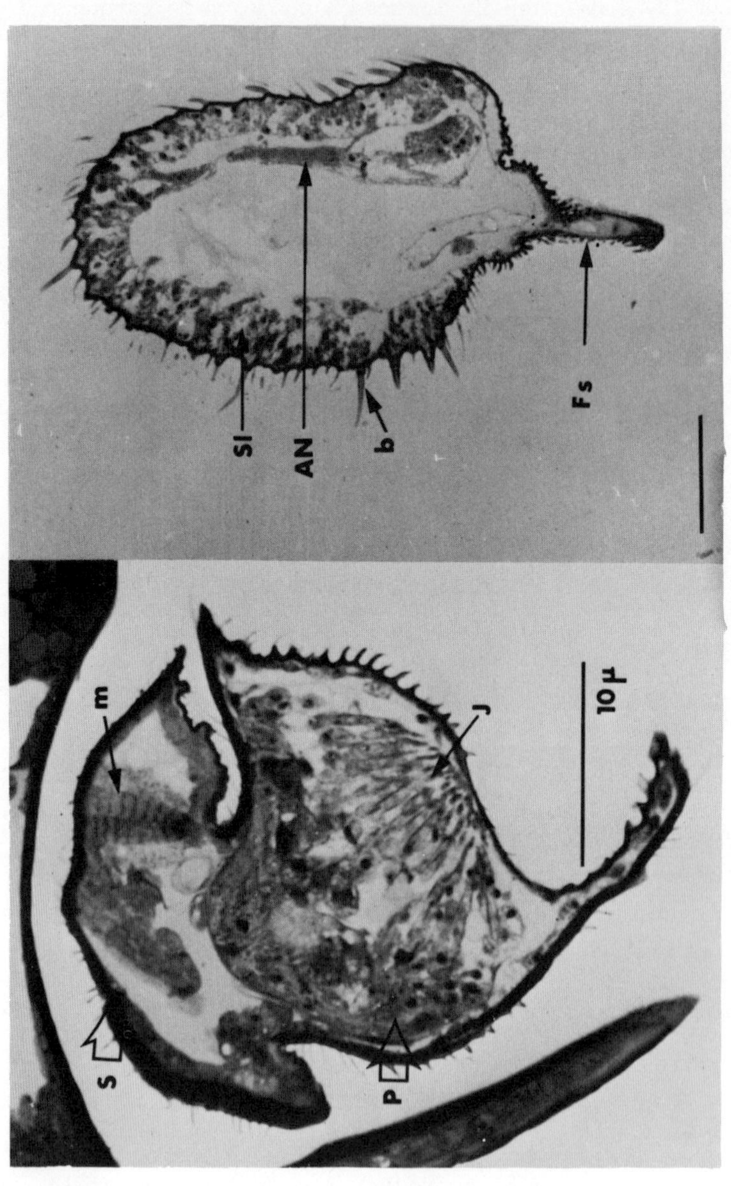


Fig. 4 Longitudinal section of antenna of *iav*/+ genotype. On the left the first two proximal segments are shown; S-Scapus and P-Pedicellus. The antennal muscles (m) are marked in the first segment and Johnston's organ (j) in the second. On the right, the Funiculus has all the components of the wild-type fly. Sl-Soma layer, AN-antennal nerve, b-sensory bristles, Fs-Funiculus stalk. Compare to Hertweck (1931) p. 631. Calibration bars are 10 μ for each plate.

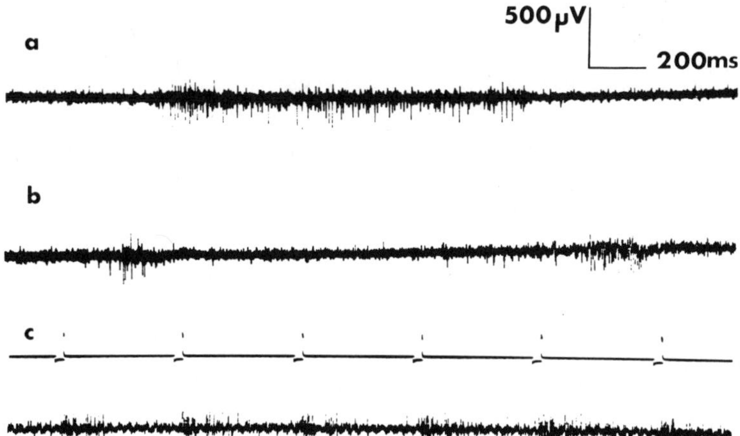


Fig. 5 Extracellularly recorded activity of antennal muscles in a male *Canton-S* fly evoked by (a) prolonged, (b) two short, and (c) repetitive air puffs applied to the arista. Top trace in (c) shows time of air puff application.

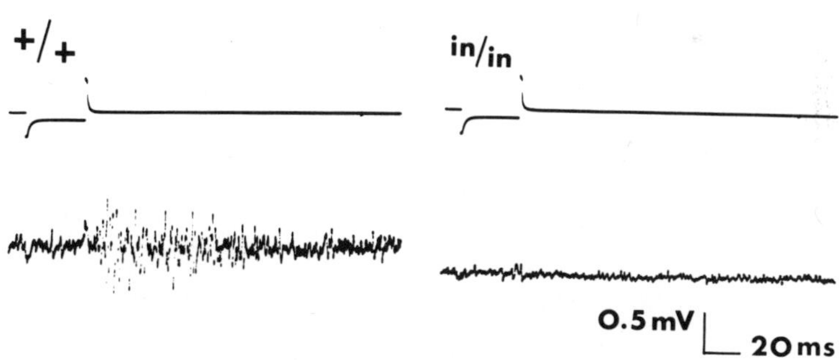


Fig. 6 (Left) Electrical responses recorded extracellularly from the antennal muscles of a *Canton-S* female fly as a response to a short air puff applied to the arista. Duration of stimulus is shown on upper trace. (Right) The same stimulus fails to evoke a response in a homozygous inactive mutant female fly.

with an air puff directed to move both antennae. The flies used were bilaterally mosaic; the antenna on the female side was heterozygous for the *iav* gene while on the male side, the antennal tissue was inactive. In 17 cases, no AM responses could be elicited from the *iav* antenna while its contralateral counterpart, having an *iav*/+ genotype, always exhibited the typical responses. Two mosaic flies showed external markers indicating that one antenna only was inactive while the rest of the head and body was normal. Here, again, no responses could be elicited from the mutant antenna whereas the other AM responded normally (Fig. 7).

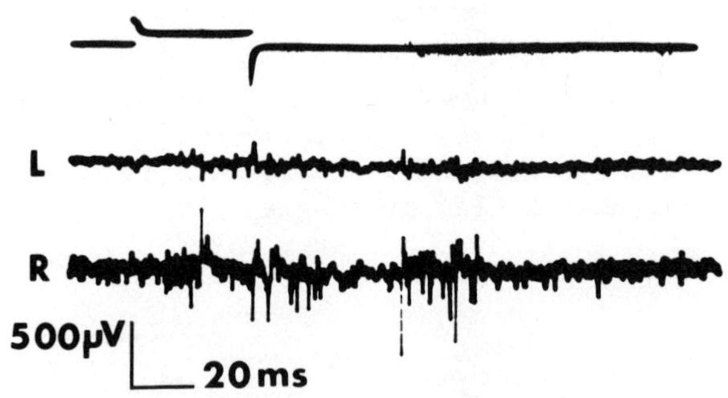


Fig. 7 Electrical responses from left and right antennae of a bilaterally mosaic gynandromorph fly. Responses were evoked by a brief air puff delivered simultaneously to both antennae. Upper trace: stimulus duration. Middle trace: left antenna shows no response to puff. Bottom trace: large responses from the right antenna. External cuticle of left antenna is mutant while the right is wild type.

One may conclude from these data that the mutation is autonomous in the genetic sense as far as the AM response is concerned and is not due to a humoral factor, nor influenced by the genotype of the contralateral antenna. Assuming the AM response to be monosynaptic the *iav* mutation defect must be localized within one of the following components involved in the response:

1) Peripheral receptors and antennal nerve
2) Motor neurons
3) Antennal muscles.

## Defect Localization

Direct activation of the motor components of the *iav* mutant, bypassing the peripheral sensory elements, may narrow down the localization of the defect. Short electrical stimuli of 0.1 msec duration delivered to the cervical connectives elicited contractions of the AM. While this indicates that the AM are capable of contracting, whether the motor neurons innervating these muscles are normal remains to be tested. Selective electrical stimulation of the AM motor neurons proved unsuccessful and an indirect method for their activation was designed.

A mutant showing hyperkinetic behavior, $Hk^1$, has been previously described (Kaplan and Trout, 1968). Among other hyperkinetic aspects of its behavior, the $Hk^1$ mutant exhibits continuous leg shaking under 3% ether (Kaplan, 1971). Ikeda has localized the neurons responsible for this shaking within the thoracic ganglia (Ikeda and Kaplan, 1970b) and later tentatively identified them as pacemaker interneurons driving the leg motor neurons which in turn innervate the leg muscles. Introduction of such pacemaker neurons into an *iav* mutant ganglion could throw light on a motor system defect in the *iav* fly.

Homozygous $Hk^1$ *iav* flies were obtained by crossing $Hk^1$ males with inactive females and isolating recombinant offsprings produced by the $F_1$ females. The resulting *iav* $Hk^1$/*iav* $Hk^1$, flies, homozygous for both traits, exhibited general inactivity. The typical $Hk^1$ leg shaking might be expected if the motor neuron and muscle components in the *iav* mutant are normal and are driven by the $Hk^1$ mutant pacemakers. On the other hand, if the *iav* defects were localized in either the motor neurons or muscles, no shaking should appear in the double *iav* $Hk^1$ mutant.

Indeed, *iav* $Hk^1$ flies in the presence of 3% ether exhibited the typical $Hk^1$ leg shaking pattern. Careful observation revealed that often the antennae of these double mutants showed spontaneous vibrations under ether anaesthesia, as is seen in $Hk^1$ flies. These results indicate that the motor components are not affected in the *iav* mutant and the absence of AM responses may be localized elsewhere, namely, in the sensory component.

## Sensory Nerve Conduction

The sensory elements are composed of the receptor part, the conducting axon and its central terminations. Direct recordings of generator potentials were unsuccessful. However, extracellular recordings of both the antennal and haltere nerves (Fig. 8) showed normal responses, indicating that the peripheral receptor parts are functioning in the *iav* mutants. Essentially the same result was

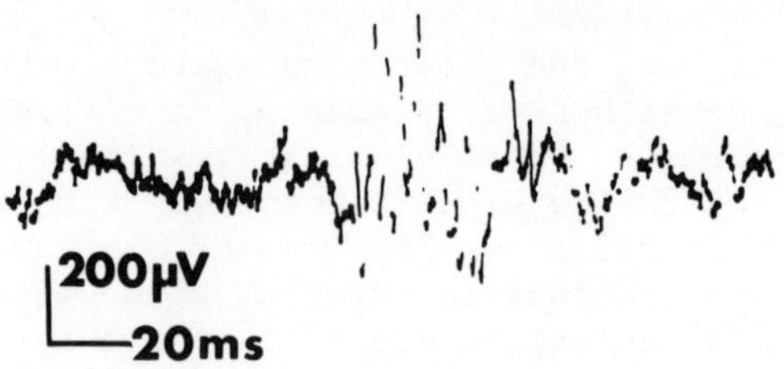


Fig. 8 Activity recorded extracellularly from an abdominal nerve of a third instar *iav* larva. The activity was evoked by a gentle touch to the caudal end of the larva while the nerve proximal to the recording point was severed, to abolish spontaneous activity.

obtained from third instar larval abdominal nerves. To abolish centrally originating activity, the nerves were sectioned near the ganglion and activity was recorded distally to the section. The results indicated that the defect is central rather than peripheral, either in the sensory to motor neuron synaptic area or, if they exist, in the interneurons between these two elements.

## Biochemical Approaches

Acetylcholine (Ach) has been stipulated as the transmitter of sensory neurons in arthropods. Both crustaceans and insects have been shown to possess cholinergic synthesising and catalysing systems and the effect of topically applied Ach to the insect's CNS has been previously studied (Pittman, 1971). In *Drosophila*, the values for choline acetyltransferase range as high as 0.5 mmoles/g protein/h (Dewhurst *et al.*, 1970). A defect in the cholinergic enzymatic system could possibly explain the *iav* phenotype. However, measurements of Ach content, Ach-transferase, and cholinesterase activities were found to be in the normal range of the wild type *Canton-S* strain (Dewhurst, 1974). These findings further limit the defect localization; if indeed the sensory components are responsible for the *iav* phenotype, the transmitter release mechanisms may be the target of the *iav* gene.

To test this hypothesis, whole heads of either *iav* or *Canton-S* male flies were incubated in tritium-labelled choline as an Ach precursor (see methods). It has been shown that the external sensory hairs of *Drosophila* have a cuticular opening (Falk, 1974) and in the cockroach uptake of choline by the CNS via the antenna was demonstrated. After incubation, both *Canton* and *iav* heads showed uptake and conversion of choline to Ach (Fig. 9). In washout experiments, where the effluent was collected in discrete fractions (see methods) the release of labelled material was monitored following pulses of either normal or high concentrations of potassium or magnesium. A 20 mM pulse of potassium caused a 150% increase in release of labelled material. If this release is synaptic due to K depolarization, it should be prevented by Mg, and indeed high Mg pulses were found to diminish the amount of radioactive material release (see Fig. 10). Following a 20 mM K pulse, no significant differences between release from *Canton* and *iav* heads were found (Fig. 11). However, at 12.5 mM K, where no release of radioactive material could be detected from *iav* heads, a small, but reproducible amount was released from the wild type *Canton* heads (Fig. 12).

Thus it appears that the release mechanism of acetylcholine, the putative sensory transmitter in insects, is at fault in the *iav* mutant.

## DISCUSSION

The results presented here center around the antennal response and point to a defect in Ach liberation from sensory neurons of the antennae. The general inactivity of the fly cannot be explained by this defect alone. Even a completely antennaless *Canton-S* fly shows normal activity. Thus, we may assume that all sensory hairs covering the *iav* fly's body have this defect. Preliminary recordings of electroretinograms from the *iav* mutant appear normal, but the visual system may not be a cholinergic sensory system and thus may function normally. Under total darkness, a fly with reduced sensory hair detection capabilities should exhibit behavior similar to total sensory deprivation responses. Preliminary observations on *iav* flies grown in the dark show that they do indeed exhibit a very reduced fertility, presumably due to lack of mating. Further observations are necessary to quantitate this phenomenon.

If our conclusion that the inactivity of the mutant flies is due to lack of Ach release from sensory axon endings is correct, it would be interesting to determine and isolate the mutant gene product. A presynaptic release protein or malformed synaptic vessicles are possible targets. Furthermore, possibly other behavioral mutants of the "strange behavior" type may also be synaptic in nature. Thus we may eventually have enough data to reconstruct processes involved in transmitter release and to understand the genic control of this mechanism.

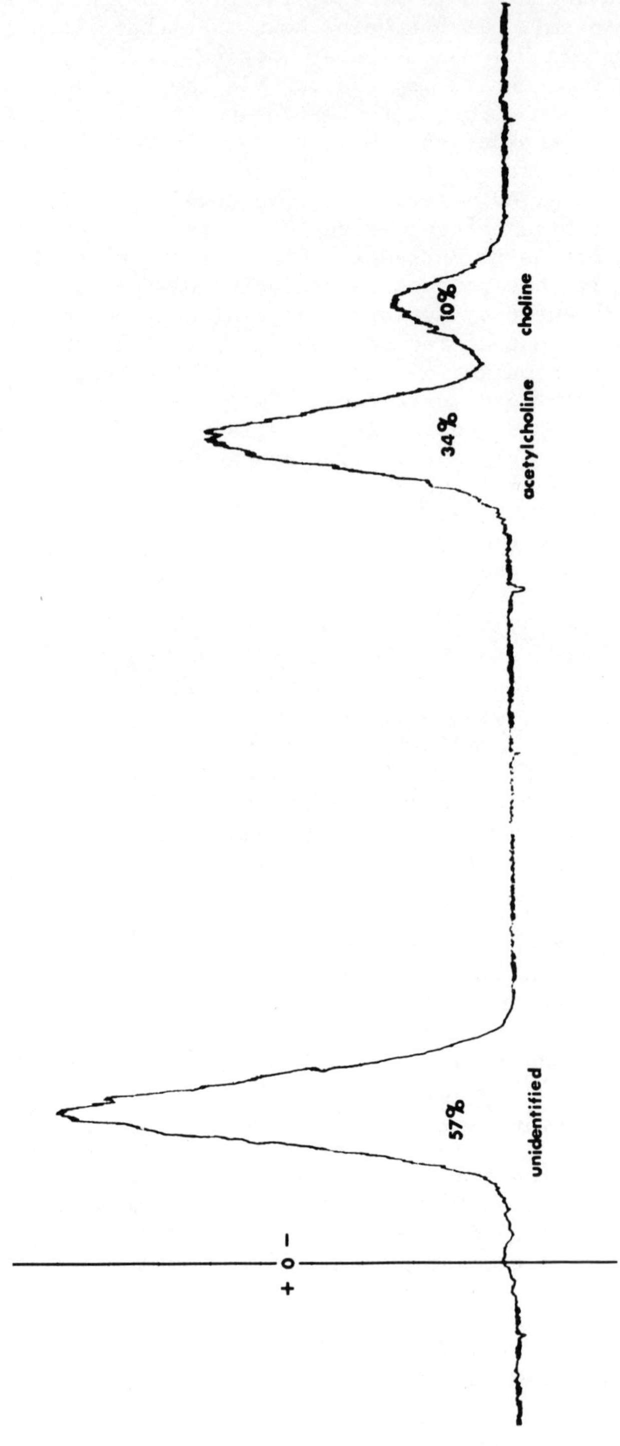


Fig. 9 Electrophoresis of *iav* fly brain extract after choline-$H^3$ incubation. Scan of the paper strip indicates a large conversion of choline to acetylcholine and an unidentified compound.

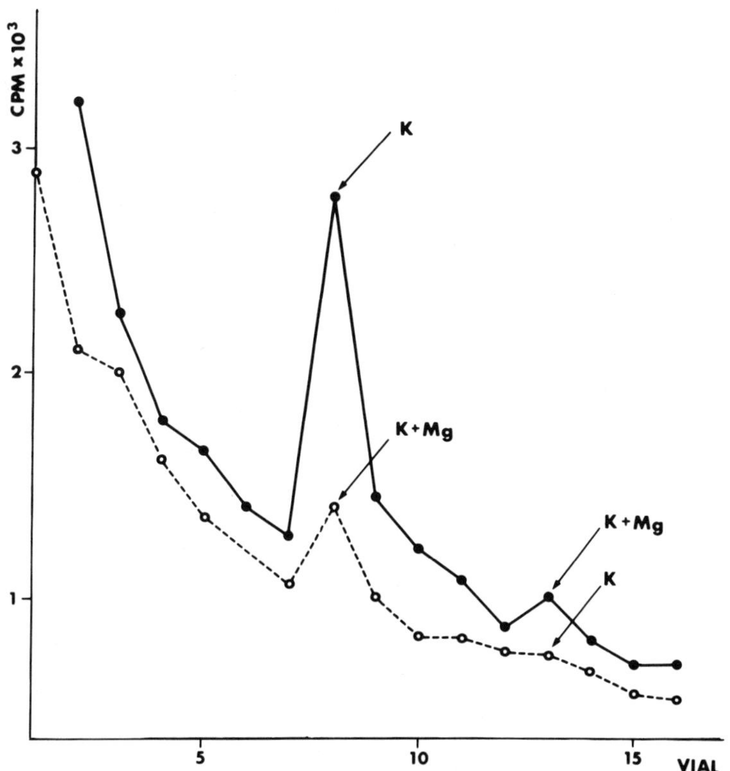


Fig. 10 Effect of a 20 mM K pulse on washout curve of fly heads incubated with choline-$H^3$. Note similar amounts of released label in inactive and wild type flies.

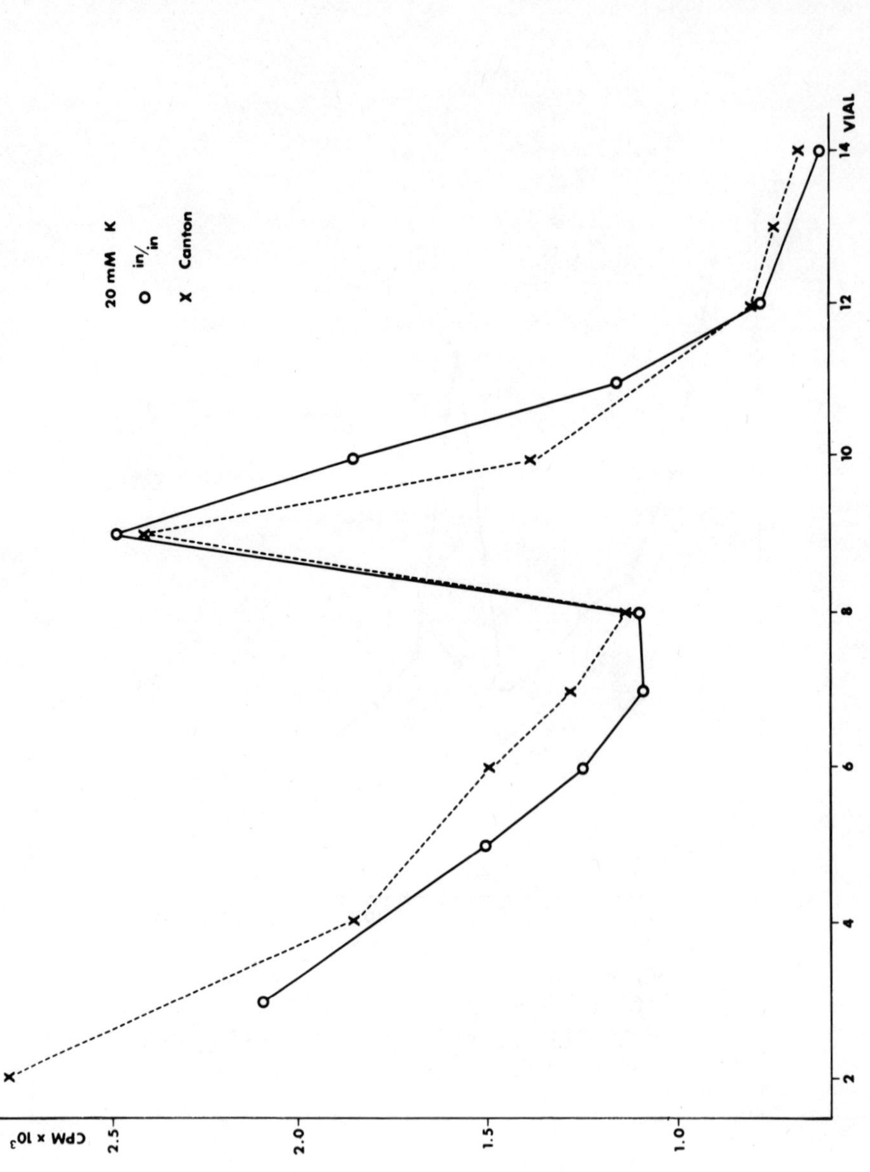


Fig. 11 Effect of K and Mg pulses on washout curves of *iav* fly heads incubated with choline-$H^3$.

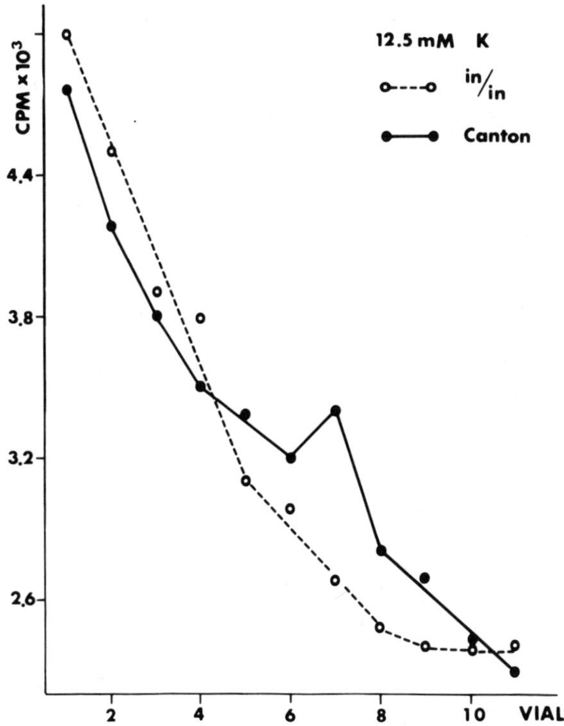


Fig. 12 Effect of a 12.5 mM K pulse on washout curves of inactive and wild type fly heads incubated with choline-$H^3$. Note the absence of release of labeled material from inactive fly heads and release of label from wild type material.

ACKNOWLEDGEMENT

We are grateful to Dr. H. Weinstein for his help in the biochemical section of this work. We also thank Ms. J. Grieshaber for her help in the morphological aspects.

## REFERENCES


1. DEWHURST, S. Unpublished results. 1974.
2. DEWHURST, S., MC CAMAN, R. & KAPLAN, W.D. *Biochemical Genetics 4:*499, 1970.
3. FALK, R. Personal Communication. 1974.
4. HERTWECK, R. *Z. wiss. Zoöl. 139:*559, 1931.
5. HOTTA, Y. & BENZER, S. *Nature 222:*354, 1969.
6. IKEDA, K. & KAPLAN, W.D. *Proc. Nat. Acad. Sci. U.S.A. 66:* 765, 1970a.
7. IKEDA, K. & KAPLAN, W.D. *Proc. Nat. Acad. Sci. U.S.A. 67:* 1480, 1970b.
8. KAPLAN, W.D. Genetic and behavioral studies of *Drosophila* neurological mutants. In: Biology of Behavior, p. 133, Proc. 32nd Ann. Biol. Colloq. (Ed. J.A. Kiger, Jr.), Oregon State Univ. Press. 1971.
9. KAPLAN, W.D. & TROUT, W.E. *Genetics 60:*191, 1968 (abstract).
10. KIKUCHI, T. *Japan J. Genetics 48: No. 2*, 105, 1973.
11. LEWIS, E.B. & BACHER, F. *Drosophila Information Service 43:* 192, 1968.
12. MANNING, A. *Behaviour 15:*123, 1959.
13. PAK, W.L., CROSSFIELD, J. & WHITE, N.V. *Nature 222:*351, 1969.
14. PARETO, A. *Z. Zellforsch 131:*109, 1972.
15. PITTMAN, R. *Comp. & Gen. Pharm. 2:*347, 1971.
16. WILLIAMSON, R., KAPLAN, W.D. & DAGAN, D. *Nature*, In press, 1974.

# LIST OF PARTICIPANTS

ABELES, MOSHE
Hebrew University, Hadassah Medical School, Jerusalem, Israel
AKOV, SHOSHANA
Israel Institute for Biolological Research, Ness-Ziona, Israel
ASSAF, JACOB
Hebrew University, Hadassah Medical School, Jerusalem, Israel
AZMON, ZVI
Hebrew University, Jerusalem, Israel
AZMON, MRS. RUTH

BAR-ZEEV, MICHA
Israel Institute for Biological Research, Ness-Ziona, Israel
BEIDLER, LLOYD
Florida State University, Tallahassee, Florida, U.S.A.
BEEMER, ABRAHAM
Israel Institute for Biological Research, Ness-Ziona, Israel
BEN-DAVID, AMNON
Israel Institute for Biological Research, Ness-Ziona, Israel
BENHAR, EFRAIM
Weizmann Institute of Science, Rehovot, Israel
BINO, TAMAR
Israel Institute for Biological Research, Ness-Ziona, Israel
BLAKEMORE, COLIN
Cambridge University, England
BLAKEMORE, MRS.

CARLEN, PETER
Hebrew University, Jerusalem, Israel
COHEN, SARA
Israel Institute for Biological Research, Ness-Ziona, Israel
CORETT, RUTH
Israel Institute for Biological Research, Ness-Ziona, Israel
DAGAN, DANY
Technion, Medical School, Haifa, Israel
DUDAI, YADIN
Weizmann Institute of Science, Rehovot, Israel

EDERY, HABIB
Israel Institute for Biological Research, Ness-Ziona, Israel
FUCHS, HAYA
Israel Institute for Biological Research, Ness-Ziona, Israel
GAINER, HAROLD
National Institutes of Health, Bethesda, Maryland, U.S.A.
GALUN, RACHEL
Israel Institute for Biological Research, Ness-Ziona, Israel
GLASS, ITZHAK
Tel-Aviv University, Tel-Aviv, Israel
GOLDSTEIN, YEHUDA
Tel-Aviv University, Tel-Aviv, Israel
GOTHILF, SHMUEL
Israel Institute for Biological Research, Ness-Ziona, Israel
GOTTLIEB, YEHEZKEL
Hebrew University, Hadassah Medical School, Jerusalem, Israel
GOTTLIEB, MRS.

GROSSOWICZ, NATHAN
Hebrew University, Hadassah Medical School, Jerusalem, Israel
GROSSOWICZ, MRS.

GRUNFELD, YONA
Israel Institute for Biological Research, Ness-Ziona, Israel
GUTNICK, MICHAEL
Hebrew University, Hadassah Medical School, Jerusalem, Israel
HANANI, MENACHEM
Hebrew University, Jerusalem, Israel
HECHT, BENJAMIN
Israel Institute for Biological Research, Ness-Ziona, Israel
HECHT, MRS.

HESTRIN, SARAH
Hebrew University, Hadassah Medical School, Jerusalem, Israel
HILLMAN, PETER
Hebrew University, Jerusalem, Israel
HOCHSTEIN, SHAUL
Hebrew University, Jerusalem, Israel
HODIS, YEHIEL
Hebrew University, Hadassah Medical School, Jerusalem, Israel
HORN, GABRIEL
Cambridge University, England
HUBEL, DAVID
Harvard Medical School, Boston, Massachusetts, U.S.A.
HUBER, FRANZ
Max Planck Institute für Verhaltensphysiologie, Seewiesen, West Germany
KATZIR, GAD
Hebrew University, Jerusalem, Israel

KAUFMANN, ELISHEVA
Israel Institute for Biological Research, Ness-Ziona, Israel
KAYE, MYRA
Israel Institute for Biological Research, Ness-Ziona, Israel
KEDEM, JOSEPH
Bar-Ilan University, Ramat-Gan, Israel
KLINGBERG, MARCUS A.
Israel Institute for Biological Research, Ness-Ziona, Israel
KLINGBERG, WANDA
Israel Institute for Biological Research, Ness-Ziona, Israel
KORN, HENRY
C.H.U., Paris, France
KOSOWER, EDWARD, M.
Tel-Aviv University, Tel-Aviv, Israel
KUTTIN, ELIEZER
Israel Institute for Biological Research, Ness-Ziona, Israel
LAIWAND, RONI
Hebrew University, Jerusalem, Israel
LENHOFF, HOWARD
University of California, Irvine, California, U.S.A.
LESHEM, BARUCH
Israel Institute for Biological Research, Ness-Ziona, Israel
LIOR, SIMA
Schneorson Institute, Tel-Aviv Municipality, Israel
MIRSKY, MICHAEL
Former Moscow State University "Lemonossov", Moscow, U.S.S.R.
NAFTALI, ARIE
Former member of the Criminology Institute, Hebrew University, Jerusalem, Israel
NITZAN, YIGAL
Tel-Aviv University, Tel-Aviv, Israel
PARNAS, ITZHAK
Hebrew University, Jerusalem, Israel
PARNAS, MRS.

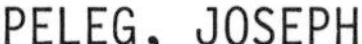

PELEG, JOSEPH
Israel Institute for Biological Research, Ness-Ziona, Israel
PENER, MEIR P.
Hebrew University, Jerusalem, Israel
PENER, HEDVA
Ministry of Health, Jerusalem, Israel
PRATT, HILLEL
Hebrew University, Hadassah Medical School, Jerusalem, Israel
RICE, MARTIN
University of Queensland, Brisbane, Australia
ROEDER, KENNETH
Tufts University, Medford, Massachusetts, U.S.A.
SCHNEIDER, DIETRICH
Max Planck Institute für Verhaltensphysiologie, Seewiesen, West Germany

SCHNEIDER, MRS.

SELTZER, ZEEV
Hebrew University, Hadassah Medical School, Jerusalem, Israel
SHATKAY, ADAM
Israel Institute for Biological Research, Ness-Ziona, Israel
SHAW, CHRIS
Hebrew University, Jerusalem, Israel
SHLOSBERG, SARA
Clinical Psychologist, Haifa, Israel
SPIEGELSTEIN, MICHA
Israel Institute for Biological Research, Ness-Ziona, Israel
STEINBERG, S.
Hebrew University, Jerusalem, Israel
STREIFLER, MAX B.
Ichilov Hospital, Tel-Aviv, Israel
SILMAN, ISRAEL
Weizmann Institute of Science, Rehovot, Israel
SIMON, GAD
Israel Institute for Biological Research, Ness-Ziona, Israel
SNIR, JOSEPH
Hebrew University, Jerusalem, Israel
SOMER, CHAIM
Hebrew University, Hadassah Medical School, Jerusalem, Israel
SPIRA, MICHA
Hebrew University, Jerusalem, Israel
TAHORI, ALEXANDER
Israel Institute for Biological Research, Ness-Ziona, Israel
TEITZ, YAEL
Israel Institute for Biological Research, Ness-Ziona, Israel
VAADIA, EILON
Hebrew University, Hadassah Medical School, Jerusalem, Israel
WALL, PATRICK
University College, London, England
WERMAN, ROBERT
Hebrew University, Jerusalem, Israel
WOLLBERG, ZVI
Tel-Aviv University, Tel-Aviv, Israel
YASSKY, DOV
Israel Institute for Biological Research, Ness-Ziona, Israel
YATHOMM, SHOSHANA
Volcani Center, Beit-Dagan, Israel
YINON, URI
Hadassah University Hospital, Jerusalem, Israel
YAFFE, DAVID
Weizmann Institute of Science, Rehovot, Israel
ZYDON, JACOB
Israel Institute for Biological Research, Ness-Ziona, Israel
ZYDON, MRS.

SUBJECT INDEX